Constantino Manuel Torres, P.
David B. Repke, BSc

Anadenanthera
Visionary Plant
of Ancient South America

Pre-publication
REVIEWS,
COMMENTARIES,
EVALUATIONS . . .

"This extensively researched, thoroughly documented, and delightfully illustrated book has a focus on psychoactive preparations made from the *Anadenanthera* genus and their role in pre-Columbian art and culture. The importance of *Anadenanthera* snuffs has probably been grossly underemphasized by many pre-Columbian anthropologists, and this book does a good job of correcting that oversight. It provides an effective integration of anthropology, archaeology, and ethnobotany that will fascinate those seeking to understand the role that psychoactive plants played in the development of New World societies as well as those with a general interest in the pre-Columbian period.

Numerous artifacts, particularly in the form of snuffing equipment and smoking pipes, clearly illustrate the importance of snuffs made from *Anadenanthera* seeds, especially in Peru, Chile, Bolivia, and Argentina. As the authors clearly document, there was a continuing association of these snuffs with the Andean cultures. The strongest case yet has perhaps been made that the alkaloid bufotenine, which occurs in relatively high concentrations in *Anadenanthera* species, is psychoactive, a subject that has been of considerable controversy among scientists for many years.

Although the focus of this book is *Anadenanthera* as a psychoactive plant, the authors do present some information on the economic value of *Anadenanthera* as a renewable resource. In addition, one chapter provides an overview of the chemistry and pharmacology of bufotenine, related tryptamines, and how they relate to the class of what would be called hallucinogenic drugs."

David E. Nichols, PhD
Department of Medicinal Chemistry
and Molecular Pharmacology,
Purdue University

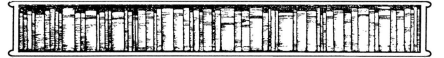

"*Anadenanthera: Visionary Plant of Ancient South America* is an encyclopedic gem of a book that draws from the fields of the humanities, the social sciences, and the natural sciences to offer the first comprehensive study on this fascinating shamanic plant. Written by art historian Constantino Manuel Torres and chemist David Repke, this in-depth examination of *Anadenanthera* covers the taxonomy, ethnobotany, archaeology, and chemistry of those species of *Anadenanthera* with seeds that, when ingested, invoke other-worldly ecstatic experiences.

Constantino Torres traces the evidence of smoking and snuffing in the archaeological record and in the early writings of Spanish chroniclers, including Christopher Columbus (Cristobal Colón), who describes its presence among the Taíno Indians of Hispañola (Cuba). He documents early use in Columbia, Peru, Bolivia, Chile, Argentina, and Venezuela as well. The highlight of Torres' contribution is the exquisitely detailed study on the iconography of *Anadenanthera*-related themes found on monuments, ceramics, and snuffing paraphernalia. Torres masterfully weaves together the shamanic imagery born from the commonality in this altered state of consciousness as evidence of the relations that existed between the Tiwanaku empire of Bolivia and the dwellers of the northern Chile desert oasis of San Pedro de Atacama.

David Repke provides a rigorous review of the chemical constituents that have been described for this plant and presents primary data on the chemical profile of *Anadenanthera* seeds. Repke reveals the chemical secret behind the allure of the seeds from this tree, pointing to bufotenine, which is a close analogue of N,N-dimethyltryptamine or DMT. According to the field and laboratory research conducted by the authors, the alkaloids from the seeds of the same trees can change according to seasonal and environmental factors. The pharmacology of bufotenine is exhaustively examined in terms of laboratory animal research, basic pharmacology including receptor interactions, and human studies including behavioral pharmacology. In the concluding chapter several bioassay studies are presented in which researchers themselves, including one of the authors, ingested ground *Anadenanthera* seeds and later described their experiences. One account details the visual effects, drawing parallels to iconographic elements found in pre-Columbian art from cultures that revered this shamanic inebriant.

As the authors aptly state in closing, we may never know the intricacies of the complex relations that have existed between South American cultures and the *Anadenanthera* plant nor whether ancient trade in the seeds of this plant were intentionally designed to sow new religious ideology and worldviews. What we do know is that there is still much for us to uncover regarding the intricate workings of our brains, and that psychoactive plants, those deemed sacred by these indigenous cultures, can provide keys for us to unlock this mysterious part of our being, our minds, and our existence. This solid, scholarly work is destined to be a classic, and will surely grace the bookshelves of a diverse reading audience."

Stacy Schaefer, PhD
Associate Professor of Anthropology,
Co-Director, Museum of Anthropology,
California State University, Chico

More pre-publication
REVIEWS, COMMENTARIES, EVALUATIONS . . .

"**A**nadenathera: *Visionary Plant of Ancient South America* is the result of an extraordinary multidisciplinary investigation. Seldom (if ever?) has a member of the plant kingdom been examined in so comprehensive a manner. With the publication of this book, Torres and Repke have set a new standard for investigations into native pharmacology, indigenous mythologies, and ancient art. Not only have they clearly documented that this remarkable tree has been—and continues to be—an integral part of South American Indian shamanic culture over a period of at least 4,000 years, they show us why.

Chemists, botanists, anthropologists, art historians, as well as specialists from several other disciplines will find this new book well worth adding to their libraries and then carefully reading. It is a model of thorough scientific, investigative research, coupled with lucid, descriptive writing."

Alana Cordy-Collins, PhD
Professor of Anthropology,
University of San Diego

"**W**hen the Western world finally found the Andean world, their food-stuff discoveries were readily utilized, with potatoes and corn rapidly becoming part of accepted agricultural science. But the mind-stuff discoveries of the Andean world have had a very different reception, with their mind-altering materials receiving little scientific attention. When this attitude begins to change, *Anadenanthera* will be considered a landmark.

Certainly the beliefs and mythologies of the Andean world were profoundly affected by their mind-stuffs, paralleling the relation between the founding mythology of the Greeks and their mushrooms. *Anadenanthera* prepares a foundation for studies of the relation between Andean mythology and Andean mind-altering materials, thus providing the basis for profound comparative studies of the Andean and the Western world."

William J. Conklin
MARCH, Harvard University,
Research Associate, Field Museum

The Haworth Herbal Press®
An Imprint of The Haworth Press, Inc.
New York • London • Oxford

Anadenanthera

Visionary Plant
of Ancient South America

THE HAWORTH HERBAL PRESS®
Titles of Related Interest

Concise Handbook of Psychoactive Herbs: Medicinal Herbs for Treating Psychological and Neurological Problems by Marcello Spinella

Herbal Medicine: Chaos in the Marketplace by Rowena K. Richter

Botanical Medicines: The Desk Reference for Major Herbal Supplements, Second Edition by Dennis J. McKenna, Kenneth Jones, and Kerry Hughes

Tyler's Tips: The Shopper's Guide for Herbal Remedies by George H. Constantine

Handbook of Psychotropic Herbs: A Scientific Analysis of Herbal Remedies for Psychiatric Conditions by Ethan B. Russo

Understanding Alternative Medicine: New Health Paths in America by Lawrence Tyler

Seasoning Savvy: How to Cook with Herbs, Spices, and Other Flavorings by Alice Arndt

Tyler's Honest Herbal: A Sensible Guide to the Use of Herbs and Related Remedies, Fourth Edition by Steven Foster and Varro E. Tyler

Tyler's Herbs of Choice: The Therapeutic Use of Phytomedicinals, Second Edition by James E. Robbers and Varro E. Tyler

Medicinal Herbs: A Compendium by Beatrice Gehrmann, Wolf-Gerald Koch, Claus O. Tschirch, and Helmut Brinkmann

Understanding Medicinal Plants: Their Chemistry and Therapeutic Action by Bryan Hanson

Ayurvedic Herbs: A Clinical Guide to the Healing Plants of Traditional Medicine by M. S. Premila

Anadenanthera

Visionary Plant
of Ancient South America

Constantino Manuel Torres, PhD
David B. Repke, BSc

The Haworth Herbal Press®
An Imprint of The Haworth Press, Inc.
New York • London • Oxford

For more information on this book or to order, visit
http://www.haworthpress.com/store/product.asp?sku=5377

or call 1-800-HAWORTH (800-429-6784) in the United States and Canada
or (607) 722-5857 outside the United States and Canada

or contact orders@HaworthPress.com

Published by

The Haworth Herbal Press®, an imprint of The Haworth Press, Inc., 10 Alice Street, Binghamton, NY 13904-1580.

PUBLISHER'S NOTE
The development, preparation, and publication of this work has been undertaken with great care. However, the Publisher, employees, editors, and agents of The Haworth Press are not responsible for any errors contained herein or for consequences that may ensue from use of materials or information contained in this work. The Haworth Press is committed to the dissemination of ideas and information according to the highest standards of intellectual freedom and the free exchange of ideas. Statements made and opinions expressed in this publication do not necessarily reflect the views of the Publisher, Directors, management, or staff of The Haworth Press, Inc., or an endorsement by them.

Cover design by Jennifer M. Gaska.
Watercolor painting on cover is by Donna Torres.

Library of Congress Cataloging-in-Publication Data

Torres, Constantino Manuel.
    Anadenanthera : visionary plant of ancient South America / Constantino Manuel Torres, David B. Repke.
        p. cm.
    Includes bibliographical references and index.
    ISBN-13: 978-0-7890-2641-5 (hc. : alk. paper)
    ISBN-10: 0-7890-2641-4 (hc. : alk. paper)
    ISBN-13: 978-0-7890-2642-2 (pbk. : alk. paper)
    ISBN-10: 0-7890-2642-2 (pbk. : alk. paper)
  1. Anadenanthera—South America. I. Repke, David B. II. Title.

QK495.L52T67 2005
615'.7883—dc22
                                                                                    2005002809

To Donna, Christina, and Miguel

C. M. T.

To my wife, Linda, for her unending patience;
to my parents, Charold and George Repke,
for a lifetime of encouragement;
to Professor David H. Kenny,
for showing me the infinite wonders
of organic chemistry.

D. B. R.

ABOUT THE AUTHORS

Constantino Manuel Torres, PhD, is Professor of Art History in the Art and Art History Department, Florida International University, Miami, Florida. His primary interest is in the art and archeology of psychoactive plant use in the Central Andes. He conducts research and archaeological work in the Atacama desert of northern Chile. He has edited and/or authored numerous articles and chapters and was editor of the special thematic issue "Archaeology of Hallucinogens in the Andean Region" in Eleusis 5, 2001.

David B. Repke, BSc, is an organic chemist specializing in the investigation of centrally active medicinal plants. He has authored numerous papers and chapters in monographs on topics such as the synthesis of new medicinal agents, the isolation, identification, and synthesis of both fungal and higher plant alkaloids, the elemental analysis of human bone from burials at Carthage, and the chemical analysis of both contemporary and archeological medicinal plant preparations from South America. His recent research interests include a number of areas involving the central nervous system and the medicinal chemistry and pharmacology of the serotonin neurotransmitter system.

CONTENTS

Foreword

My first meeting with Constantino Manuel Torres was almost twelve years ago, just before the initial International Conference for the Study of Modified States of Consciousness, which was held in the city and state of San Luis Potosí, in central Mexico. That was many years ago, and it was the story of Manuel's research that led me to appreciate just how ancient the history of psychoactive drug use really is. He is a professor with Florida International University, in Miami, in the area of art history. But his true love is pre-Columbian art and culture, and he has been the source of much of our knowledge of the pre-Christian history of the Andean area of South America.

It was several years earlier that I had first met David Repke. At that time he was an organic chemist with a northern California pharmaceutical company, and I quickly appreciated that he was a master in the area of tryptamine chemistry. He was interested in the synthesis of plant alkaloids and their analogues, and this fit beautifully with my own curiosity about psychoactive compounds. Our interaction has led to our co-authoring of a couple of publications in the scientific literature. At that time, our mutual interests were focused on the N-alkylated analogues of the active ayahuasca component dimethyltryptamine and the four-substituted counterparts such as psilocin and psilocybin that are the major contributors to the activity of the magic mushrooms of the *Psilocybe* genus.

The third component of this remarkable confluence was yet earlier, back in the late 1950s, when I learned of the sources, structure, and possible activity of a simple but largely unknown compound called bufotenine or mappine. It had the reputation of being a potent hallucinogen, but through my own preliminary exploration with it I had come to the conclusion that it was not a psychedelic material. Indeed, some activity could be assigned to it, but I had decided that these observations were an extension of neurological stimulation outside of the brain, and casually dismissed the compound as active, but not centrally active. The published reports on the action of bufotenine in clinical trials over the intervening forty years have presented much conflicting data that have not satisfactorily answered this question. There has been a continuing contradiction between the two conflicting conclusions: one stating, "Yes, it is active," and the other, "No, it is not active." This book neatly summarizes all this earlier published data and brings it up to date. The inescapable conclusion—bufotenine is indeed a psychoactive alkaloid.

To the curious reader, this presentation is a remarkable interdisciplinary integration. It presents, with thorough documentation, the anthropological, botanical, chemical, and pharmacological worlds that contain our scientific knowledge of a most remarkable group of trees. But this book, for me personally, is a pleasant bringing together of the worlds of three old friends, two of them remarkable scientists and the third one a mysterious white crystalline solid.

Alexander T. Shulgin
Independent Researcher
Lafayette, California

Preface

At the outset, it must be appreciated how inextricably entwined are various plant species in the story of the New World visionary drug complex. That this is so attests to two rather amazing facts: (1) the Western Hemisphere contains what seems to be a vast array of plants that possess the means to open doors to other worlds, yet when the numbers are tallied, approximately 100 species (Schultes and Hofmann 1980) out of a global estimate of 600,000 to 800,000 have been discovered to have been so used; and (2) the resourcefulness of pre-Columbian indigenous peoples at discovering and utilizing just the right plant or, even more intriguing, the right plant mixtures for use in their traditional healing practices is compelling. We have tried not to stray too far from the path when telling the story of the species of arborescent legumes with which this monograph is concerned. However, the inescapable interconnection of *Anadenanthera* with other plant species and families used for the same or similar purposes compels the occasional discussion of them to preserve continuity.

The genus *Anadenanthera* was, together with tobacco, one of the most widely used shamanic inebriants. It is primarily South American in distribution and includes two species with two varieties each. The earliest evidence for the use of psychoactive plants in South America is provided by remains of seeds and pods recovered from archaeological sites four millennia old. Seeds are roasted, pulverized, and inhaled through the nose, or smoked in pipes or as cigars. *Anadenanthera* also serves as an ingredient for *chicha* (a fermented drink) or similar preparations. The archaeological and ethnographical record have provided a wealth of information concerning the use of *Anadenanthera*. This is particularly true for regions of Peru, Chile, Bolivia, and Argentina where the climate has favored preservation of ancient artifacts and human remains. Study of these materials has provided evidence of the continuous association of *Anadenanthera* with emerging Andean cultures. Such findings are indicative of its central role in the cultural development of indigenous New World societies.

In addition to cultural and ideological issues, there are scientific and economic concerns that a study of this genus makes apparent. In the age of sophisticated chemical synthesis in which modern methods of analysis have made possible the development of hundreds of new potential therapeutic agents in a single year, we forget that many of our widely used life-saving medications are either natural products or artificial compounds derived synthetically using natural products as starting points or design templates. The medicinal properties of totally artificial drugs have often been discovered using time-honored natural agents in classic pharmacological studies. Many of these wonder drugs have had their origin in the folk remedies of past centuries. As R. E. Schultes has pointed out on many occasions, there is some urgency in the study of indigenous (some would say "primitive") natural product use and their plant sources, particularly in the New World. This is because many of these plants and the people who use them are sadly disappearing, the former by large-scale destruction of habitats, the latter because of inevitable enculturation by modern societies.

The scientific study of the visionary tryptamines has not only advanced our knowledge in the neurosciences but has also had a direct impact upon the development of antimigraine medications. The use of these materials (and synthetic agents derived from them) as tools in the study of central nervous system function, although well on its way, is still in its infancy. Those who discount the utility of these agents in such endeavors would do well to ponder the words of Mandell and Geyer (1976: 730):

> [H]allucinogenic drugs produce massively awesome phenomena in man that can and do become prepotent over any of our trivial theories of how drugs may work and caution us not to become too grandiose in our feelings that we understand how man's brain functions.

Although much discussion has been allocated to the botany, chemistry, and anthropology of *Anadenanthera,* we have endeavored to provide information on other uses of the genus, such as in lumber and paper production. Such economic botany is an important consideration for the emerging nations of South America, especially in light of the fact that these trees are a renewable resource that grow well under cultivation in otherwise marginal soils. Reforestation projects are sorely needed in the Western Hemisphere, as elsewhere.

This book provides a detailed study of the genus *Anadenanthera* and its role in the construction and subsequent modifications of native American ideologies. The first chapter focuses on botanical aspects, taxonomy, and geographical distribution; distinctions between *Anadenanthera* and *Piptadenia* species are also discussed. In Chapter 2 we investigate the use of *Anadenanthera* by pre-Columbian cultures, while in Chapter 3 we discuss ethnographical, historical, and traditional aspects of *Anadenanthera* use. These two chapters include formal and iconographic analyses of artistic expressions inherent in the associated ritual and ceremonial paraphernalia. Subsequently, Chapters 4 and 5 describe the chemical and pharmacological investigations of the genus and the various visionary preparations derived from it, with emphasis on the biologically active constituents. Theories of the mechanisms of action of the active tryptamines and carboline alkaloids are presented as well as the possible synergism between the two classes of compounds. Finally, Chapter 6 provides a comparative review of the evidence. Comparisons of wood anatomy, morphology, and percentage of alkaloid content attest to the broad range of variability of the genus. Stylistic and iconographic traits are evaluated and provide new insights into mechanisms of ideological interaction. Evidence provided by investigations into the shamanic use of *Anadenanthera* in the Amazon during the postconquest period is compared with the archaeological evidence. We conclude with a comprehensive bibliography.

Acknowledgments

We acknowledge gratefully the generous assistance of Dr. Alexander Shulgin for reviewing Chapters 4 and 5, and for writing the foreword. We are beholden to Dr. Jonathan Ott for discussion and advice, and for carefully reviewing the manuscript. Dr. María Antonietta Costa, Dr. Agustín Llagostera, Dr. Robert Montgomery, and Dr. Christian Rätsch provided invaluable field assistance; their generosity and enthusiasm, together with that of J. Ott and D. Torres, contributed greatly to the success of our journeys of research. We thank our friend and colleague, Dennis McKenna, for many shared years in the pursuit of common interests, for 25 years of friendship, and for many hours of scholarly discussions on matters pertaining to the study of traditional healing practices in the Americas.

We would like to express our appreciation to the following specialists for support, insightful input, hospitality, and encouragement in this endeavor: Dr. Richard Evans Schultes, Professor Emeritus and Curator, Botanical Museum, Harvard University, Cambridge, Massachusetts; Dr. Robert F. Raffauf, Professor Emeritus, Northeastern University, Boston, Massachusetts; Dr. Bo Holmstedt of the Karolinska Institute, Stockholm, Sweden; Nicole Grinder; Dr. Hans Maag; William and Barbara Conklin, Washington, DC; Linda Repke, Milpitas, California; Dr. Alexander Muehldorf; Dr. Richard Eglen, Senior Vice President, Assay Technologies, LJL BioSystems, Sunnyvale, California; Reddy Chamakura, Forensic Laboratory, New York City Police Department; Dr. Jace Callaway, Kuopio, Finland; Dr. Luis Eduardo Luna, Swedish School of Economics, Helsinki, Finland; Professor William Maguire, Art and Art History Department, Florida International University, Miami; Dr. Lautaro Núñez, Francisco Téllez, Macarena Oviedo, Timoteo Cruz, Santiago Ramos, Luis Ramirez, and Tomás Cruz of the Instituto de Investigaciones Arqueológicas y Museo R. P. Le Paige, San Pedro de Atacama, Chile; Pedro Tolaba and Dr. Fortunato Ruiz, Misión Wichi, General Mosconi, Salta, Argentina; Dr. Carlos Aldunate, Dr. José Berenguer, Luis Cornejo, Carole Sinclaire, Julia Arriagada, and Francisco Gallardo, Museo

Chileno de Arte Precolombino, Santiago, Chile; Dr. Alicia Fernandez Distel, Jujuy, Argentina; Luis Alberto Lucas, Jujuy, Argentina; Alberto Lopez Viñals, Salta, Argentina; Dr. Carlos Aschero, Universidad Nacional de Tucumán, Argentina; Dr. Javier Escalante and Eduardo Parejas, Museo Tiwanaku, La Paz, Bolivia; Ricardo Cespedes, Museo de Antropología y Arqueología de la Universidad de San Simón, Cochabamba, Bolivia; and the late Dr. S. Henry Wassén, Gothenburg, Sweden.

Chapter 1

The Botany of *Anadenanthera*

TAXONOMIC BACKGROUND

The genus *Anadenanthera* Spegazzini is in the section Mimosoideae of the family Fabaceae, order Fabales. Its first scientific description appeared in 1737 in the *Hortus Cliffortianus,* from a specimen growing in the Clifford Garden in Holland. Safford (1916) and Reis Altschul (1964) are of the opinion that the seed from which the type specimen was grown came from the West Indies or northern South America. The earliest valid name is *Mimosa peregrina,* from Linnaeus's *Species Plantarum* (1753; Safford 1916). Linnaeus did not specify why he applied the epithet *peregrina.* His description was based on the more complete entry in the *Hortus Cliffortianus* (Reis Altschul 1964). The 1806 Willdenow edition of *Species Plantarum* identified as *Inga niopo* the material collected by Humboldt and Bonpland along the Orinoco River. In 1814, Humboldt corrected Willdenow and identified the plant as an *Acacia* and not an *Inga,* labeling it *Acacia niopo* (Humboldt and Bonpland 1971). In her taxonomic study of the genus, Siri von Reis Altschul (1964) considers this specimen to be equivalent to *Anadenanthera peregrina* var. *peregrina* (see Appendix).

The genus *Anadenanthera* as established by J. P. M. Brenan (1955) and Reis Altschul (1964, 1967, 1972) was originally conceived by Bentham (1840, 1841-1842, 1874-1875) as section *Niopa* of the genus *Piptadenia.* Bentham placed 25 species under *Piptadenia,* all of them American. He divided the genus into three sections, *Eupiptadenia* and *Pityrocarpa* with spicate inflorescences, and *Niopa* with globose inflorescences (Reis Altschul 1964; Brenan 1955). Bentham originally distinguished five species in section *Niopa: Piptadenia peregrina, P. macrocarpa, P. falcata, P. colubrina,* and *P. microphylla.* Bentham (1874-1875) later proposed only four species, placing *P.*

microphylla in synonymy with *P. macrocarpa*. Brenan (1955) indicated that *Niopa* is a natural group, whereas the species included in the other two sections were very mixed and should not be classified as proposed by Bentham.

In 1922, Carlos Spegazzini founded the genus *Anadenanthera* to accommodate *P. peregrina* and *P. falcata*. He based the genus on the flowers lacking anther glands, and on the elliptical and elongated anthers that differ from those found in the species with anther glands (Spegazzini 1922). According to Reis Altschul (1964) and Brenan (1955), this is insufficient to justify generic separation. In 1927, Britton and Rose proposed section *Niopa* as a genus (Reis Altschul 1964). However, *Anadenanthera* antedates *Niopa* as a generic name.

In 1955, Brenan revised the genus *Piptadenia* according to criteria that included the mode of dehiscence of the pod and the structure of the seed. Brenan proposed eight genera with species formerly included in *Piptadenia*. The genus *Anadenanthera* as proposed by Brenan (1955) consists of the four species formerly in section *Niopa* of *Piptadenia*. He distinguished *Anadenanthera* by the following characteristics: globose inflorescence; dehiscence of the pod along one suture; suborbicular, narrowly or not winged seeds lacking endosperms; and strictly American distribution (see also Reis Altschul 1964). Differences in wood anatomy coincide with the eight genera proposed by Brenan and support the distinctiveness of *Anadenanthera* as a genus (Reis Altschul 1964; Brazier 1958; see also Tortorelli 1948).

Siri von Reis Altschul (1964), in her taxonomic revision of the genus, considered *Anadenanthera* to consist of two species, *A. peregrina* (L.) Speg. and *A. colubrina* (Vell.) Brenan, each species having two varieties. The two varieties of *Anadenanthera peregrina* are *A. peregrina* (L.) Speg. var. *peregrina* Reis Altschul and *A. peregrina* (L.) Speg. var. *falcata* (Benth.) Reis Altschul. The varieties of *A. colubrina* are *A. colubrina* (Vell.) Brenan var. *colubrina* Reis Altschul and *A. colubrina* (Vell.) Brenan var. *Cebil* (Griseb.) Reis Altschul.

Reis Altschul distinguished these two species by means of a few consistent morphological characters and their correlation with particular geographical locations. The taxonomy was based partly on the presence or absence of a gland on each anther, and on the position of the involucre surrounding the peduncle. The two species can be identified most easily on the basis of the pod texture, since the flowers of the different genera that compose the Mimosoideae are so similar. *A. peregrina* has dull, scurfy to verrucose pods and it is the more northerly of the two species. *A. colubrina* has nitid, smooth to reticulated pods, and it is limited to the southern hemisphere (Reis Altschul 1964). *A. peregrina* var. *peregrina* (Plates 1, 2) and *A. colubrina* var. *Cebil* (Plates 3-5) are the two species employed as the source of psychoactive preparations, most notably in the form of snuff powders.

The genus *Anadenanthera* has a wide distribution on the South American continent and in the Greater Antilles. The two species have a preference for savanna habitats, although they seem to be adaptable to a variety of altitudes. Siri von Reis Altschul (1964: 40) stated:

> Neither species of *Anadenanthera* is represented, to my knowledge, in western Amazonas nor in the Andes of northern Peru, Ecuador and Colombia. This circumstance is probably due to an inability of the representatives of *A. peregrina* var. *peregrina* to tolerate the true rain-forest conditions through which they would have to pass in a westward dispersal. There is equally little reason to believe that representatives of *A. colubrina* var. *Cebil* would descend from the Andes into lowland rain-forest.

In a study of plant domestication among the Yanomamö, Napoleon Chagnon reported the presence of *A. peregrina* var. *peregrina* in the upper Orinoco region. Chagnon emphatically stated that in this region *Anadenanthera* is a jungle plant ("*hisioma* es una planta selvática en esta región"). All Yanomamö groups know this tree and refer to it using the same term, *hisioma,* suggesting a wide distribution of *Anadenanthera* in the upper Orinoco region (Chagnon et al. 1970: 188-189).

SPECIES DESCRIPTIONS

Anadenanthera peregrina (L.) Speg. (Reis Altschul 1964: 45-46):

> Shrub to tall tree, 3-27 m high. Trunk 20-40 cm in diameter at breast height, usually leaning, twisted, sometimes divided at the base into several shafts; more frequently the contorted, irregular branches spread out above the middle of a solitary trunk into an

umbrella-like crown. Bark gray to nearly black with many small lenticels; unarmed or lower trunk producing conical thorns or wedge-shaped projections, sometimes intensely so when young, becoming tubercular-verrucose, corky, rugose and, in drier climates, very thick. Young twigs and foliage puberulent, occasionally glaucescent; mature foliage glabrous or nearly so. Leaves, including petioles, 12-30 cm long, the main rachis more or less channeled ventrally. Petioles somewhat darkened at their bases, 5-15 mm above which each bears a flattish, oval or oblong gland .5-5 mm long; 1-4 similar, smaller glands borne one between or just below each of the ultimate pinna pairs. Pinna pairs 10-30 or more, each pinna 2-5 cm or more long, opposite or subopposite leaflets usually imbricate 25-80 pairs, 2-8 mm long, .5-1.5 mm wide, linear, oblong or lanceolate, straight to falcate, at the base oblique or truncate, at the apex acute to acuminate to apiculate; venation obscure except for a single, nearly straight, slightly excentric mid-vein; membranaceous to coriaceous and nitid, sometimes differing in color and texture dorsiventrally. Heads 10-18 mm in diameter, including stamens, greenish white to creamy yellow, in fascicles of 1-5, puberulous to glabrous in the bud; the heads axillary to the leaves and subterminal, rarely becoming arranged in racemose patterns in the branch apices. Peduncles 1.75-4 cm long, puberulous, filiform or thicker, each bearing about three-quarters of the way up the axis a puberulous bi-dentate, campanulate involucre which becomes detached and slides down to encircle loosely the base of the peduncle. Calyx .5-2.6 mm long. Corolla 2-3.5 mm long stamens 5-8 mm long; anthers eglandular in the bud. Legume 5-35 cm long (including the stipe but not the peduncle), 1-3 cm wide, straight to falcate, oblongish to elongated, regularly to irregularly, vaguely or not at all contracted between the seeds, more or less flattened with margins slightly thickened; at the base attenuate to obtuse, at the apex mucronate to acuminate to cuspidate or, if the tip has broken off, rounded; surface scurfy to verrucose, and dull; dark brown with rufous scales in dried specimens. Seeds 8-16, very thin, flat, orbicular to suborbicular, dark chestnut brown to black, shiny, 10-20 mm in diameter.

Compared to *A. colubrina*, *A. peregrina* has a wider north-south distribution and is found from 20 degrees N latitude to 26 degrees S latitude (Reis Altschul 1964). *A. peregrina* var. *peregrina* can be found in the Greater Antilles, most notably on the islands of Hispaniola and Puerto Rico. It is likely that humans are responsible for the introduction of *Anadenanthera* into the Greater Antilles (Reis Altschul 1964). The distribution of the tree in the Greater Antilles coincides with Taíno occupation, early inhabitants of Hispaniola and Puerto Rico (see Chapter 2). The snuff prepared from *A. peregrina* seeds was of great importance to Taíno spirituality. *A. peregrina* var. *peregrina* is less frequently represented in the Lesser Antilles. These islands were occupied by Caribs, who arrived in the islands relatively late and are not known to have used *Anadenanthera* preparations. On the other hand, the tree is represented in Trinidad and Tobago, islands considered to be similar floristically to the adjacent South American mainland. In northern South America, var. *peregrina* is present in Colombia, Venezuela, British Guiana, and northern Brazil. This is the most widespread and north-ranging of the two varieties, occurring from 20 degrees N latitude to 15 degrees S latitude (Reis Altschul 1964). *A. peregrina* var. *falcata* is a much shorter tree than var. *peregrina*. The pod, usually falcate, is shorter and narrower than in var. *peregrina*. It is found in the southern Brazilian states of Minas Gerais, Mato Grosso, Paraná, and São Paulo, and in Paraguay. This is the most southern-ranging variety of *A. peregrina* and is found from 15 degrees S latitude to approximately 26 degrees S latitude (Reis Altschul 1964).

Anadenanthera colubrina (Vell.) Brenan (Reis Altschul 1964: 51-52):

> Shrub to tall tree, 3-30 m high. Trunk 30-50 cm in diameter at breast height, commonly erect. Bark 2-5 cm thick, grayish, smooth or rugose, sometimes striated with small longitudinal fissures; unarmed or with mammillose protuberances. Young twigs and foliage partly puberulent, sometimes tomentellose, usually becoming glabrous with maturity. Leaves, including petioles 4-20 cm long, the main rachis channeled ventrally. Petioles scatteredly pubescent, at their bases horizontally wrinkled and each commonly bearing, somewhere below the first pinna pair, a flattened or erect, oval to disciform more or less centrally depressed gland 1-5 mm long; 1-3 (rarely to 7) similar, smaller glands borne one between or just below each of the ultimate pinna pairs. Pinna pairs 7-35 or more each pinna 1.2-7 cm long,

usually opposite. Leaflets not always borne to the tip of the pinna, which may end in a fine point 1.5-2 mm beyond the ultimate pair of leaflets. Leaflets imbricate or expanded, 20-80 pairs, .9-6 mm long, .5-1.5 mm wide, linear or slightly dilated in the middle, oblong to lanceolate, usually straight (not falcate), and the base oblique or truncate, at the apex acute to apiculate or obtuse; venation obscure, or with a straight or nearly straight, slightly excentric mid-vein, and more or less prominent secondary reticulated veins; membranaceous to coriaceous and nitidulous above, sometimes differing in color and texture dorsiventrally. Heads 15-20 mm in diameter, including stamens, white to whitish yellow to orangey, in fascicles of 1-7, minutely whitish-tomentose to nearly glabrous in the bud; the heads axillary to the leaves and subterminal, or becoming arranged in racemose-paniculate patterns in the branch apices with the leaves reduced or absent. Peduncles 2-4 cm long, puberulous to glabrous, thicker than filiform, each bearing just below the receptacle and often hidden by the mature head a narrow, more or less glabrous annular involucre. Calyx .6-3 mm long. Corolla 2.5-4 mm long. Stamens 5-8 mm long; anthers each with a caducous gland. Legume 10-32 cm long (including the stipe but not the thickened peduncle), 1-3 cm wide, straight to sometimes falcate, oblongish to very elongated, regularly contracted to sinuate, or irregularly contracted where seeds have aborted, sometimes very flattened and thin, with margins often strongly thickened, even though sometimes narrow; at the base attenuate to obtuse or truncate, at the apex mucronate to acuminate to cuspidate or, if the tip has broken off, rounded; surface smooth to reticulated, and nitid; light, dark or reddish brown or dark gray in dried specimens. Seeds 8-16, thin, flat, orbicular to oblong, dark chestnut brown, very shiny, 12-20 mm in diameter.

A. colubrina is only present south of the equator, and has an approximate distribution from 0 to 30 degrees S latitude (Hunziker 1973; Reis Altschul 1964). It has adapted to a wider variety of environments than the other species and can be found on river banks or dry slopes up to altitudes of 2700 m. *Anadenanthera colubrina* var. *Cebil* is the more variable of the two varieties and has the wider east-west distributional range. It is found from the equator to 30 degrees S latitude (Hunziker 1973; Reis Altschul 1964) and is a taller tree than var. *colubrina,* from which it may also be distinguished by the pods, which are shorter, wider, and more thickly margined. It is found in Argentina in the provinces of Salta, Jujuy, Catamarca, Tucumán, and Misiones. It grows most abundantly in Salta and Jujuy provinces—in some areas of western Salta it is a dominant tree. It can also be found in Paraguay, Bolivia, and Peru where it grows as far north as the Marañón River valley on the western slopes of the Andes (Reis Altschul 1964).

Anadenanthera colubrina var. *colubrina* is the less widespread variety, found from 12 to 27 degrees S latitude. It is the most easily recognized variety of the genus owing to the distinctive arrangement of the inflorescences, which are borne in paniculate patterns and have fewer flowers (Reis Altschul 1964). The pod is more elongated and darker than in var. *Cebil.* This variety tends to have a coastal distribution, limited to the Brazilian states of Bahia, Paraná, Rio de Janeiro, and São Paulo; it is also found in Misiones, Argentina (Reis Altschul 1964). *A. colubrina* var. *colubrina* overlaps in its distribution with *A. peregrina* var. *falcata.* The information available for var. *colubrina* is sparse consequently our understanding of its ecology and distribution is limited (Reis Altschul 1964). The areas shared by *A. peregrina* var. *falcata* and *A. colubrina* var. *colubrina* are within the locus proposed by Reis Altschul (1964) for the origin of the genus *Anadenanthera,* located in the southern part of the Brazilian highlands.

APPENDIX:
SYNONYMS AND INDIGENOUS NAMES

Anadenanthera *Synonymy*

Anadenanthera peregrina (L.) Speg. var. *peregrina* von Reis Alt. (Reis Altschul 1964):

Mimosa peregrina L. (earliest valid name, 1753)
Inga niopo Humb. & Bonpl. ex. Willd.
Acacia niopo (Humb. & Bonpl. ex. Willd.)
Piptadenia peregrina (L.) Benth.
Piptadenia niopo (Humb. & Bonpl. ex. Willd.)
Niopa peregrina (L.) Britton & Rose
Acacia microphylla Willd.

Acacia angustiloba (*Acacia angustifolia* might be a synonym)
Acacia peregrina (L.) Willd.
Mimosa parvifolia Poir.

Anadenanthera peregrina (L.) Speg. var. *falcata* (Benth.) von Reis Alt. (Reis Altschul 1964):

> *Piptadenia falcata* Benth.
> *Piptadenia peregrina* (L.) var. *falcata* (Benth.)
> *Anadenanthera falcata* (Benth.) Speg.

Anadenanthera colubrina (Vell.) Brenan var. *colubrina* von Reis Alt. (Reis Altschul 1964):

> *Mimosa colubrina* Vell.
> *Acacia colubrina* (Vell.) Mart.
> *Piptadenia colubrina* (Vell.) Benth.
> *Anadenanthera colubrina* (Vell.) Brenan

Anadenanthera colubrina (Vell.) Brenan var. *Cebil* (Griseb.) von Reis Alt. (Reis Altschul 1964):

> *Acacia Cebil* (Griseb.)
> *Piptadenia macrocarpa* Benth. (*cebil colorado* and *cebil moro*)
> *Piptadenia macrocarpa* Benth. var. *vestita* Chod. & Hass.
> *Piptadenia macrocarpa* Benth. var. *genuina* Chod. & Hass.
> *Piptadenia macrocarpa* Benth. var. *Cebil* (Griseb.) Chod. & Hass.
> *Anadenanthera macrocarpa* (Benth.) Brenan
> *Piptadenia Cebil* (Griseb.) Griseb.
> *Piptadenia microphylla* Benth.
> *Piptadenia Hassleriana* Chod.
> *Piptadenia Hassleriana* Chod. var. *fruticosa* Chod. & Hass.

Indigenous Names for Anadenanthera Species

Acujá: Yecuaná, Upper Ventuari river; *A. peregrina*. Koch-Grünberg 1917-1928; Wassén 1965; Wassén and Holmstedt 1963; Wurdack 1958.

Aimpä, Aimpë: Tupari, Rio Branco, and Guaporé, W. Brazil; *A. colubrina*. Caspar 1956; Wassén 1965, 1967b.

Akiri: Bororo, upper reaches of the Paraguay River and its effluents, Matto Grosso, Brazil; *A. colubrina*. Fabian 1992.

Akuá: Tunebo, Arauca River, E. Colombia; *A. peregrina.* Cooper 1949; Márquez 1979; Uscátegui 1961.

Cebil, Cébil, Cevil, Cibil, Sebil, Sevil: Northwest Argentina, Paraguay, Uruguay, southeast Brazil; *A. colubrina* var. *Cebil.* Lozano 1941; Reis Altschul 1972; Sotelo de Narvaez 1965 (first mention: ca. 1583—*Sebil*).

Cohoba, Cogioba, Cohobba, Cojoba: Taíno, Greater Antilles; *A. peregrina* var. *peregrina.* Bourne 1906; Las Casas 1909; Oviedo y Valdés 1959; Pané 1974 (first mention: Christopher Columbus, ca. 1496); Safford 1916; Wassén 1967a.

Curupa, Curupá, Curuva, Curuba: Otomac, Orinoco area, Omagua, mouth of the Napo; *A. peregrina* var. *peregrina.* La Condamine 1778; Métraux 1948b; Reis Altschul 1964. See Reis Altschul 1972 and Wassén 1965 for discussion of etymology of *curupa*.

Hatáj, Hatax, Ha'tax, Jatáj, Jatáj-ilé: Wichi (Mataco); *A. colubrina* var. *Cebil.* Arenas 1992; Califano 1976; Dasso 1985; Dijour 1933.

Hisioma, Hisiomi, Sisioma: Yanomamö (Waika); *A. peregrina* var. *peregrina.* Brewer-Carias and Steyermark 1976; Chagnon et al. 1970; Chagnon et al. 1971; Plotkin 1993; Wassén 1965; Wassén and Holmstedt 1963.

Kurupá, Kurupaî, Curupay: Guaraní (S. Brazil); *A. colubrina* var. *Cebil.* Pardal 1937; Reis Altschul 1972.

Morí: Kaxúyana, Trombetas River, Brazil; *A. peregrina.* Frikel 1961; Polykrates 1960.

Vihó: Tukano, Vaupés River, Colombia. Reichel-Dolmatoff uses the word *Vihó* to refer to *Anadenanthera* (Reichel-Dolmatoff 1971) and *Virola* snuff powders (Reichel-Dolmatoff 1978).

Vilca, Huilca, Huillka, Villca, Willka: Peru, Bolivia; *A. colubrina* var. *Cebil.* Acosta 1985; Reis Altschul 1967, 1972; Duviols 1967 (quoting a *Relación* by Cristobal de Albornoz, ca. 1580); Larraín Barros 1976; Ondegardo 1916 (first mention: 1571—*Villca,* referring to Inca use); Yacovleff and Herrera 1934-1935.

Yopo, Jopa, Yop, Yopa, Niopo, Ñopo: Colombia: Muisca, Tunebo, Pijao (Alto Magdalena), Guahibo, Guayupe (Guaviare River); Venezuela: Piaroa; *A. peregrina* var. *peregrina.* Aguado 1956; Gumilla 1984; Humboldt and Bonpland 1971; Oviedo y Valdés 1959 (first mention: ca. 1535—*Yop,* referring to Muisca use); Smet and Rivier 1985; Spruce 1970 (Guahibo); Vargas Machuca 1892.

Chapter 2

Archaeological Evidence
for *Anadenanthera* Preparations

Archaeological evidence for the use of psychoactive plants exists in several forms. The most direct evidence is actual plant remains in an archaeological context. *Anadenanthera* seeds have been found in archaeological sites in northwestern Argentina and in northern Chile (see Fernández Distel 1980; Llagostera et al. 1988). Tobacco and *Ilex guayusa* (a caffeine-containing plant) leaves were excavated at the site of Niño Korin in Bolivia (Wassén 1972b; Schultes 1972). Remains of the psychoactive cacti known as San Pedro and huachuma *(Trichocereus pachanoi)* have been found at archaeological sites on the central Peruvian coast (Fung 1972; Polia Meconi 1996). However, these are rare occurrences possible only in dry environments with good preservation of organic materials.

The most frequent category of evidence consists of the implements utilized in preparation and ingestion of psychoactive plants. Snuffing paraphernalia and smoking pipes provide the best evidence of this type. The equipment for the inhalation of psychoactive powders consists of a distinct set of implements: a small tray, a snuffing tube, a spoon, and leather pouches as containers for the powders (Plates 6, 7). Snuffing, the nasal inhalation of very fine powders, was a widely distributed practice throughout South America and the Caribbean. It was generally accomplished in the following two modes: self-administered and collaborative. Self-administration is performed via a variety of inhalers, usually made of bird bone or wood. The shapes include single tubes and double parallel tubes, as well as Y- and V-shaped inhalers. The collaborative modality is usually achieved via a long bamboo or bird bone tube that is preloaded with the powder, one individual blowing the snuff into the nose of another; this method is most frequent among the Yanomamö of the Orinoco basin. Snuffing tubes in pre-Columbian times are mostly single cylinders intended for self-administration. Archaeological evidence for the collaborative method is scarce.

Bone, ceramic, or stone smoking pipes are also frequent in archaeological sites throughout the south central Andes. Among formative cultures of northwestern Argentina, particularly those in the Puna de Jujuy, such pipes have been associated with *Anadenanthera* seeds (Fernández Distel 1980; Pérez Gollán and Gordillo 1994).

Enemas represent another category of implements for the ingestion of ritual inebriants. Enema syringes generally consist of a reed or bone tube to which is attached a bulb made out of a bladder or leather. Implements of this type have been found in Argentina, Bolivia, and Chile (Nordenskiöld 1930; Rosen 1924; Smet 1985; Wassén 1972b). Rectal ingestion of *Anadenanthera* seed potions is widespread in the Amazon basin (Smet 1985).

Plants that are prepared as beverages, such as San Pedro cactus *(Trichocereus pachanoi)* and *Brugmansia,* present particular difficulties that complicate their identification in an archaeological context. Ingestion or preparation of such plants requires no paraphernalia that might be identified with certainty, and conjecture of such practices based solely on presence of elaborate drinking vessels is insubstantial and unwise.

Artistic representation of plants constitutes a third type of archaeological evidence for shamanic inebriants. San Pedro cacti are represented in the stone sculptures and ceramics of the Chavín culture of the Peruvian highlands (ca. 1000-300 B.C.; Burger 1995; Mulvany de Peñaloza 1984; Sharon 2000). Probable mushroomic representations are seen in pre-Hispanic Colombian goldwork of the Darién style (ca. A.D. 900-1500s; Schultes and Bright 1979). *Anadenanthera* depictions are seen in the pottery of the Moche (ca. A.D. 100-800), a coastal culture of northern Peru (Furst 1974b). Psychoactive plants are nevertheless rarely represented in pre-Columbian Andean artifacts. The ingestion of psychoactive plants and the instruments employed in their preparation and use are sometimes depicted. Snuffing implements, for example, are prominently displayed by the monumental stone figures at San Agustín, Colombia, and Tiwanaku, Bolivia (Berenguer 1987; Torres 1981).

Early colonial documents offer a fourth category of evidence. Chroniclers such as Ramón Pané (1974), Bartolomé de Las Casas

(1909), Gonzalo Fernández de Oviedo y Valdés (1959), and Fray Pedro de Aguado (1956), writing in the late fifteenth and early sixteenth centuries, clearly described the preparation and ingestion of psychoactive snuff powders and smoking mixtures derived from seeds and herbs. The plants are often referred to by their indigenous names, and the rituals related to psychoactive plant use are briefly delineated. The resulting primary evidence is of crucial importance to the understanding of ancient ritual inebriants.

Documentation of ancient use of *Anadenanthera* is founded on all the methods described. As previously mentioned, however, archaeobotanical remains of *Anadenanthera* are rare; representations of the genus in Andean artifacts likewise are restricted to Moche pottery. The Moche occupied the arid north coast of present-day Peru between ca. A.D. 100 and 800. Depictions of *Anadenanthera* in Moche ceramics were first identified by Peter Furst (1974b), based on the design of a Moche IV pottery dipper painted with a deer-hunting scene (Plate 8). The bipinnately compound leaves and the sinuate, irregularly contracted pods with cuspidate apices are all characteristic of *Anadenanthera* (see Donnan 1976, 1978; Furst 1974b). In addition, in Moche ceramics this tree is represented with its typical slightly arched branches. All these features clearly distinguish this genus from other leguminous trees abundant throughout the western slopes of the Andes and Pacific coast such as *algarrobo (Prosopis chilensis)* and *espino (Acacia macracanta)*. Usually the tree is represented in Moche pottery, but in some instances only pods or seeds are shown.

Anadenanthera representations are restricted to painted stirrup-spout vessels and pottery dippers, where it is usually associated with a deer identified by Christopher Donnan (1982) as the white-tailed deer (*Odocoileus* sp.). Male and female animals are depicted, although male representations are twice as common as female (Donnan 1982). *Anadenanthera* trees generally form part of deer-hunting scenes. These scenes appear ritualistic in character since the hunt is conducted by elaborately dressed individuals, sometimes with supernatural attributes (Plates 8, 9). Several other factors reinforce the ritualistic or symbolic connotations of the hunt. Donnan (1982) remarked that evidence for eating deer meat was totally absent from the Moche archaeological record. The deer on Moche pottery are usually spotted (Plate 10). This is a rare feature on white-tailed deer, and a white spot that is sometimes painted on the deer's neck does not seem to occur in nature. In addition, deer are the only animals anthropo-morphized in Moche art (Donnan 1978, 1982). The ritualistic nature of these scenes is reinforced by the constant presence of fruiting *Anadenanthera* trees.

We have no evidence for snuffing among the Moche, although several scenes involving deer depicted on stirrup-spout vessels suggest the possibility that *Anadenanthera* preparations might have been administered orally. In one of these scenes, two female figures are associated with large vessels with domed lids and attached tree branches that, when compared to those on the vessels with deer hunting scenes, could tentatively be identified as *Anadenanthera*. The domed lids of two of the vessels represented on these vases are replaced by deer heads (Plate 11). The constant association and identification of the deer with fruiting *Anadenanthera* trees and their association with these ceramic vessels and ladles underscore the possibility of oral administration among the Moche. A thorny, columnar cactus and a plant with a single flower are sometimes represented in these deer hunting scenes (Donnan 1976, 1982). The cactus could possibly be a *Trichocereus* species. The flowering plant has been tentatively identified by Christopher Donnan (personal communication, 1998) as a bromeliad, and there is suggestive evidence for psychoactive bromeliads in Brazil and Mexico (Ott 1996).

The most abundant evidence for ancient *Anadenanthera* use consists of snuffing equipment and smoking pipes, although chroniclers were reliable in describing the use of *Anadenanthera* by cultures they contacted during the early colonial period. The Taíno of the Greater Antilles were meticulously documented by Columbus, Pané, and Las Casas. The Taíno were the first people observed by the European conquerors to snuff and smoke both *Anadenanthera* and *Nicotiana* preparations.

The following sections place evidence for the use of *Anadenanthera* spp. within its proper cultural context. The detailed documentary and archaeological evidence related to the Taíno are discussed first. Snuffing was of great importance to the Taíno, and rituals surrounding its use and preparation, and the related cosmology, affected every aspect of their life. If *Anadenanthera* use by the Taíno was as important as the archaeological record and the early documents indicate, the question must be asked as to the antiquity and geographical distribution of this practice. Discussion of Taíno *Anadenanthera* use is accordingly followed by an inquiry into the earliest archaeological evidence and its chronological development.

THE TAÍNO

The earliest descriptions of the use of visionary plants in the Americas refer to smoking of tobacco and inhalation of powdered seeds of *Anadenanthera peregrina* by the Taínos of the Greater Antilles (Plate 12; Colombo 1992; Las Casas 1909; Oviedo y Valdés 1959; Pané 1974). Taíno is the appellation given to the Arawakan speakers that occupied the Bahamas, most of the Greater Antilles, and the Virgin Islands at the time of first contact with Europeans (1492). Irving Rouse (1992) divided the Taíno into three groups. The habitat of the Western Taíno included Jamaica, most of central Cuba, and the Bahamian archipelago. The Eastern Taíno inhabited the Virgin and Leeward Islands. The Classic Taíno occupied Puerto Rico, Hispaniola, and the eastern tip of Cuba. For the purpose of this work emphasis is placed on the Classic Taíno, since most of the documentary evidence refers to them.

The Arawak language family is widespread in northern South America, and it is generally accepted that the ancestors of the Taíno originated in that area. The initial migratory movements of Arawak speakers into the islands of the Caribbean are defined by a ceramic type known as Saladoid, which derives its name from the type-site of Saladero, located near the Orinoco River delta. These ceramics have the form of inverted bells and are decorated with white-on-red designs (Rouse 1964). Saladoid peoples reached Puerto Rico around 200 B.C. and by A.D. 250 had settled the eastern half of Hispaniola (Rouse 1992). The Saladoid peoples displaced the Casimiroid and Ortoroid, the original inhabitants of the Greater Antilles (Rouse 1992). By A.D. 600 they occupied the islands from Guadeloupe to eastern Hispaniola, and consequent to new migratory waves evolved into a culture known as Ostionoid. Ostionoid (ca. A.D. 600-900) groups are defined by a ceramic known as Ostiones, first reported from the site of Punta Ostiones, near Cabo Rojo, Puerto Rico (García Arévalo 1982). This ceramic type is characterized by its polished surface and cylindrical shape, with convex walls having red decorations (Rouse 1964). The Ostionoid are generally classified as Subtaíno, since they shared cultural traits with the Taíno of Columbus's time. The next pottery type in the cultural sequence is known as Chicoid. It was first excavated at the site of Boca Chica in the Dominican Republic, with an early occupation of ca. A.D. 850. This ceramic continues the Saladoid-Ostionoid tradition, although it differs in its decoration, which includes linear incisions and relief (Rouse 1964). The latter Chicans (after A.D. 1200) could, according to Rouse (1992), be identified as the Classic Taínos, and as the ethnicity that first came in contact with Columbus.

Our knowledge of Taíno religion and mythology, and consequently of snuffing practices, is based on the writings of Columbus, Pané, and Las Casas. Taíno religion centered on a category of supernatural beings and spiritual forces known as *zemís*. The term referred to formal deities but could also be applied to features of the landscape, such as caves, rocks, streams, and trees. *Zemís* also served as intermediaries between the worlds (Pané 1974; Saunders and Gray 1996; Stevens-Arroyo 1988). Some *zemís* were related to the ancestors, others to agriculture, meteorological phenomena, and healing practices. They were represented in a wide variety of media, including stone, wood, and cotton (see Rouse 1992). Although the Taíno shared many elements with South America, *zemí* worship seems to be unique to this culture. In order to communicate with the *zemís,* the Taínos snuffed a psychoactive powder they referred to as *cohoba.*

Evidence for snuffing is present in the settlements of the early Saladoid, who snuffed a powder from small ceramic vessels with two lateral, parallel tubular projections. The Ostionoid continued this practice. The custom of placing the snuff on a platform atop anthropomorphic or zoomorphic figures, then inhaling it through parallel or forked tubes, originated with the Chicoid peoples (Plates 13, 14; Rouse 1992).

The first description of snuffing practices in the Americas was written by Christopher Columbus from observations made during his second voyage (1493-1496). During his brief period of residence on the island of Hispaniola, Columbus observed that the natives engaged in a religious ceremony in which the snuffing of a psychoactive powder was an integral part:

> I was able to discover neither idolatry nor any other sect among them, although their kings, who are many, not only in Hispaniola but also in all the other islands and on the mainland, each

have a house apart from the village, in which there is nothing except some wooden images carved in relief which are called
zemis. . . . In this house they have a finely wrought board, round
like a wooden dish in which is some powder, and is placed by
them on the heads of these *zemis* in performing certain ceremonies; then with a cane that has two branches which they place in
their nostrils they inhale this dust. The words they say none of
our people understand. With this powder they lose consciousness and become like drunken men. (Bourne 1906: 311-312;
Colombo 1992: 289; Pané 1974: 88-89)

We know of Columbus's description only through the writings of his
son Fernando, who copied his father's words from a now lost original
manuscript (Colombo 1992). Fernando's work, written in Spanish,
had not been published at the time of his death in 1539. His account
was translated into Italian by Alfonso Ulloa and published in Venice
in 1571. The original Spanish manuscript is now lost, and all we
know of Fernando's writings is Ulloa's Italian version (Bourne 1906;
Pané 1974).

The work of Fernando Colombo (1992) also includes the manuscript of a friar, Ramón Pané (English version: Bourne 1906; Spanish
version: Pané 1974), whom Christopher Columbus commissioned to
collect information on all the ceremonies and antiquities of the is-
landers (Bourne 1906; Pané 1974). Fray Ramón Pané, a member of
the order of Saint Jerome, arrived on the island of Hispaniola on January 2, 1494, and stayed on the island until the end of 1498, conducting
what could be considered the first ethnographic research in the Americas (Pané 1974). He recorded creation myths, beliefs about the supernatural, and names and attributes of deities. Pané obtained most of
his information from the Taíno who lived in the vicinity of Isabela, a
town on the north coast of Hispaniola, near the Cibao gold mines
(Rouse 1992). His original manuscript is no longer extant, but Fernando Colombo included the entire work by Ramón Pané in his
Historie, Chapter 61. This manuscript was used by Bartolomé de Las
Casas, who included the data on the Taíno religion in his *Apologética
Historia de las Indias* (Chapters 70, 166, 167) and had known Pané
personally (Pané 1974).

Pané first referred to the Taíno practice of snuffing in Chapter 11 of
his treatise, and his descriptions deserve to be quoted extensively.
The first mention occurs while Pané is relating the activities of mythi-

cal twins who had caused great havoc on the island. According to his account, the twins met an old man whom they addressed as "grandfather" and from whom they requested *casabe* (a manioc bread). Instead of *casabe* the old man gave them *cohoba* snuff:

> As soon as they came to the door of Bayamanaco and noticed that he carried *cazabe,* they said: "Ahiacabo guáracoel," which means "Let us know this our grandfather" (literal trans. "Hablemos con nuestro abuelo"). In like manner, Deminán Caracaracol, seeing his brothers before him, went in to see if he could have some *cazabe,* and this *cazabe* is the bread that is eaten in this country. Caracaracol having entered the house of Bayamanaco, asked him for *cazabe*. . . . And he put his hand in his own nose and threw at him a *guanguayo* (?) hitting him in the back; said *guanguayo* was full of *cohoba,* which he had made that day; the *cohoba* is a certain powder, which they take sometimes to purge themselves, and for other effects you will hear of later. This they take with a cane half-an-arm's length, they put one end in the nose and the other in the powder; and in this manner they inhale it through the nose and this purges them thoroughly. . . . Caracaracol, after this, returned to his brothers and told them what had happened to him with Bayamanacoel, and of the blow he had received with the *guanguayo* on his back, and that it pained him very much. Then his brothers looked at his back and saw that it was much swollen . . . and taking a stone axe they opened it, and there came out a live turtle, female; and so they built their cabin and cared for the turtle. (Bourne 1906: 324-325; Colombo 1992: 302-303; Pané 1974: 30-31)

This account gives for the first time a reference to a snuff powder by a specific name, as well as a description of a snuffing activity. This story tells us about the introduction of *cohoba* to the Taíno and how it could be used to communicate with the ancestors. The introductory statement "let us speak with our grandfather" eventually leads Caracaracol to acquire *cohoba*. The association of the snuff with a turtle should also be noted, as a *zemí* in the British Museum represents a bird with a turtle serving as a base (Plate 16; Rouse 1992; Wassén 1965). Aspects of this narrative are apparently represented on a *zemí* (Plate 17) carved with two figures seated on the low wooden benches known as *duhos* (see page 23 in this chapter; Plate 18), and on a ceramic figurine depicting a human with a turtle embedded on his back (Plate 19).

In his discussion of Taíno healing practices, Pané made the following observation about the *cohoba* powder:

> When one is ill they bring the *behique* to him as a physician. The *behique* is obliged to observe a diet like the sick man himself and to play the part of a sick man. This is done in the way which you will now hear. He must purge himself like the sick man; and to purge himself he takes a certain powder, called *cohoba,* inhaling it through the nose, which inebriates them so that they do not know what they do; and in this condition they speak many things, in which they say they are talking to the *zemis,* and that by them they are informed how the sickness came upon him. (Bourne 1906: 327; Colombo 1992: 307-308; Pané 1974: 35)

Pané also gave an interesting account that, among other things, illustrated the relationship between the carving of the wooden idols known as *zemís* and the snuffing of the *cohoba* powder:

> Those of wood are made in this fashion: When someone is going along on a journey he says he sees a tree which is moving its roots; and the man in a great fright stops and asks: "Who is it?" And the tree replies "Call a *behique* and he will tell you who I am." And the man goes to the physician and tells him what he has seen; and the enchanter or wizard runs immediately to see the tree . . . and sits down by it and inhales *cohoba.* . . . And when the *cohoba* is made he stands up on his feet and gives it all his titles as if it were some great lord, and he asks: "Tell me who you are and what you are doing here, and what you want of me and why you have had me called. Tell me if you want me to cut you or if you want to come with me, and how do you want to be carried, and I will build you a house with heritage." Then that tree or *cemí* . . . replies to him telling him the shape in which it wants to be made. And he cuts it and carves it as it was ordered; he builds the heritage house, and many times a year performs the *cohoba.* This *cohoba* is to pray to it and to please it and to ask and to learn some things from the *cemí* . . . Consider what state their brains are in, because they say the cabins seem to them to be turned upside down and that men are walking with their feet

in the air. (Bourne 1906: 330-331; Colombo 1992: 314-315; Pané 1974: 41-42)

This text illustrates the manner in which the carving of a shamanic implement was closely related to the ingestion of a psychoactive substance among the Taíno, and how the ecstatic state thus produced dictated the form the object adopted. Consequently, the black wood out of which these highly polished objects (*zemís, duhos,* snuff trays, and forked tubes) are usually manufactured contain power in the form of the spirit presumably residing in it. Polished black wood artifacts such as these were seen as indicators of status and its allied elite prerogatives (Helms 1986).

Fray Bartolomé de Las Casas also refers to the snuffing of a psychoactive powder, and gives an excellent account of its use. Las Casas resided in the Greater Antilles from 1502 to 1514, when he renounced his estates and became an activist in defense of the Indians. He was the first to provide a description, however brief, of the nature of the powder, as well as a detailed discussion of the use of the tray and the tube:

> They had some powders made of certain herbs very dry and finely ground and of the color of cinnamon or powdered henna; these they placed on a wooden dish, not flat but somewhat deep and with a slight curvature, so beautiful, smooth and pretty that it would not be any more beautiful if it were made of gold or silver; it was almost black and polished like Jet. They had an instrument made of the same wood and material, and of the same polish and beauty; said instrument was the size of a small flute, after two thirds of its length it divides into two hollow tubes. . . . These two tubes are placed on the two nostrils, and the beginning of the flute, so to say, on the powders that were on the dish, they would inhale to the inside with their breath, and in so inhaling they would receive the amount of powder they desired; once inhaled, they came out of their senses as if they were drinking strong wine. . . . These powders and these ceremonies or acts were known as *cohoba,* the middle syllable elongated, in their language; there they spoke like Arabs, or like Germans, I do not know what things or words. (Las Casas 1909: 445)

Las Casas's detailed description of the intricate carving of the snuffing implements suggests that the ingestion of *cohoba* and the resulting visionary state were an important element in the interactions between human beings and the supernatural. Las Casas's use of the plural to refer to the powders and the component herbs suggests that several types of snuff powder were used. The Yanomamö, for example, use both *Virola* and *Anadenanthera* snuffs (see Chagnon et al. 1971).

The first association of the word *cohoba* with the seeds of a leguminous tree was made by Gonzalo Fernández de Oviedo y Valdés early in the sixteenth century (ca. A.D. 1520-1533):

> And this *cohoba* holds some beans inside pods about a hand's length and more or less long, with some inedible lentils as fruit, and the wood is very good and strong. (Oviedo y Valdés 1959, 1: 292)

Oviedo y Valdés (1959, 1: 116; 5: Plate 1, Fig. 7) also describes a Y-shaped snuffing tube similar to that of Las Casas:

> The *caciques* and other important men have some hollow sticks the size of a *xeme,* more or less the thickness of the little finger, and these two tubes converged into one . . . all in one piece. (1: 116)

From this point on, Oviedo's description of the function of this utensil differs from that of Las Casas. Oviedo proceeds:

> . . . and the two ends they would place in the nostrils, and the other single end in the smoke or herb that was flaming or burning; these being very smooth and well carved . . . and they inhaled the smoke . . . until they lost their senses for a long time, lying on the ground inebriated . . . (1: 116)

The previous statement has created a great deal of confusion between the uses of tobacco and *cohoba*. Oviedo's description of smoke inhalation through a Y-shaped tube is unique and is not mentioned in the earlier observations of Pané and Las Casas. Oviedo y Valdés (1959) makes no mention of snuff powders in his work, and his description of the use of the bifurcated tubes is, apparently, not derived from personal observations. The illustration accompanying Oviedo's description depicts the two ends too far apart to be placed in the nostrils simultaneously. *Nicotiana* species have been widely used for their psychoactive properties and snuffing is a common method of administration. In his comprehensive study of tobacco and shamanism in South America, Johannes Wilbert (1987: 165) stated, "Tobacco is . . . clearly experienced as a sight- and vision-altering drug that permits the tobacco shaman to behold the numinous world." It is difficult to determine the exact distribution of tobacco snuff, since it is often used as an admixture to powders prepared from *Anadenanthera* or *Virola*. According to Wilbert (1987) the five major areas of tobacco snuff utilization include the Orinoco basin, the northwest Amazon, the Montaña-Río Purús, the Guaporé River area, and the central Andes. Nevertheless, the ingestion of tobacco and *Anadenanthera* smoke through the nose and mouth has been reported from the Achagua by Aguado (1956) during the early 1500s, and by Wilbert (1987) during the mid-twentieth century.

The source of *cohoba* was identified definitively as *Anadenanthera peregrina* var. *peregrina* (then classified as *Piptadenia*) by the North American ethnobotanist William E. Safford (1916). It should be noted that this genus had been previously suggested as a probable source of archaeological snuff powders by Max Uhle (1898, 1915), and Eric Boman (1908). Safford identified the source of *cohoba* by posing a series of questions: he asked whether the practice of snuffing by means of bifurcated tubes was still extant in any part of America; if so, from what plant was the snuff prepared; and was this plant to be found growing in the Greater Antilles? Safford answered the first question in the affirmative and identified the plant as *Piptadenia peregrina,* noting further that the name *cohoba* is still applied to it in the Antilles. He then went on to cite Gumilla (1984), La Condamine (1778), and Humboldt and Bonpland (1971) in further support of his argument (Safford 1916). It is likely that the Taíno introduced *Anadenanthera peregrina* into the Caribbean from South America (Reis Altschul 1964; Safford 1916). The distribution of the tree in the Greater Antilles coincided with Taíno occupation. Clear evidence of Taíno trade with South America is seen in the presence of gold and copper alloy artifacts (Rouse 1992).

The practice of snuffing among the Taíno can be reconstructed through archaeological finds and the descriptions of Columbus, Pané, and Las Casas (see also Dieve 1978; Franch 1982). *Cohoba* inhalation rituals are represented in several pictographs in the Cuevas del Borbón complex (Perdomo 1978). Columbus, Pané, and Las Casas related that the *cohoba* was deposited on a round tablet or tray. The dish with the powder was then placed on the platform surmounting the head of a *zemí* (Plates 15-17). According to Columbus, the powders were then inhaled through "a cane that has two branches." Double, parallel snuffing tubes are a frequent occurrence in the Amazon (Wassén 1965). Las Casas (1909) described a Y-shaped snuffing tube similar to those that form part of Amazonian snuffing paraphernalia (Wassén 1965). Snuffing tubes of this type (Plates 13, 14) have been found in Taíno archaeological sites in Haiti and the Dominican Republic (Arrom 1975; Caro Alvarez 1977; Kerchache 1994; Wassén 1965).

Most *zemís* associated with snuffing practices depict a seated anthropomorphic figure with a small table or platform above its head (Plate 15). Wooden images of this type have been found in Cuba, Hispaniola, Puerto Rico, and Jamaica (see Arrom 1975; Caro Alvarez 1977; Fewkes 1907; Rouse 1992; Saunders and Gray 1996). The representation is usually male, and exhibits clear skeletonized features such as ribs and vertebrae (see Kerchache 1994). The process of skeletonization is intimately related to shamanism (Halifax 1979) and suggests a modified state of consciousness, propitiated in this case by snuffing *cohoba*. According to Mircea Eliade (1964) this reduction to a skeleton and the acquisition of new flesh could be seen as a rebirth into a shamanic or mystical state. This interpretation agrees with the observations of Columbus, Pané, and Las Casas and clearly establishes the shamanic character of this type of *zemí*. In addition to the human representations, two other *zemís* of this type include bird representations as part of the base. One of these is the bird and turtle *zemí* from the British Museum previously mentioned in relation to the story of the origins of *cohoba* (Plate 16). The second was found at Aboukir, Jamaica (Saunders and Gray 1996). Birds are frequently associated with the use of psychoactive plants throughout South America.

Duhos (Plate 18), highly polished low benches with curved or vertical backs carved out of a single piece of black wood, are a third category of objects related to *cohoba* rituals (Arrom 1975; Kerchache 1994). Las Casas (1909: 445-446; see also Safford 1916) described the use of *duhos* as follows:

> I saw these people on several occasions celebrate their *cohoba,* and it was an interesting spectacle to witness how they took it and what they spake. The Chief began the ceremony, and while he was engaged all remained silent. When he had taken his *cohoba* . . . being seated on certain handsomely carved low benches which they called *duhos* (the first syllable elongated), he remained silent for a while with his head inclined to one side and his arms placed on his knees. Then he raised his face heavenward uttering certain words. . . . He described to them his vision, saying that the *zemís* had spoken to him. . . .

These small benches were part of the paraphernalia utilized to contact the supernatural. Often they were engraved with complex curvilinear designs on the back and legs. The bench was frequently carved in the round with human or animal attributes (Rouse 1992). Small wooden seats are used for similar purposes by the Desana of the Vaupés region of Colombia. Reichel-Dolmatoff (1971) notes that the benches provide physical rest and contribute to mental concentration during the trance, in addition to being symbols of stability and wisdom. The Creators allegedly possessed such benches during the time of creation; while seated on them, one is protected by such benevolent forces.

A vomiting stick or spatula is a fourth category of objects related to *cohoba* rituals. It is composed of a handle usually carved with human or animal motifs, and a curved blade; size ranges from 20 to 50 cm in length (Garcia Arevalo and Chanlatte 1976; Kerchache 1994). Generally, these objects are manufactured out of wood, shell, or bone. Their use within the context of *cohoba* rituals is described, ca. 1511, by Pietro Martire d'Anghiera, also known as Peter Martyr (Anglería 1964-1965). Although he never traveled to the New World, Anghiera collected the latest information arriving from the New World; his friendship with Columbus gave him access to firsthand information as well as to Pané's manuscript (Bercht et al. 1997). Anghiera tells that to make himself agreeable to the divinity, previous to the *cohoba* ritual, the *behique* purified his body by introducing a curved stick into the epiglottis in order to provoke vomit. A similar event is described by Gómara (1965-1966) in his *Historia General de Las Indias* (written ca. 1540-1550).

The previous discussion demonstrates that snuff powders were used for specific purposes and occasions. The early chronicles coincide as to the intensity of the inebriation and insofar as the shaman under the influence of the snuff spoke words unintelligible to the Spaniards. According to these reports, the snuff served as an interme-diary between shaman and supernatural; he or she acquired oracular capacities via *cohoba* snuff. This is evident from Pané's account of Taíno healing practices, and of the *behique* snuffing *cohoba* to com-municate with the tree. Taíno art, having been conceived in a state of communication with the supernatural, is intimately bound to the na-tive cosmology. Every artifact of Taíno shamanic art (snuffing tubes, *zemí* representations, *duhos,* vomit sticks), are complex symbolic manifestations that reflect social, political, and religious ideologies. All such objects are characterized by subtle fluidity of form, and are engraved with intricate designs that exhibit the same fluid and curvi-linear shapes. In this manner, Taíno representations foster a dual ap-proach. A first reading centers on the perception of the whole object and its thematic manifestation, while a second reading focuses on the incised linear designs. If use of visionary plants by the Taíno were as important as the archaeological record and the early documents indi-cate, the question must be asked as to the antiquity and geographical diffusion of this practice. The following sections place evidence for the use of visionary inebriants within its proper cultural context.

THE CENTRAL ANDES

The importance of *Anadenanthera* use among the Taíno, and its complex role in the shaping of Taíno cultural elements, prompts us to ask questions regarding its origins, development, and temporal distri-bution. In the Andes, early colonial documents provide clear evi-dence for the use of psychoactive plants (Plate 20; see Appendix). These writings most commonly refer to the use of *vilca* (*A. colubrina* var. *Cebil*), the most widespread botanical source for archaeological visionary preparations in the central Andes. Consequently, a discus-sion of the significance of the nominative *vilca* could contribute to a better understanding of the function of *Anadenanthera* in the pre-Columbian world. In the central Andes, numerous accounts mention its use as a purgative and as an ingredient in psychoactive potions. *Vilca* signifies in Quechua and Aymara the quality of sacredness

(Polia Meconi 1999). The first reference to *vilca* as a psychoactive
plant was made in 1571 by Polo de Ondegardo (1916, 3: 29-30):

> Those who wish to know an event of things past or of things that
> are to come . . . invoke the demon and inebriate themselves and
> for this practice in particular make use of an herb called *vilca,*
> pouring its juice in *chicha* or drinking it by another way. Note
> that even though it is said that only old women practice the craft
> of divination and of telling what happens in remote places and to
> reveal loss and thievery, it is also used today by Indians not only
> by the old but also by the young.

In 1582, the *Relaciones Geográficas de la Provincia De Xauxa*
(Hinestrosa 1965, 1: 170) referred to *vilca* as a bean and as a purgative; its use in association with tobacco snuff was also noted: "[I]n antiquity they did not know how to heal, until after the Inca became
their lord . . . and they purged themselves with some small beans
known as *vilca,* and they took powdered tobacco by the nose." But the
term *vilca* seems to have connotations that go beyond its description
as a psychoactive medicine. In *The Huarochirí Manuscript,* a series
of Quechua narratives and mytho-historical events compiled ca. 1598,
vilca seems to be a quality or a state of being, someone who has
achieved the status of *huaca* (Salomon and Urioste 1991). This is further reaffirmed in the following tale regarding the origins of *vilca* as a
medicine by Santa Cruz de Pachacuti (1993: 220), an early sixteenth-
century native chronicler. It is a quality transferred to the tree by the
slain captain Villca Quire:

> . . . and on the road to Apurimac he meets the enemies where the
> Changas kill a much spirited captain. . . . And then the captain
> *Villca Quire* tells the infantryman: "Is it possible that without a
> struggle I must die, without having left any fruits?" And *Villca
> Quire* spoke, it was said, "Here remains and its left the body."
> And he has himself buried next to a tree with the trunk carved so
> as to fit all of his body. And he tells that the grain that this tree
> shall bear will be a medicine called *villca* that would expel all
> sicknesses and humours and choleras from all persons.

According to Zuidema (1979), this battle with the Chancas took
place by the Apurimac River, at the site of the famous hanging bridge

popularized by Thornton Wilder in his novel *The Bridge of San Luis Rey.* The bridge provided access to the northwest quadrant of the Inca Empire. The Apurimac River represented the separation between the two cosmic worlds of the civilized highland cultures and the uncivilized Chancas and their lowland connections (Zuidema 1979). An important oracle, most probably related to the mythic origins of *vilca,* was located on the Cuzco side of the bridge. This oracle was described by the Spanish chronicler Pedro Pizarro during the mid-sixteenth century as an elaborately painted shrine, within which was located the thick trunk of a tree ornamented with gold and silver objects and delicate female garments. The shrine was tended by a sister to the Incas, who later jumped into the river canyon foreseeing the impeding advance of the Spaniards. In Pedro Pizarro's description, the Apurimac spoke through the tree trunk effigy. Zuidema (1979) concluded that this oracle marked the location of the death of captain Villca Quire and consequently designated the mythic origins of *vilca.* Siri von Reis Altschul (1972) examined herbarium specimens of *A. colubrina* var. *Cebil* from the Department of Apurimac; this area lies within its habitat. A Jesuit mission to the province of Vilcas (Ayacucho Dept.) documented ca. 1592 the worship of a *vilca* tree, including the placing of offerings (Polia Meconi 1999).

The Aymara dictionary compiled by Ludovico Bertonio (1984: 386), ca. 1612, provides additional information concerning its association with prophecies and sacred places:

> *Villca:* The sun as it was said in antiquity, and now they say *inti.*
> *Villca cuti:* The solstice when it begins to deviate from the tropic of Capricorn to Cancer.
> *Villca:* Shrine dedicated to the sun, and other idols.
> *Villcanuta:* Renowned shrine located between Sicuana and Chungara: It means the house of the sun according to the indian barbarians.
> *Villca:* It also is a medicinal thing, or thing given to drink as a purge, for sleeping, and in the sleep would come the thief who had taken the estate belonging to the one that drank the purge, and recover his estate; it was a sorcerer's deception.

In the sixteenth century, evidence for the prohibition of snuff use is seen in several church documents. In a *Relación* by Cristobal de

Albornoz, written ca. 1580 (Duviols 1967: 22), is found the following order for the destruction of snuffing paraphernalia:

> They have another kind of *huacas* that are called *vilcas*. . . . They heal and purge themselves with it and are also buried with it in most provinces of this kingdom. It should be noted that some wood or stone carvings resembling sheep, and with a hole as in an inkwell (which is where this *vilca* is pulverized), must be found and destroyed. This is called *vilcana,* and it is adored and revered. This *vilcanas* are made out of many different beautiful stones and strong woods. They have, in addition to this *vilca,* many other types of *vilcas,* especially purgatives.

Another example of religious sanctions is included in a trilingual (Aymara-Quechua-Spanish) set of sermons for the instruction of the native population, published in Lima in 1584 (Acosta 1985: folio 104). One of the sermons explains the first commandment thus: "By this commandment you are ordered not to worship the sun, nor the moon, nor the bright star . . . not to possess *villcas,* or guacas, or human effigies. . . ."

Guamán Poma de Ayala, in his *El primer nueva corónica y buen gobierno* (1980: 57), written ca. 1612-1616, provided the following recipe for the preparation of a potion with *vilca* as one of its basic ingredients:

> They had the custom of purging themselves each month with a purge known among them as *bilca tauri*. Three pairs of weighed grain are mixed with *macay,* ground and drunk by mouth and the other half is ingested below with a medicine [*melecina* in the original] and a clyster called *vilcachina*. This gave them much strength for battle and enhanced their health, and their lives lasted the time of two hundred years and they ate with much delight.

This particular oral preparation includes two other ingredients in addition to *vilca* seeds. The appellative *bilca tauri* suggests that *tauri* or *tawri* was used as an ingredient in the preparation of this purge. *Tawri* usually refers to the seeds of *Lupinus mutabiles,* a highland cultivar (Ayala 1980), with no psychoactive properties attributed to it. The third ingredient, *macay,* is described by Albornoz (in Duviols

1967) as a substance so powerful that a small amount added to a drink would cause a strong inebriation. Albornoz further stated that this plant was frequently used in ancient native rites and ceremonies.

Bernabé Cobo (1964), writing ca. 1653, identified *vilca* as a tree the size of an olive tree, which produced flat pods containing shiny brown seeds shaped like small coins. He noted that its seeds were added to *chicha*. In the course of her herbarium search, Siri von Reis Altschul (1967) found two specimens labeled *vilca,* both belonging to *A. colubrina* var. *Cebil*. According to Safford (1916), seeds labeled *huillca,* purchased from an herb vendor in Peru in 1915, were identified as *Anadenanthera*. Vilca (*huillca;* see Appendix in Chapter 1) is still used in the Andes, and it is presently sold for medicinal and ritual purposes in native markets in La Paz. Such seeds are essential ingredients of *llampu,* a potent concoction used in ceremonial payments to mountain deities known as *wamanis;* it wards against illnesses caused by these deities. In addition to *vilca* seeds, *llampu* includes grains of corn (only large-grain white corn is used), *wayluru (Cytharexylon herrerae)* seeds, coca seeds, one pair of white carnation flowers, and last, pieces of two minerals. There must be pairs of all ingredients, which are ground to a powder and added to the ceremonial drink (Isbell 1978). I know of no reports commenting on the potential psychoactivity of this preparation.

From the previous information it can be concluded that *vilca* refers to a quality analogous to the state of a person who in life has achieved the status of *huaca* (see Salomon and Urioste 1991). It is shared and transferable, as evidenced by the tale related by Santa Cruz de Pachacuti (1993: 220) in which Villca Quire transforms the seeds of *Anadenanthera* into "a medicine called *villca*." Archaeological sites located in the northern and southern sectors of the central Andes (Plate 20; Appendix) provide clear evidence for its ancient use. The south central Andes is the region of South America having the most ancient and extensive evidence for the use of *Anadenanthera* preparations. It extends from the Lake Titicaca basin to the south and includes southern Peru, Andean Bolivia, the Atacama Desert, and northwestern Argentina. Northwestern Argentina is the area with the earliest evidence, and is considered first. This section concludes with a comparative review of all archaeological evidence. Various iconographic and stylistic differences, as well as divergences in chronology, suggest shifts in patterns of interaction between the different areas.

Northwestern Argentina

The northwestern Argentina archaeological zone is not home to a homogenous culture, as it is composed of distinct regional developments. This vast mountainous area extends from the Chaco in the east to the Chilean border in the west, and from San Juan Province in the south to the border with Bolivia in the north (Bennett et al. 1948; Boman 1908; Debenedetti 1930). The Puna de Jujuy, the Quebrada de Humahuaca, and the Calchaquí Valley provide ample evidence for ancient use of *Anadenanthera* snuffs and fumatories.

A chronology of this south-central Andean area has been proposed that consists of three broad cultural periods. The Formative Period (600 B.C.-A.D. 300) encompasses the San Francisco and Vaquerías ceramic styles, which include some of the earliest smoking pipes found in the central Andes. The Regional Integration Period (A.D. 300-900) is defined by the presence of artifacts from La Aguada culture in the Catamarca Valley, and La Isla Polychrome ceramics in the Quebrada de Humahuaca. The Regional Development Period (A.D. 900-1538) is characterized by the proliferation of fortified villages. The Santa María culture is notable during this phase owing to its bronze metallurgy and large ceramic urns with geometric decorations (Pérez Gollán and Gordillo 1994).

The earliest evidence for the use of psychoactive plants in South America consists of materials found at the sites of Inca Cueva (IC c7) and Huachichocana (CH III), both located in the Puna de Jujuy, northwestern Argentina, at an altitude of 3860 m above sea level (Aguerre et al. 1973). Inca Cueva (IC c7) is a small cave with no stratification and no associated human remains (Fernández Distel 1980). The archaeological materials were deposited on top of a straw floor in the rear of the cave. Two smoking pipes (Plate 21, top) made of puma bone *(Felis concolor)* were found in association with knotted bags, gourds, spiral baskets, and *Anadenanthera* and *Prosopis* seeds (Aguerre et al. 1973; Aschero and Yacobaccio 1994; Fernández Distel 1980). Chemical analysis of the pipe residue indicated the presence of tryptamine alkaloids (Fernández Distel 1980). Radiocarbon testing yielded dates of 4080 ± 80 B.P. (2130 B.C.; T-1773; Aguerre et al. 1975), and 4030 ± 80 B.P. (2080 B.C.; Beta 64938; Aschero and Yacobaccio 1994).

A nearby cave divulged additional evidence for the smoking of tryptamine-containing plants. The site of Huachichocana is located in the Puna de Jujuy, northwestern Argentina (Fernández Distel 1980). The Huachichocana cave exhibits clear cultural stratification. The material related to smoking psychoactive plants was found in stratigraphic layer E2, dated by C_{14} to 3400 ± 130 B.P. (ca. 1450 B.C.; GAK-6357; Fernández Distel 1980). Remains of a male adolescent about 15 years old were found in association with four stone pipes (Plate 21, bottom; Fernández Distel 1980). Two pipes were found near the mouth and lying parallel to the body, the other two on each side of the body next to the lower legs and close to two turtle shells *(Geochelone chilensis),* two rattles with camelid kidney-stone noisemakers, and two staffs (probably spear throwers) decorated with turquoise inlays (Fernández Distel 1980). Abundant traces of red pigment remain on the surface of two of the pipes (Fernández Distel 1980). No *Anadenanthera* seeds were found, although tests for alkaloids in the pipe residue indicated the presence of tryptamine alkaloids (Fernández Distel 1980). It should be noted that nicotine has never been detected in material from northwestern Argentina.

Subsequently, ceramic pipes appear in the formative levels of agricultural societies in the Argentine northwest. The earliest clay pipes correspond to the initial moments of the San Francisco complex. Angular pipes with high bowls, biomorphic decorations, and supporting legs were found at the site of Saladillo Redondo, near El Piquete in the San Francisco River basin, and have a radiocarbon date of 620 ± 80 B.C. This is one of the earliest ceramic period dates in northwestern Argentina (Dougherty 1972; Pérez Gollán and Gordillo 1994). These also are the earliest ceramic pipes known from the central Andean area. Such angular pipes have been found at several sites in the Quebrada del Toro, the upper Calchaquí Valley, and the Puna de Jujuy. The extensive basins of the Pilcomayo and Bermejo rivers facilitated their distribution to the Puna area and its eastern fringes (Pérez Gollán and Gordillo 1994). Similar pipes have been found in San Pedro de Atacama, northern Chile, but chemical analysis of the pipe residue has not detected the presence of any alkaloids (James C. Callaway, personal communication, 1999). Ceramic pipes are widely distributed throughout northwestern Argentina in association with polychrome pottery known as Vaquerías (200 B.C.-A.D. 400). Pipe fragments associated with Vaquerías ceramics, with radiocarbon dates of A.D. 230 and A.D. 250, have also been excavated in Chile in upper Loa River archaeological sites (Aldunate et al. 1986).

Evidence for snuffing practices is lacking from the Formative Period (ca. 600 B.C.-A.D. 300), and appears for the first time toward the end of the Regional Integration Period (ca. A.D. 300-900). Most of the extant snuff trays and snuffing tubes from northwestern Argentina probably belong in the Regional Development Period (ca. A.D. 900-1538), in contrast to neighboring San Pedro de Atacama, Chile, where snuff trays and tubes are a frequent occurrence after ca. A.D. 200. Climatic differences between the Atacama and northwestern Argentina might partially account for the paucity of finds of wooden snuffing implements on the eastern slopes of the Andes. However, this argument is compromised by the relative frequency of such instruments in this same geographical area after ca. A.D. 900. The total absence of such artifacts during most of the Regional Integration Period suggests a later adoption of snuffing practices in northwestern Argentina (cf. Dougherty 1972; Pérez Gollán and Gordillo 1994).

The late adoption of snuffing practices in this area contrasts with the situation in other regions of the central Andes. The oldest snuff trays and tubes known from all of South America are those excavated by Junius Bird (1948; Bird and Hyslop 1985) and Frédéric Engel (1963) along the central Peruvian coast (Plate 22). In excavations conducted at the site of Huaca Prieta, Chicama Valley, as part of the Virú Valley Project of 1946, Junius Bird (1948) unearthed two whalebone snuff trays and a bird and fox bone tube, dated ca. 1200 B.C. (Wassén 1967a). Frédéric Engel excavated four snuff trays and eighteen tubes of the same approximate date as those found by Bird. The trays, tubes, and snuff powder containers were found at the site known as Asia in a mound referred to by Engel as Unit 1 (Engel 1963). One of the snuff trays was associated with a bottle-shaped gourd that contained a grayish powder and black seeds (Engel 1963). Snuff trays and tubes were found subsequently in similarly dated archaeological sites along the Pacific coast (Bird 1943; Dauelsberg 1985; Uhle 1915).

Once snuffing appeared in northwestern Argentina ca. A.D. 800-900, it spread rapidly and became a frequent occurrence at Regional Development Period sites. The areas with the most extensive and frequent evidence for snuffing are located in the Puna de Jujuy, the Quebrada de Humahuaca, and the Yocavil Valley. In the southern part of northwestern Argentina, snuffing paraphernalia is not found as frequently, and it indeed marks the southern limit of the diffusion of this type of implement (Gambier 2001). Notably, this coincides with the southern limits of the distribution of *A. colubrina* (30 degrees S). The evidence from each of these areas is discussed next.

The Puna de Jujuy is a high barren area (over 3500 m), with little or no rainfall, which extends from Bolivia through Jujuy Province and further south. Sites with snuffing implements in this area include Cusi Cusi, Casabindo (Ambrosetti 1906), Pucará de Rinconada (Boman 1908), San Juan Mayo (Bennett et al. 1948), and Santa Catalina (Lehmann-Nitsche 1902). These are all late pre-Hispanic sites, and some include evidence of Spanish contact. Casabindo and Pucará de Rinconada ceramics are in the Cuzco Polychrome style and are considered to date from the period of Inca occupation (Bennett et al. 1948). The site of Cusi Cusi, located high in the Puna near the Chile-Bolivia border, has yielded a snuffing kit and *Anadenanthera* seeds (Luis A. Lucas and Alicia Fernández Distel, personal communication, 1998). Associated tunics and bags have embroidered borders similar in style and technique to textiles from San Pedro de Atacama which have radiocarbon dates of ca. 890 ± 60 B.P. (ca. A.D. 1060; Beta-64389). This is the earliest available evidence for snuffing in the Puna de Jujuy.

The Quebrada de Humahuaca is one of the best-known archaeological regions in the Argentine northwest. Several sites in this area, including Pucará de Tilcara, Angosto Chico (Bennett et al. 1948), Los Amarillos (Marengo 1954), La Huerta (Lafón 1954), and Ciénaga Grande (Salas 1945), have yielded snuff trays that exhibit homogenous characteristics. All trays are ornamented by one, two, or three appendages carved in the round with anthropomorphic or zoomorphic motifs. Low-relief carvings are restricted to the site of Calilegua located to the northeast of the city of Jujuy, on a tributary of the Bermejo River. Nothing is known about this site in terms of ceramic associations or other objects that presumably may have been found with the trays. Calilegua is not included in Bennett et al.'s (1948) study of the archaeology of northwestern Argentina, and the catalog of the National Museum of the American Indian does not provide any information related to grave lots from this site. It is probable that the provenience given in the museum catalog is erroneous. The Pucará de Tilcara and Ciénaga Grande were occupied during the Regional Development Period (ca. A.D. 900-1538) and were operational until after Spanish contact (Debenedetti 1930; Salas 1945). This is an interesting factor, as snuffing paraphernalia in northern Chile, as will be seen, is practically absent during Inca domination.

The highest concentration of snuffing paraphernalia in northwestern Argentina occurs at the ruins of La Paya, situated at the confluence of La Paya and Calchaquí rivers, in the Department of Cachi, Salta Province. Juan Ambrosetti conducted extensive excavations in the city of La Paya during 1906 and 1907 and unearthed a total of 24 snuff trays and several snuffing tubes (Ambrosetti 1907-1908). These snuffing implements are of probable Calchaquí affiliation (ca. A.D. 700-1000) and are certainly pre-Inca in origin (Bennett et al. 1948).

The sites of Tolombón and Quilmes are located in the Yocavil Valley, to the south of La Paya (Ambrosetti 1899). The two sites are contemporary, as indicated by the association of Santa María urns and La Paya polychrome ceramics characteristic of late Regional Integration Period sites in the area (after A.D. 800). Only one snuff tray is known from the site of Tolombón (Plate 23); however, it is of importance to this study because of its close similarities to snuff trays from the Middle Loa region discussed later. A snuff tray from Quilmes was one of the first to be described in the archaeological literature (Ambrosetti 1899). On this tray, which has an unusual variation of the "double" theme, a central feline figure supports a human personage, as opposed to the common representation of feline above human. The flanking individuals, both facing frontward with hands clasped over their chests, are human beings surmounted by human heads. This representation is the only case in which the figures are both humans—again, not the usual alter ego representations of feline over human.

The southern sector of northwestern Argentina marks the limits of the archaeological evidence for snuffing. Snuff trays have been found at Guandacol (Alanís 1947), in the province of La Rioja, and at Calingasta (Ambrosetti 1902) in the province of San Juan. Two additional snuff trays were found at the sites of Tudcum and Angualasto in the Iglesia Valley, also in San Juan Province (Plate 24; Gambier 2001). The snuff trays from this area mark the limit of the evidence for the nasal inhalation of visionary powders. Again, this coincides with the southern extreme of the distribution of *A. colubrina* var. *Cebil* (Hunziker 1973; Reis Altschul 1964).

To summarize, northwestern Argentina demonstrates the earliest evidence for psychoactive plant use in the central Andes; bone pipes from the site of Inca Cueva are approximately 4000 years old. In addition, San Francisco–style ceramic pipes are among the oldest ceramic objects in the south central Andean area. The evidence clearly indicates *Anadenanthera colubrina* var. *Cebil* as the primary component of snuff powders and smoking preparations. The most frequent subjects depicted in snuff trays from northwestern Argentina are birds, human beings with probable feline characteristics such as a fanged mouth, the double or alter ego, and the decapitation theme. Snuff trays have been found at several sites showing evidence of Inca occupation, such as Ciénaga Grande, Casabindo, and Rinconada. Although the evidence is not clear as to whether the trays were associated with the Inca material or not, it suggests the possibility of the use of snuff trays and tubes during this late period (after A.D. 1480). This situation contrasts with that of northern Chile, where snuffing paraphernalia was a rare occurrence during late pre-Hispanic times.

Tiwanaku

A distinct pictorial configuration begins to appear relatively early (ca. 300 B.C.) in the Lake Titicaca basin, and later (ca. A.D. 200) in southern Bolivia, San Pedro de Atacama, and the Arica archaeological zone. Its most complex and monumental manifestations occur at the site of Tiwanaku (ca. A.D. 100-900), located in the Bolivian highlands, approximately 30 kilometers south of Lake Titicaca. Icons and motifs equivalent to those on Tiwanaku monumental stone sculpture are carved on 84 snuff trays and 23 tubes. Discussion of this iconography as expressed on the snuffing equipment is followed by an analysis of its relationship with monolithic sculpture and architectural elements at the site of Tiwanaku. Monumental stone sculpture and public architecture represent established forms and conventions and form the basis upon which Tiwanaku art has been defined. Snuffing paraphernalia is present in practically every archaeological site in which this iconography is known; because of its portability, it could be proposed that the snuffing equipment was partially responsible for the distribution of this iconographic system. In localities such as San Pedro de Atacama and Niño Korin, the snuffing equipment was carved with the most complex and varied manifestations of Tiwanaku iconography.

A thermoluminescence date of ca. A.D. 190 ± 140 (UCTL-224) obtained from tomb 4229-30, Toconao Oriente, San Pedro de Atacama, northern Chile, represents the earliest date associated with snuffing implements bearing Tiwanaku icons (Plate 25). This date is consistent with the funerary context, which includes three San Pedro Rojo Pulido ceramic vessels. This pottery type is diagnostic of Phase II (ca. 300 B.C.-A.D. 100; Berenguer et al. 1986, 1988) of the San Pedro de Atacama cultural development. A snuff tray with a camelid representation from the site of Solcor 3, tomb 5, San Pedro de Atacama, dated by thermoluminescence to ca. 920 ± 120 (UCTL-48; Phase V, Berenguer et al. 1986), has the latest date associated with Tiwanaku snuffing paraphernalia (Plate 26).

Tiwanaku snuff trays are generally manufactured out of wood. However, due to low preservation of organic materials at the site of Tiwanaku, nine of the extant ten snuff trays from this site are of stone and one of bone. Most have a convex longitudinal profile and consist of two clearly defined sections: a rectangular cavity area and a flaring panel-like sector. The cavity area usually carries no decoration, while the flaring panel supports complex and proliferous carvings. Most Tiwanaku snuffing tubes are wooden perforated cylinders (Plate 27). Notable exceptions are the Y-shaped tubes excavated by Alfred Kidder in Pukara (Chávez and Torres 1986) and a bifurcated camelid bone snuffer found on the surface at the site of Tiwanaku (Uhle 1898).

Snuff trays with probable southern Lake Titicaca basin provenance include two in the collection of the Roemer Museum, Hildesheim (Boetzkes et al. 1986; Uhle 1912). The Museo Etnográfico, Buenos Aires, owns one stone tablet purchased by the Argentine archaeologist Salvador Debenedetti in La Paz in 1910 (Posnansky 1957; Wassén 1967a). There are two fragments (Plate 28b) and a complete tray (Plate 28a) in the University Museum, Philadelphia. A seventh tray was in a private collection in Oruro at the time Uhle published his study in 1912; its present location is unknown. In 1894, two additional stone snuff trays from Tiwanaku belonged to Dr. Ernesto Mazzei, whom Uhle had met in La Paz (Uhle 1912). Dr. Mazzei was a Florentine scholar who traveled in South America during the late 1800s collecting pre-Columbian and ethnographic artifacts for the

National Museum of Anthropology and Ethnology of Florence (Ciruzzi 1992). The present whereabouts of these two snuff trays are not known; they are not currently in the collection of the Florence museum. A bone snuff tray was excavated at the site of Tiwanaku and is presently in the collection of the Tiwanaku site museum. It can be inferred from the presence of nine stone snuff trays that wooden equivalents were most likely used in Tiwanaku; climatic conditions in this area, as previously mentioned, are not conducive to the preservation of wood. This is also suggested by the fact that all snuff trays with Tiwanaku iconography in San Pedro de Atacama, Niño Korin, and elsewhere are made out of wood.

Other trays in the Tiwanaku style have been found near the town of Niño Korin in northeastern Bolivia (Oblitas Poblete 1963; Wassén 1972b; Wassén 1973). The site itself, known as Caliicho (or Qalliichu), is located to the east of Lake Titicaca on the eastern slopes of the Cordillera Oriental of the Andes, at an altitude of 3500 m (Wassén 1972b). Five wooden snuff trays (Plate 29), bamboo tubes and containers, enema syringes, several spoons and spatulas, baskets, and fur and skin pouches were found in a multiple grave. The objects found at this site have been studied by S. Henry Wassén and are now part of the collection of the Gothenburg Ethnographical Museum, Sweden. The find was made in June 1970 (Wassén 1972b), but apparently not as the result of controlled excavations. Wassén (1972b) had obtained three radiocarbon dates from this site: A.D. 355 ± 200, A.D. 375 ± 100, and A.D. 1120 ± 100.

A snuffing kit was found in a rock shelter near the locality of Amaguaya, Depto. de La Paz, in the western range of the Andes (Rendón 1999). The kit included a large wooden snuff tray inside a tight-fitting leather sheath (Plate 30), a bone spoon with a bird carved on its handle, and a pouch made of animal fur. The tray is carved with a profile upward-looking genuflecting figure, and it is decorated with gold and spondylus shell inlays. Other snuff trays bearing Tiwanaku iconography have been reported from Ilo (Alcalde Gonzáles 1995), and from the site of La Real, Valle de Majes, in southern Peru (García and Bustamante 1990).

The San Pedro de Atacama archaeological zone is the area with the largest sample of Tiwanaku snuffing implements and represents the southernmost manifestations of this type of iconography. Because of poor preservation of organic materials at the site of Tiwanaku, San

Pedro de Atacama offers the most complete and best-preserved examples of Tiwanaku wooden objects, woolen textiles, and engraved bones. These include three mantles, five tunics, several bags with embroidered borders, one headband, two wristlets, six ceramic vessels (e.g., Llagostera and Costa 1984), and ten engraved bones (Le Paige 1965). Snuffing implements represent the largest category of Tiwanaku objects in San Pedro de Atacama (Plates 27, 31, 32). Tiwanaku designs are carved on 63 snuff trays and 22 snuffing tubes, and represent approximately 10 percent of the local snuffing equipment. In addition, many of the objects decorated with Tiwanaku elements found in San Pedro de Atacama are associated with the snuffing equipment (i.e., textile bands and bags). In San Pedro de Atacama, sectors of some archaeological sites (e.g., Solcor 3, Coyo Oriente, Quitor 6) have yielded Tiwanaku objects. However, no complete Tiwanaku burials are known from the area, only graves with occasional Tiwanaku artifacts. Snuffing equipment from San Pedro de Atacama that does not exhibit Tiwanaku characteristics is discussed in the next section.

The apparent homogeneity of the so-called Tiwanaku style masks a system of extreme variability. A detailed study of Tiwanaku iconography on snuff trays and tubes reveals significant differences in representational conventions and thematic emphasis, as well as variables in the interrelation of individual motifs. Most of the themes represented on the snuff trays consist of principal figures with no subsidiary attendants. Tiwanaku iconography, as represented on the snuffing paraphernalia, can be categorized into several themes:

1. Frontal figure (Plate 33a): consists of a frontal anthropomorphic figure with outstretched arms holding staffs. Notable differences include the presence or absence of cephalic projections and staff composition.
2. Disembodied rayed head over a stepped platform (Plate 33b).
3. Profile, genuflecting, staff-bearing figures (Plate 33c): This is the most frequently represented theme. Several distinct personages can be identified, but they all share the genuflecting stance (except one from Niño Korin), the upward-looking crowned head, the presence of an object protruding from the mouth, and a staff held in the right hand. The types of being represented differ in the cephalic configuration and in the nature of the objects

held. This type of profile figure could be the oldest Tiwanaku iconographic theme in the San Pedro de Atacama area, since on two occasions it is associated with Roja Pulida ceramics (ca. 300 B.C.-A.D. 100).

4. Condors (Plate 33d): This avian representation can be identified as a condor by the crest, hooked beak, and distinctive collar. One of the condor representations is similar to the profile genuflecting figures previously discussed. On this tray, a profile upward-looking condor with an object protruding from its mouth is carved in low relief over a stepped platform. Other snuff trays have profile condor representations, but they do not have the heads turned upward nor an object emanating from the mouth.

5. Anthropomorphized camelid representations (Plate 33e): These trays share the depiction of a two-legged profile personage with a bundle on its back and a noose around its neck. The figure stands over a stepped platform flanked by either avian or feline heads. The being represented is apparently a human wearing a costume with animal characteristics. This is suggested by the textile-like nature of the designs covering the body and the band that flows down its back. This band is similar to a Pucara textile sash illustrated by William Conklin (1983) in a study of Pucara and Tiwanaku tapestry. The zoomorphic traits present seem to be those of a camelid, as indicated by hooflike feet, slightly undulating mouth, bulging forehead, and prominent ears and teeth.

6. Miscellaneous representations (Plate 33f): The five themes enumerated in this list are frequently represented wherever this type of iconography is found. However, there are also several snuff trays that represent unique or infrequent iconographic themes. These include four snuff trays, each depicting a human wearing a headdress with tassels descending on both sides of the face, three showing a reclining figure with raised knees and torso, another with a condor devouring a human head, and another with two rampant felines.

These iconographic themes are articulated through a series of individual signs that form the raw material for the thematic formulation (Plate 34). These individual signs do not seem to be hierarchical in nature, each sign interacting and combining with another, constantly changing places and serving in turn primary and auxiliary functions.

Three formal tendencies can be identified: one with predominantly geometric characteristics (Plate 34a), and the other two predominantly biomorphic (Plate 34b, c). The basic organizational device for the individual signs is the body, human or animal. The functions served by these basic or primary signs seem to be determined by their design, association, and location within the body. Some signs serve as terminators, such as the undulating tripartite element. Others usually occupy interior positions in the cluster (e.g., zigzag within rectangle as body of staff), and others seem to function as connectors of the different component elements (rectangular elements in headdress, head/neck connectors). These motifs cluster (Plate 35) to form elements of the body, or expansions (e.g., winged eyes, wings, tails) or attachments (e.g., headdresses, staffs, elbow pendants).

These clusters in turn construct the basic thematic formulations previously enumerated, thus allowing the creation of numerous structural changes in every theme. These changes become evident when variations of the same theme are compared, such as the frontal figure holding staffs engraved in a wooden snuff tray from San Pedro de Atacama, the central personage carved in low relief in a monumental gateway at the site of Tiwanaku, and the figure incised on the back of the Bennett monolith (Plate 36). The three personages share the frontal pose with outstretched arms carrying scepters and tunics decorated with a row of heads in the lower border. Apart from this basic thematic formulation, these three frontal personages greatly differ. The lithic representations both have a rayed head, whereas the one from San Pedro de Atacama (Plate 36 upper left) exhibits instead an elaborate headdress. The scepters held by the figures differ in shape and also in component signs. The configuration of eyes, tunics, and elbow pendants demonstrate a great variability. These variations suggest that the individual signs derive meaning from affiliation with other signs, from the position within the anatomy, and from the theme being expressed; the sign itself is modified by the thematic change.

The themes constructed by these signs, however, have clear hierarchical connotations (Plates 33a-f). The arrangement of these themes within the body of the monolithic stone sculpture suggests a hierarchical structure and also further demonstrates the idea of the body as the basic organizational device. In the Bennett and Ponce monoliths (Plates 37, 38), two of the more iconographically complex sculptures at the site of Tiwanaku, the individual thematic units are placed

within the anatomy in central and subsidiary positions. The spatial relationship between the two rayed disembodied heads and the staff-
bearing figure depicted at the base of the spinal column of the Bennett
monolith (Plate 37b) invest the dorsal area of this sculpture with a
certain degree of frontality. Winged profile personages and packed
camelids converge on the pendants on the chest and abdomen of the
stone figure. Thematic clusters envelop the monolith, articulated by
its anatomy, acquiring an affinity with our notion of text.

Several layers of meaningful activity can be tentatively proposed:

1. Individual component signs (Plate 34)
2. Clusters of signs within the composition (e.g., stepped platforms with lateral projections, headdresses, staffs; Plate 35)
3. Individual themes (e.g., staff-bearing frontal figures, profile
   genuflecting individuals, anthropomorphized packed camelids;
   Plates 33a-f)
4. Thematic configurations—pictorial compositions that combine
   the different thematic units and comprise the most complex expression of the iconography (Plates 37, 38)

Thematic configurations are mostly restricted to monumental stone
sculpture and architectural decoration. In most cases, the snuff trays,
textiles, ceramics, and engraved bones represent only individual
themes. In this manner, numerous variations in style as well as iconography can be identified at the different sites in which the so-called
Tiwanaku style is found.

The snuffing paraphernalia shares most of its basic components
with the monolithic sculpture at Tiwanaku. The themes represented
on the snuff trays, including frontal personages, disembodied rayed
heads, profile staff-bearing figures, and packed camelids, are represented on the Bennett and Ponce monoliths (Plates 37, 38), and on
monumental gateways and lintels. The relationship between Tiwanaku iconography and the use of *Anadenanthera*-based visionary potions and inhalants is also apparent in other aspects of the megalithic
sculpture. Several of these depict human beings holding two objects
against the abdomen. Most researchers agree that one of the objects is
a *kero,* a vessel with divergent sides of widespread use in the Andes
(Berenguer 1987). The identification of the second object has remained elusive. Berenguer (1987, 2001) tentatively identified it as a

snuff tray, partially basing his argument on stylistic and iconographic comparisons. In addition, the pectoral carved on the Bennett monolith is suggestive of an anthropomorphized *vilca* tree (Plate 39a). Knobloch (2000), in her work on power and ritual in Conchopata, has identified an icon suggestive of the leaves, pods, and seeds of *Anadenanthera*. This is an icon occasionally represented on the snuff trays from San Pedro de Atacama (see Plate 34b). Its presence as part of the chest pendant on the Bennett monolith is notable because of its central position and proximity to the proposed *kero* and snuff tray (Knobloch 2000). If Knobloch's identification of the *Anadenanthera* signifier is correct, it can be proposed that the pendant describes an anthropomorphized *vilca* tree. Its association with a *kero* and a snuff tray might indicate the drinking of a potion, as well as nasal inhalation of formulations including *Anadenanthera* seeds. A variable of this anthropomorphized *vilca* tree is incised on the arms of the Ponce monolith (Plate 39b).

In addition, the right hand of the Bennett and Ponce monoliths is depicted in the gesture usually referred to as *half-fist*. This term denotes a hand position with the thumb erect on the side and the four fingers bent so that the nails are still visible (see Sharon and Donnan 1974). A frontal personage with both hands performing the same gesture is seen on a snuff tray from San Pedro de Atacama (see Plate 33f bottom left). A snuff tray from Niño Korin and another from San Pedro de Atacama are carved in this shape (Plate 40). Both trays were directly associated with Tiwanaku artifacts (Wassén 1972b). This prominent display of visionary imagery on public monumental sculpture and architecture suggests an active role for visionary preparations derived from *Anadenanthera* in the development of Tiwanaku ideology.

Evidence for the use of *Anadenanthera*-based visionary preparations by the Tiwanaku is supported by other factors in addition to snuffing implements and iconographic evidence. The seeds of *A. colubrina* var. *Cebil* were readily available since its habitat includes the Tiwanaku sphere of influence (Reis Altschul 1964). Detection of bufotenine in snuff powder samples from San Pedro de Atacama (see next section) indicates *A. colubrina* as its botanical source. The burial where the snuff powders were found was part of a distinct group of three graves within the Solcor 3 cemetery, which included the following artifacts carved with Tiwanaku motifs: a snuff tray, a snuffing tube (Plates 6, 7), a carved bone, and a bag with an embroidered border. Other burials in the same cemetery included small leather pouches containing *Anadenanthera* seeds (Llagostera et al. 1988).

Because of its complexity, diversity, and variability throughout a wide geographical and temporal sphere of influence, it can be proposed that the formation, evolution, and dispersion of the Tiwanaku pictorial configuration were not centrally controlled activities. Outside the Tiwanaku core area, this iconographic system is discreet and coexists with local artifacts and other foreign objects. As mentioned previously, no predominantly Tiwanaku burials are known from San Pedro de Atacama, only graves with occasional Tiwanaku artifacts. A brief comparison of Wari and Tiwanaku will emphasize the independence of this iconographic system from specific and exclusive political entities. Notwithstanding marked differences, it is evident that both of these contemporaneous societies shared basic iconographic elements (Torres and Conklin 1995). In Tiwanaku it is expressed on monumental sculpture and architecture, while no such monuments are known at Wari. Textiles identified as Wari are superficially similar to those from Tiwanaku, differing in technique and in emphasis on specific themes and component signs. Tiwanaku architecture with its gateways and carved lintels has no equivalent in Wari constructions. Tiwanaku iconography is closely linked to snuffing paraphernalia (Berenguer 1987; Uhle 1898, 1912), while that of Wari suggests instead psychoactive potions (Knobloch 2000).

This differentiation is accentuated when peripheral areas such as Arica and San Pedro de Atacama are compared. Arica has extensive textile evidence in the form of woolen tunics and four-pointed hats, a typical Tiwanaku headdress. However, in San Pedro de Atacama four-pointed hats are not present. In San Pedro de Atacama there are numerous Tiwanaku snuff trays and tubes; in Arica, an area with excellent preservation of organic materials, there is no evidence of Tiwanaku iconography on snuffing utensils (Chacama 2001).

The wide temporal and geographic distribution of this iconography, in addition to regional shifts in thematic emphasis and media, prompt an inquiry into its development and dispersion. Was it motivated by social, religious, or political interaction, through conquest, or through mercantile exchange? The diversity of media, form, and type of expression seems to contradict all of these models for expansion. The manner in which this iconography is shared by such diverse cultures, over such a long span of time, suggests mechanisms of inter-action not necessarily dependent upon a central administrative site. All these variables indicate that there is not necessarily a direct and uniform correspondence between iconographic representation and significance in every geographic and temporal locality.

It can be postulated that San Pedro de Atacama, Niño Korin, and Arica, among others, were part of numerous south central Andean communities that contributed responsively, in accordance with re-sources and location within patterns of ideological exchange, to the formation and development of the iconographic system. The impor-tance of the body, of the various gestures and poses that define the dif-ferent thematic units, and of the signs that articulate these ideologies, indicate a transmission of information dependent on performative ac-tivities. Direct and early association of snuffing paraphernalia with Tiwanaku iconography indicates that ecstatic experiences provoked by visionary inhalants and potions contributed significantly to the formation and development of Tiwanaku style and iconography.

San Pedro de Atacama

The archaeological region of San Pedro de Atacama is located in the Atacama Desert of northern Chile at an altitude of 2450 m above sea level. San Pedro de Atacama is composed of settlements within oases clustered together at the end of the San Pedro River. The associ-ated pre-Hispanic cemeteries and habitation sites are referred to by the present names of the settlements near which they are located (e.g., Coyo Oriente, Quitor 5, Quitor 6, Sequitor Alambrado Oriental, Sol-cor 3).

One of the unique aspects of the San Pedro artifactual assemblage is the frequent presence of snuffing implements (Le Paige 1964, 1965; Núñez 1963; Llagostera et al. 1988; Torres 1987a). A total of 614 snuffing kits have been found in 42 of the approximately 50 sites excavated in the area. Investigations conducted by Ana María Baron (1984) and María Antonietta Costa (Llagostera et al. 1988) have de-termined that the snuffing kits are generally found with adult male re-mains. The size, chronology, and gender bias of the sample indicates that approximately 20 to 22 percent of the adult male population was using psychoactive snuffs ca. A.D. 200-900. All of the snuff trays and tubes have been found in funerary contexts and demonstrate a wide range of stylistic and iconographic diversity.

The cultural development of this area has been divided into eight phases, San Pedro I-VIII, based on a seriation of ceramic types (Berenguer et al. 1986; Tarragó 1968). The ceramic type known as San Pedro Roja Pulida is diagnostic of Phase II (ca. 300 B.C.-A.D. 100; Berenguer et al. 1986). Only seven snuff trays are associated with this early pottery type. The majority of the snuffing implements are associated with the pottery types known as San Pedro Negra Pulida and San Pedro Negra Casi Pulida. These ceramic types define Phase III (ca. A.D. 100-400) and IV (ca. A.D. 400-700) respectively. The practice of snuffing seems to diminish considerably during the early stages of Phase VII (ca. A.D. 1000-1470), since only three snuff trays are associated with San Pedro Roja Violácea, the pottery diagnostic of this phase. The latest radiocarbon measurement associated with snuffing paraphernalia is a date of ca. A.D. 1050 ± 80 obtained from tomb 3236, Quitor 9, in a context that included a Bolivian highland ceramic type known as Huruquilla (Núñez 1976). During Phase VIII (ca. A.D. 1470-1530), which is characterized by Inca presence, snuffing paraphernalia is completely absent from the archaeological record.

The gradual disappearance of snuff trays and tubes from the San Pedro de Atacama archaeological record ca. A.D. 1100 suggests that the practice of snuffing itself might have diminished. At the site of Quitor 6 in its middle phase (ca. A.D. 400-800), approximately one out of every three individuals had snuffing paraphernalia in the burial (123 snuff trays). Excavations conducted by María Antonietta Costa (1988) in the later phases of this cemetery (after A.D. 1200) produced only one snuff tray and one tube. The presence of foreign objects also notably lessened during the later phases. This gradual disappearance coincides with the appearance of similar snuffing kits in northwestern Argentina, where these continued to be used well into late pre-Columbian times, and in some sites such as Casabindo, probably into the early colonial period.

All the snuffing tubes from San Pedro de Atacama are single perforated cylinders (Plate 41). So far no Y-shaped or double snuffing tubes, such as those from the Amazon or the Greater Antilles, have been found. The collection of the San Pedro de Atacama archaeological museum includes approximately 140 snuffing tubes. Structurally, a tube consists of two clearly defined sections, the nosepiece and the shaft; a third section is sometimes delineated in the distal end of the tube. The snuffing tubes are generally manufactured out of wood, sometimes from bird bone, and very rarely out of a fragile local reed or cane. Those of wood are generally carved in one piece, although on some occasions they have separate nosepieces made out of wood, bone, or stone. The bone snuffing tubes always consist of two separate pieces: the nosepiece and the shaft. The nosepiece attached to a bird-bone shaft was carved from a separate piece of the same material, or sometimes out of wood or stone.

The majority of the snuff trays and tubes from San Pedro de Atacama are carved with local and Pan-Andean motifs and do not exhibit Tiwanaku characteristics. Most of these are ornamented with regional variations of widely distributed themes, such as Heraldic Woman, and alter ego representations (Plates 42, 43). Frequently, motifs of a more local or regional nature, such as human figures with cylindrical headdress and ear pendants, are depicted on the trays. It is difficult to determine any foreign affiliations to this group of implements.

Animal and human characteristics are often associated in alter ego representations (Plate 43). In most representations of this type, a human figure is surmounted by a feline. This configuration of motifs, in an ethnographical context, likely refers to the shaman's ability to acquire zoomorphic characteristics, most often while under the influence of psychoactive plants. This is a frequent theme in snuffing paraphernalia, which is common in Amazonia and in trays and tubes from northwestern Argentina. In northern Chile, alter ego representations are seen in tubes from archaeological sites located in the Middle Loa region, including Calama, Chiu-Chiu, and Toconce. This theme is also present in other pre-Hispanic objects throughout the Andes, most notably in the sculpture of San Agustín, Colombia (Preuss 1974).

Zoomorphic representations are relatively frequent and include birds, camelids, and felines (Plate 44). Snuffing paraphernalia with this type of ornamentation is present in other areas, most notably in the middle Loa River valley and in northwestern Argentina. On the snuffing tubes, felines or birds are usually carved in the round on the midpoint of the shaft (see Plate 41c, d). In addition to the snuff trays and tubes, small spoons or spatulas that form part of snuffing kits have avian representations carved on the handles. The association of birds with snuffing equipment is also evident in the innumerable tubes made of bird bone. These tubes have been found together with the earliest known trays, as evidenced by the material excavated at Huaca Prieta, Peru, by Junius Bird (1948).

Camelid representations include zoomorphic depictions and anthro-pozoomorphic beings holding an axe and a trophy head (Torres 1987b). It could be argued that feline characteristics are depicted on these artifacts. Nevertheless, if these personages are compared with other feline representations from San Pedro de Atacama, several differences become apparent. The snouts of the felines are not as prominent, nor the ears as large and pointed as they are on the personages on the snuff trays and tubes under consideration. When these images are compared to those of camelids, it can be seen that the snout, the nose, and the slightly curved and pointed ears are closer to those of a llama than to a feline. This long-snouted Sacrificer, as well as the alter ego, persist late into the sequence (ca. A.D. 900-1100) and are among the few thematic units shared by the snuffing paraphernalia from San Pedro de Atacama, the Loa River valley, and northwestern Argentina. The distal end of the snuffing tubes is occasionally carved with a representation of an open-mouthed animal head. This zoomorphic representation could be identified tentatively as a camelid because of the pointed ears, slightly undulating mouth, and prominent nose. The head is represented as if it were strapped to the end of the tube. This is clearly seen in the way that the ears are depicted as if they were tied to the tube's end; when a camelid head is not present the end is undecorated. Camelids are also of great importance in the rupestrian art of northern Chile (Mostny and Niemeyer 1983).

Smoking was not as important in San Pedro de Atacama as in northwestern Argentina. Approximately 60 ceramic smoking pipes (over 50 percent are fragments) are in the collection of the archaeological museum in San Pedro de Atacama. These pipes have all been found in an early context (before A.D. 400). Most are angular pipes with a high bowl and two-legged supports (Plate 45). The smoking material has not yet been determined. Analysis of several samples has yielded negative results for alkaloids. Only five pipes are known to have been associated directly with snuffing equipment. Evidence from neighboring areas in northwestern Argentina suggests the smoking of *Anadenanthera* seeds. There is a strong probability that several of the pipes found in San Pedro de Atacama originated in northwestern Argentina. The pipes with biomorphic decoration have many features in common with pipes of the San Francisco complex (ca. 650 B.C.-A.D. 300) and other formative ceramic styles of the Argentine northwest (Pérez Gollán and Gordillo 1994; see also Westfall 1993-1994). According to Tarragó (1980), the majority of the San Pedro de Atacama pipes demonstrate notable similarities with those found at Campo Colorado (ca. 100 B.C.-A.D. 100), in the Calchaquí Valley, Argentina. Campo Colorado is contemporary with Phases II/III of the ceramic sequence proposed for San Pedro de Atacama by Berenguer et al. (1986). In San Pedro de Atacama, pipes gradually disappeared during Phase III (ca. A.D. 100-400) as snuff trays became more common (after A.D. 200). This contrasts with northwestern Argentina, where smoking remained the preferred modality for consumption of psychoactive plants.

One notable feature of the San Pedro culture is the relative abundance of artifacts from diverse areas in the south central Andes. The presence in this area of numerous exotic artifacts must be taken into account for an understanding of the importance of San Pedro in processes of cultural interaction. In this work, an object is considered to be of foreign provenience if it has a direct equivalent in other areas. In San Pedro de Atacama, these foreign objects coexist with each other and with local artifacts.

The most cohesive category of foreign objects in San Pedro de Atacama, as previously discussed, is those decorated with Tiwanaku designs. Objects from northwestern Argentina, although not as unified in provenience as those from Tiwanaku, are relatively frequent. Some are of probable La Aguada provenience. These include wooden carvings (Berenguer 1984; González 1964; Llagostera 1995), and a well-preserved tie-dyed tunic found at the site of Quitor 2 (Llagostera 1995). Llagostera (1995) attributed 17 baskets with polychrome woolen thread decoration found in San Pedro to the Aguada culture. On two occasions, Le Paige (1964, 1974) mentioned the presence of fragments of Aguada ceramics in San Pedro de Atacama. Radiocarbon dates associated with the Aguada culture in northwestern Argentina range from A.D. 650 to 900. In this context, it should be noted that snuffing utensils have not been found in Aguada archaeological sites in northwestern Argentina, and ceramic pipes are not common there.

The lower levels of occupation of Tulor village yielded fragments of San Francisco Negro Grabado pottery, an early ceramic type from the Argentine northwest (ca. 650 B.C.-A.D. 300). Surface collections in the southernmost sectors of San Pedro de Atacama have yielded additional San Francisco fragments (Agustín Llagostera and Francisco Téllez, personal communication, 1995). Several ceramic smoking pipes of evident San Francisco affiliation have been found in the area (see MChAP 1994; Pérez Gollán and Gordillo 1994). Condorhuasi ceramics (ca. 200 B.C.-A.D. 600) are present at the sites of Tulor Algarrobo and Tchaputchayna (Le Paige 1974; Llagostera and Costa 1984). Isla Polychrome ceramics (ca. A.D. 600-1050) have been excavated at the sites of Quitor 5 and Quitor 6 in association with a local ceramic type, San Pedro Negra Pulida (Pérez 1978; Tarragó 1977). Snail shells were frequently used as containers (MChAP 1984). These snails, *Strophocheilus intertextus* (Parkinson et al. 1987), are abundant in the *cebil* forests in the eastern sector of Salta Province.

Marked differences distinguish the objects of local manufacture from the intrusive artifacts. For example, the local ceramics are monochromatic, black, gray, or red, while those attributed foreign provenience have polychrome decorations. Local tunics and other textiles are characteristically warp faced and warp patterned, utilize the natural colors of camelid yarns or at times black or red dyes, and only to a limited extent other colors. These local textiles contain no representational imagery, although they sometimes have striping and repetitive warp patterning. The foreign textiles differ from their local equivalents in use of decorations and multicolored yarns. The Aguada tunic, a bag with Peruvian south coast designs, and the Tiwanaku textiles are technically different from anything found locally. The local and foreign snuff trays also exhibit notable differences in style, iconography, and execution. Tiwanaku snuff trays are generally carved in low relief or with linear incisions and describe quite complex images. Snuff trays decorated with local or Pan-Andean themes are carved in the round, and only rarely have low-relief decoration on flat panels. Notable exceptions to this are snuff trays with flat panels and geometric motifs, and those with the Heraldic Woman theme (Plate 42a; Torres 1987a).

Chemical analyses of two samples of archaeological snuff powders from the site of Solcor 3 (Plates 46-48), dated ca. A.D. 780, have detected the presence of 5-hydroxydimethyltryptamine (bufotenine), dimethyltryptamine (DMT), and 5-methoxy-DMT (Torres et al. 1991). The finding of bufotenine in these samples suggests that the plant source of this material was a species of the genus *Anadenanthera*. Small pouches containing *Anadenanthera* seeds have been found in several burials in Solcor 3. This is the only genus implicated in the snuffing complex that contains bufotenine, although it has been found in purported *Virola* snuffs from the upper Orinoco (Holmstedt and Lindgren 1967a). The species of *Anadenanthera* with a south central Andean habitat is *A. colubrina* var. *Cebil,* present in north-western Argentina in western Salta, Jujuy, and Tucumán provinces. This tree is not present today in the San Pedro de Atacama area, or in other areas of northern Chile. If this leguminous tree, with its profuse seed production, once existed in ancient San Pedro de Atacama, it is probable that it could still be found in the area today. So far, this has not been the case.

A tree superficially similar to *A. colubrina* and referred to locally as *vilca* is found in San Pedro de Atacama and throughout northern Chile. Chemical analyses of the seeds of this tree, probably *Acacia visco* Lorentz ex Griseb. (see Santos Biloni 1990), have yielded negative results for the presence of tryptamines or any other known psychoactive alkaloids. This confusion has probably arisen from the fact that foliage and flowers of the different genera that compose the Mimosoideae are so similar. The pods of *A. colubrina* have a woody, reticulated texture, and are considerably larger than the parchment-like pods of *Acacia visco,* the so-called *vilca* from northern Chile. The most obvious distinguishing trait is that the pod of *A. visco* opens along both sutures, while that of *A. colubrina* opens only along one suture.

The presence in San Pedro de Atacama of such a wide variety of foreign objects, some of a relatively early date, suggests the possibility of a vast network of interaction in the south central Andes dating from the early stages of the Formative phase. Many of the exotic objects are carved with iconographic themes, such as the alter ego and Sacrificer, which are of Pan-Andean distribution. Given the high incidence of snuffing paraphernalia in San Pedro de Atacama, the trade in *cebil* seeds with northwestern Argentina must have been of considerable importance (see also Núñez 1994). The importance of Tiwanaku iconography and of snuffing in San Pedro de Atacama, together with its insignificance in northwestern Argentina, suggest that exchange of complex ideological traits did not necessarily follow established trade patterns.

The Middle Loa River Basin

Seventy kilometers north of San Pedro de Atacama, several sites are found with a high incidence of snuffing implements. These sites are located on tributaries of the Loa River in its middle course. Approximately 188 snuff trays have been unearthed in the settlements of Caspana, Chiu-Chiu, Toconce, Lasana, and Chunchurí (Dupont), among others. The majority of the snuff trays from this area have a rectangular cavity with one, two, or three figures carved in the round. Trays with Tiwanaku iconography are virtually absent, suggesting a post-Tiwanaku date for the snuffing paraphernalia from this area (after A.D. 900). Stylistic and iconographic features suggest a connection with similar developments in northwestern Argentina.

Caspana, located about 100 kilometers to the north of San Pedro de Atacama, has the highest rate of snuffing implements in the region, a total of 78 snuff trays (Allende 1981; Baron 1979; Le Paige 1959). Trays carved with three figures projecting from one of the narrow sides are frequent in Caspana (Plate 49). These typically depict two seated profile individuals flanking a third frontward-facing figure seated in the same manner. The lateral beings exhibit prominent snouts and fangs and are apparently human beings wearing masks. Chiu-Chiu, located at the confluence of the Loa and Salado Rivers, is second in frequency of snuff trays in the area of the middle Loa River. Approximately 32 trays have been found at this site, but in most cases ceramic and cultural associations are not known. Eighteen trays have been reported from Toconce, 50 kilometers to the east of Chiu-Chiu; two of these are ornamented with representations of a human being playing a panpipe. In northern Chile, this motif is seen in a tray from Caspana and another found by Spahni (1967) at the mouth of the Loa River. The alter ego is also represented on several tubes from Toconce. At the site of Chunchurí (also known as Dupont), Max Uhle (1913) excavated 30 trays. At this site, Lautaro Núñez (1964) found a snuffing tube carved with a representation of an individual holding an axe and a trophy head. Núñez (1976) obtained a radiocarbon date of A.D. 1390 from this site. Other sites in the middle Loa area and from which snuff trays and tubes have been reported are Lasana, Paniri, and Turi, but the salient information is paltry.

The snuffing paraphernalia at these sites seems to postdate that from San Pedro de Atacama, and rather to be contemporary with that of northwestern Argentina. Work by Carlos Aldunate and colleagues (1986) suggested a relatively late date for these developments in the Loa region (after A.D. 900). Structural and iconographic similarities between the snuff trays and tubes from the middle Loa and northwestern Argentina indicate some degree of interaction between these two areas (cf. Plates 23 and 49). The evidence points to a shift, ca. A.D. 900-1000, from San Pedro de Atacama to the Loa region, in the interaction between northwestern Argentina and the neighboring western slopes of the Andes. The iconography of the snuff trays from the Loa River has several features in common with those from northwestern Argentina. Both areas share the ornament consisting of two vertical crescents united by a horizontal bar, human beings playing panpipes, a frontal fanged personage flanked by seated profile figures, and Sacrificer depictions. Rampant felines are present on snuff trays from the Pucará de Tilcara in northwestern Argentina and Chiu-Chiu in northern Chile (Uhle 1913).

The iconographic and stylistic similarities between the Loa and northwestern Argentina contrast with the situation in San Pedro de Atacama, where the interchange of iconographic elements with the Argentine northwest does not seem to have been so direct. Tiwanaku influence is totally absent in the trays from northwestern Argentina. Planiform extensions are present only at the site of Calilegua, but these lack Tiwanaku-style incisions. The lack of Tiwanaku elements in the Loa region also suggests a low level of ideological interaction between the Loa and San Pedro de Atacama ca. A.D. 400-900.

THE NORTHERN ANDES

In the Colombian Andes, use of visionary snuffs is evident in the stone sculpture of San Agustín (ca. A.D. 400-1100s) in the upper Magdalena River and in Muisca (ca. A.D. 500-1500s) metallurgy (Plate 50). In Ecuador, snuffing implements have been recovered, without associated plant material, from Valdivia and Chorreras archaeological contexts (Stahl 1985; Zeidler 1988). Snuffing practices apparently persisted until late in the preconquest period, as evidenced by the Guancavilca (Manteño) archaeological site of San Marco in the Colonche Valley (Stothert and Cruz Cevallos 2001). Excavation of a group of undisturbed graves, dated ca. A.D. 1470-1550, produced four wooden snuffing tubes similar to those found in late prehistoric contexts in northern Chile and northwestern Argentina. Chemical analysis of residue from one of the wooden inhalers produced negative results for alkaloids (Stothert and Cruz Cevallos 2001). In the Colombian Andes, evidence for the use of *Anadenanthera* preparations is primarily found in the writings of the early chroniclers (e.g., Oviedo y Valdés 1959; Vargas Machuca 1892). Due to the high relative humidity of this area, perishable materials have disappeared from the archaeological record. The evidence provided by snuffing equipment, which is so prevalent in the drier environment of the south central Andes, is restricted to Muisca metallurgy. Additionally, the stone sculpture of San Agustín provides ample iconographic support for snuffing in the upper Magdalena area.

The archaeological region of San Agustín is located in southern Colombia, on the eastern slopes of the Colombian Massif. The basic motif in San Agustín sculpture is the representation of a human being who usually exhibits zoomorphic characteristics. Although most of the stone sculpture consists of freestanding figures, there are also carved boulders, relief slabs, and bedrock carvings. Iconographically, the fanged mouth is the most widely distributed trait. The alter ego concept, bird-snake associations, and animal transformation are common thematic units.

The argument for the probable use of *Anadenanthera* preparations in San Agustín is indirect and inconclusive. It is suggested by some iconographic elements such as alter ego representations, figures with feline and avian characteristics, and by depictions of probable snuffing implements. Several statues hold a shell in one hand and a stick in the other, as is clearly seen in the main figure from the east mound of Mesita A (Reichel-Dolmatoff 1972) and on a similar sculpture from Alto de los Idolos (Plate 51). It is known that snail shells are used as snuff containers by many tribes of the Amazon basin (Wassén 1965). The size of these shells ranges from 12 to 17 cm, or slightly larger than the palm of the hand. It seems highly likely that the shell in these two sculptures represents a snuff container. The object held in the right hand could then be tentatively identified as a snuffing tube.

In addition to iconographic similarities of Andean and Amazonian snuffing paraphernalia with the sculpture of San Agustín, the use of *yopo* (*A. peregrina* var. *peregrina*) was described for the upper Magdalena area during the sixteenth century. Bernardo de Vargas Machuca (1892), writing ca. 1599, described the use of *yopo,* tobacco, and *coca* to attain an ecstatic state among Pijao shamans *(mohans)* of the upper Magdalena River. He defined *yopo* as the fruit of a leguminous tree:

> *Jopa* is a tree that produces certain small pods, similar to vetches, and the seeds inside are likewise, but smaller. These the Indians take ground in the mouth in order to speak with the Devil. (Spanish orig. in Vargas Machuca 1892, 2: 111)

However, it is unlikely that the ancient people of San Agustín were exclusively utilizing *Anadenanthera* as the source of their snuffing mixtures, since this genus has a sparse distribution in northwestern Amazonia and the northern Andes. In contrast, evidence for Muisca use of *Anadenanthera* seeds in psychoactive preparations is conclusive and is considered next.

The Muisca

At the time of European contact, the Muisca, a Chibcha-speaking tribe of central Colombia, were utilizing a variety of psychoactive plants including tobacco, *Brugmansia, coca,* and *Anadenanthera* (Reichel-Dolmatoff 1965). The Muisca developed a complex gold-working tradition that includes unique examples of snuffing paraphernalia and related objects. Most of these were cast in gold or *tumbaga* (a gold and copper alloy) by the lost wax method (Pérez de Barradas 1958).

Approximately 20 Muisca gold snuff trays have been reported in the literature (Bray 1978; Kunike 1916; Pérez de Barradas 1958). These trays are similar in form to those from the south central Andes in the rectangular shape of the receptacle and in the relief figures on a flat panel. The iconography comprises avian, feline, and ophidian motifs; human beings are sometimes represented. Trays with known provenances include one found near the town of Gachancipá, another at Guatavita, and two near Cogua, all in the present-day Department of Cundinamarca (Plates 52a, b). These three sites are located within 25 kilometers of each other within the Muisca core territory.

The first description of a snuff tray in the archaeological literature is that of a Muisca artifact made by Liborio Zerda in 1883; he did not attempt to specifically determine its function. The snuff tray was found together with 12 *tumbaga* objects deposited inside an anthropomorphic urn. The find was made in 1882, at the site of Chirajara, Hacienda Susumuco, near the town of Quetame, Cundinamarca (Zerda

1972). Quetame is located on the southern frontier of Muisca territory. This is an area with easy access to the lowlands of the Guaviare,
Vichada, and Meta Rivers, where extensive use of snuffs has persisted up to the present.

In addition to the snuff trays, Muisca gold work includes numerous
trapezoidal figurines, known as *tunjos*. These figurines sometimes
represent a human being snuffing via a tube and a rectangular tray
(Plate 53; Kunike 1916; Pérez de Barradas 1958); similar scenes were
depicted in ceramic effigy vessels (Bray 1978). All extant Muisca
snuff trays are rectangular in shape, although one of the ceramic effigy vessels holds a circular dish and a tube.

The writings of sixteenth-century Spanish chroniclers suggest *Anadenanthera* as one probable botanical source of Muisca snuff powders. Oviedo y Valdés (1959, 3: 122), writing ca. 1514-1548, briefly
mentioned the use of *yopo (yop, jopa, niopo)* among the Muisca and
its relation to divinatory practices:

> These Indians have another idolatry or sorcery, and they will
> not take to the road, or accept war, nor do any other thing of im-
> portance, without knowing, or at least trying to inquire, what
> will be the outcome of their enterprise. In order to do so they
> have two herbs which they ingest, called *yop* and *osca* which
> when taken separately, beginning from a certain time and at in-
> tervals, they say that the Sun tells them what they must do in
> those things about which they have inquired.

The first specific reference to use of visionary snuffs among the
Muisca was made by Fray Pedro Simón (1882-1892, 5: 60) in the
early 1600s:

> Not so long ago, finding myself in the Sogamoso valley, in one
> of our curacies called Tota, immediately after saying Mass, I
> met an old man by name of Paraico next to the church door . . .
> and knowing he was a sorcerer I had him show me what he was
> carrying under the rags he was wearing, and found on him a
> knapsack with the tools of his trade, which were a small gourd
> which contained the powder of certain leaves they call *yopa*, to-
> gether with some of the same leaves not yet pulverized, and a
> piece of a mirror of ours imbedded in a little stick, and a small
> broom . . . and a deer bone cut lengthwise in a slant and very well

adorned, made like a spoon with which . . . they take these powders and put them in their noses and because of their pungency, make the mucus flow down to the mouth, and they observe this in the mirror, and if it runs straight it is a good sign, but if crooked, the contrary, for everything they endeavor to divine.

Fray Pedro de Aguado documented the use of *yopo*, ca. 1560, by native groups of the lowlands east of the Muisca heartland. Aguado identified the source of *yopo* as the seed of a tree and observed its use among the Guayupe of the Guaviare:

> They are accustomed to take *yopa* and tobacco, and the former is the seed or pip of a tree, and the latter is a certain leaf they keep, broad, long and fuzzy, and these they smoke, sometimes by mouth or sometimes through the nose, until it inebriates them and deprives them of their judgment. . . . This custom of taking *yopa* and tobacco is widespread in the New Kingdom and, so I understand, in most of the Indies, and more so than any other occupation . . . with the smoke the Indians take of these things they become inebriated and deprived of their natural faculties. (Aguado 1956, 1: 599)

According to Wilbert (1987), the Guayupe smoked tobacco and *Anadenanthera* cigars both through the nose and mouth. The observations by Aguado and Wilbert are of importance, since the preceding evidence suggests *Anadenanthera peregrina* as a source of Muisca snuff powders. The Guayupe were situated on the southeast boundary of Muisca territory, and sites such as Quetame would have had easy access to the region; the presence of *Anadenanthera* in the Muisca heartland was at best sparse. All of the Muisca interphase with the Orinoco lowlands was inhabited by native groups such as the Achagua and the Tunebo (Márquez 1979; Rivero 1956; see Chapter 3), well known for their intensive use of psychoactive inhalants. However, Oviedo, an experienced observer who had described the use of *cohoba* snuff among the Taíno and identified its source as the beans of a tree (Oviedo y Valdés 1959), described Muisca snuff as composed of herbs. The possibility then remains that the Muisca could have also had a locally available snuff source and were not exclusively dependent on the importation of *Anadenanthera* seeds from adjacent areas.

APPENDIX: ARCHAEOLOGICAL EVIDENCE FOR ANADENANTHERA USE

Name	Location	Use	References
Amaguaya	Depto. de La Paz, Bolivia	Snuffing	Escalante and Parejas, personal communication, 1999; Rendón 1999
Ancachi	II Región, Chile	Snuffing	Latcham 1938
Angosto Chico	Quebrada de Humahuaca, Argentina	Snuffing	Bennett et al. 1948; Casanova 1942
Angualasto	Argentina	Snuffing	Pérez Gollán and Gordillo 1994
Aplao	Valle de Majes, Peru	snuffing	García Márquez and Bustamante Montoro, 1990
Arica	I Región, Chile	Snuffing	Bird 1943; Dauelsberg 1985
Asia	Omás River basin, Peru	Snuffing	Engel 1963
Calama	II Región, Chile	Snuffing	Latcham 1938; Uhle 1915
Caleta Huelén	Mouth of the Loa River, II Región, Chile	Snuffing	Núñez, personal communication, 1983; see also Spahni 1967
Calilegua	Eastern Jujuy Prov., Argentina	Snuffing	Torres 1987a
Calingasta	San Juan, Argentina	Snuffing	Ambrosetti 1902
Campo Colorado	Calchaquí Valley, Salta Prov., Argentina	Smoking	Tarragó 1980
Casabindo	Puna de Jujuy, Argentina	Snuffing	Ambrosetti 1906; Lehmann-Nitsche 1902

Caspana	Middle Loa River basin, II Región, Chile	Snuffing	Allende 1981; Baron 1979; Le Paige 1959
Chañaral	III Región, Chile	Snuffing	Evans and Southward 1914
Chavín de Huantar	Mosna River valley (Marañon tributary), Peru	Snuffing	Burger 1995; Cordy-Collins 1980, 1982
Chiu-Chiu	Middle Loa River, II Región, Chile	Snuffing	Latcham 1938; Oyarzún 1931; Rydén 1944; Uhle 1913
Ciénaga Grande	Quebrada de Humahuaca, Argentina	Snuffing	Salas 1945
Cobija	II Región, Chile	Snuffing	Latcham 1938
Copiapó	III Región, Chile	Snuffing	Núñez 1963
Coquimbo	III Región, Chile	Snuffing	Castillo 1984, 1992
Cusi Cusi	Puna de Jujuy, Argentina	Snuffing	Lucas and Fernandez Distel, personal communication, 1998
Guandacol	La Rioja, Argentina	Snuffing	Alanís 1947
Huaca Prieta	Chicama Valley, Peru	Snuffing	Bird 1948; Bird and Hyslop 1985
Huachichocana	Puna de Jujuy, Argentina	Smoking	Fernandez Distel 1980
Huari (Wari)	Ayacucho, Peru	Snuffing, potion	Lavalle 1984
Inca Cueva	Puna de Jujuy, Argentina	Smoking	Aguerre et al. 1973; Fernandez Distel 1980
La Huerta	Quebrada de Humahuaca, Argentina	Snuffing	Latón 1954
La Paya	Calchaquí Valley, Salta Prov., Argentina	Snuffing	Ambrosetti 1907-1908

Lasana	Middle Loa River, II Región, Chile	Snuffing	Spahni 1964; Torres 1987a
Los Amarillos	Quebrada de Humahuaca, Argentina	Snuffing	Marengo 1954
Moche	Moche and Chicama valleys, no. Peru	Potion?	Donnan 1976, 1978; Furst 1974b
Moquegua	Moquegua Valley, Peru	Snuffing	Asociacion Contisuyo 1997
Muisca	Central Colombia	Snuffing	Bray 1978; Pérez de Barradas 1958
Niño Korin	Depto. de La Paz, Bolivia	Snuffing, enema	Oblitas Poblete 1963; Wassén 1972b
Paniri	II Región, Chile	Snuffing	Torres 1987a
Paposo	II Región, Chile	Snuffing	Latcham 1938
Patillos 1	Iquique, Chile	Snuffing	Núñez 1969
Pisagua	I Región, Chile	Snuffing	Latcham 1938; Uhle 1915
Pucara	North Lake Titicaca, Peru	Snuffing(?)	Chávez and Torres 1986
Pucará de Rinconada	Puna de Jujuy, Argentina	Snuffing	Bennett et al. 1948; Boman 1908; Rosen 1924
Pucará de Tilcara	Quebrada de Humahuaca, Argentina	Snuffing	Becker-Donner 1953; Casanova 1950; Debenedetti 1930
Quillagua	I Región, Chile	Smoking, snuffing	Latcham 1938
Quilmes	Yocavil Valley, Salta Prov., Argentina	Snuffing	Ambrosetti 1899, 1902

Saladillo Redondo	El Piquete, Jujuy Prov., Argentina	Smoking	Dougherty 1972; Pérez Gollán and Gordillo 1994
San Agustín	Upper Magdalena River, Colombia	Snuffing	Reichel-Dolmatoff 1972; Torres 1981
San Juan Mayo	Puna de Jujuy, Argentina	Snuffing	Lehmann-Nitsche 1902
San Pedro de Atacama	II Región, Chile	Smoking, snuffing	Le Paige 1965; Llagostera et al. 1988; Núñez 1963; Torres et al. 1991
Santa Catalina	Puna de Jujuy, Argentina	Snuffing	Lehmann-Nitsche 1902
Santa María Miramar	Extreme south coast (near Mollendo), Peru	Snuffing	Vescelius 1960; Wassén 1967a
Taltal	II Región, Chile	Smoking, snuffing	Latcham 1938
Tarija	Southern Bolivia	Snuffing	Torres 1987a
Tebenquiche	Argentina	Smoking	Pérez Gollán and Gordillo 1994
Tiwanaku (Tiahuanaco)	Southern Lake Titicaca basin, Bolivia	Snuffing	Berenguer 1987; Posnansky 1957; Uhle 1898, 1912
Toconao	II Región, Chile	Smoking, snuffing	Latcham 1938; Le Paige 1972
Toconce	Middle Loa River basin, II Región, Chile	Snuffing	Aldunate et al. 1986; Torres 1987a
Tolombón	Yocavil Valley, Salta Prov., Argentina	Snuffing	Bennett et al. 1948; Torres 1987a

Chapter 3

Anadenanthera in Non-Andean South America

Outside of the Andean area, the evidence for *Anadenanthera* use can be divided into three major regions: the Orinoco River system, the Amazon basin, and its southern periphery (see Plate 50; Appendix). The use of psychoactive plants has been noted in the Amazon-Orinoco basin since the second half of the 1600s (Aguado 1956). During the mid-1700s, missionaries such as Joseph Gumilla (1984) and Juan Rivero (1956) provided the earliest descriptions of the use of *Anadenanthera*. Accurate and detailed information mostly refers to the postcolonial period when explorers such as La Condamine (1778), Humboldt and Bonpland (1971), and Spruce (1970) identified the tree and described preparation of its seeds as a snuff powder.

THE ORINOCO BASIN

The Orinoco River system is subdivided into two sections, with detailed descriptions of *Anadenanthera* use provided for representative native groups selected from each area. The first area includes the basins of the Apure, Arauca, Meta, Vichada, and Guaviare rivers, leftside tributaries of the Orinoco that drain the open savanna areas of Colombia and Venezuela. The second area comprises the upper Orinoco and its right-bank tributaries such as the Ventuari and the Parguaza. Intensive use of *Anadenanthera* preparations has been documented for several groups from this region (Chagnon et al. 1970, 1971; Wilbert 1958, 1963; Zerries 1964).

Left-Bank Tributaries of the Orinoco River

The open and grassy plains of the Colombian *llanos* provide a favorable habitat for *A. peregrina* var. *peregrina*. This area is occupied by the Tunebo, the Otomac, and the Guahibo (Gumilla 1984; Márquez 1979; Rivero 1956; Reichel-Dolmatoff 1944; Spruce 1970). Substantial documentation is available relating use of *Anadenanthera* snuffs.

The Tunebo

The Tunebo, Chibcha speakers, inhabited a territory that extended from the northern borders of Muisca territory on the eastern slopes of the Cordillera Oriental, along the Arauca River in the present-day Departamentos de Boyacá and Norte de Santander in Colombia (Márquez 1979). In 1634, the proceedings of an accusation of idolatry first documented the use of *yopo* snuff among the Tunebo. Father Pedro Guillén de Arce accused several Tunebos, including a chief, of using *yopa (yopo)* to contravene Spanish attempts to convert the Tunebo to Christianity:

> That night, in spite of their being Christian and having received Holy Baptism, they summoned the devil and called him up in their rites and ceremonies, complaining to him that the Spaniards had come to convert them and that the priests had deprived them of *yopa*. . . . And in this manner, all night long the *cacique* and the Indians that were with him were taking *yopa* until they were seeing the Devil and were talking to him, taking the ground *yopa* out of a snail shell stopped up with a puma's tail, and an old man distributing with a spoon made out of puma bone . . . so they went on until dawn. The Devil was to foretell all the good and evil events, diseases or deaths . . . according to the filthy liquid that was running from their noses through which they take *yopa,* and which they watch in certain small mirrors. (quoted in Reichel-Dolmatoff 1978: 26-27, from a manuscript by Guillén de Arce, *Visitas de Boyacá,* in the Archivo Histórico Nacional, Bogotá)

Several observations made by Guillén de Arce are of importance, because of their commonality, in understanding the use of snuffs.

Yopo snuff is seen as an intermediary, and it is the element that allows access to the extra-human. The ceremonies were all-night sessions involving continuous use of the snuff. Throughout Orinoquia and Amazonia, as is described in this chapter, snuffs are usually administered repeatedly over a period of several hours. The use of a snail shell as a snuff container is widespread, as is association with feline imagery. The practice of divination by observing the flow of mucus via small mirrors had been observed, as previously mentioned, by Pedro Simón in the Sogamoso Valley.

A century after Guillén de Arce, the Jesuit missionary Juan Rivero (1956: 108), writing ca. 1736, described a similar method of prognostication among the Achagua, an Arawak-speaking group that inhabited the area along the Meta River, to the south of Tunebo territory:

> One of the deceits they practice consists in the use of certain powders which they obtain from the small seeds of certain trees which are tall and abundant in foliage; these powders they call *yopa,* and with these they prophesy. . . . For this they gather and convoke many and begin to give them *yopa,* which use is through the nose, in the manner of tobacco, and it is of such strength, that in a short while deprives them of their judgment; its strength brings forth humors from the nose and here enter the divination and the signs of his presages. . . . They usually snuff *yopa* for an entire day, with their doubt, until the effect is revealed by one of the nostrils.

Rivero was one of the Jesuits missionizing the area, and traveled extensively over this territory between 1720 and his death in 1736 (Rivero 1956). He observed the use of *yopo* snuff among other neighbors of the Tunebo, including the Airico (Rivero 1956). Airico and Jirara shamans, to the southeast of Tunebo territory, snuffed *yopo* to see the future and for healing. Among these two groups, the snuff was blown over a patient's body to counteract the illness (Hernández de Alba 1948b). It is clear, despite the bias of the Christian missionaries, that the use of *yopo* snuff played an essential role in communicating and manipulating the supernatural. The use of *yopo* appears as a deeply ingrained and widespread cultural trait.

The Tunebo today refer to the snuff powder as *akuá* and not by the term *yopo* preferred by the Achagua and the Guahibo (Márquez 1979; Uscátegui 1961). Rivero (1956) uses the term *yopa* to refer to

Anadenanthera snuff use by indigenous cultures throughout the Colombian and Venezuelan savannas regardless of their respective language. Nestor Uscátegui (1961), in his comprehensive work on the use of psychoactive plants by native populations of Colombia, identifies *A. peregrina* as the source of the *akuá* snuff of the Tunebo. María Elena Márquez (1979), who resided among the Tunebo for several years, described in detail their use of psychoactive inebriants. She also identified the source of *akuá* snuff as *A. peregrina* and described its preparation and ritual use. In addition to *yopo,* the Tunebo also used *coca (Erythroxylon* sp.), known as *asa,* and tobacco, which the Tunebo call *baka* (Márquez 1979).

The Tunebo engaged in long journeys to the Tame River, a tributary of the Meta, to collect *Anadenanthera* seeds (Márquez 1979). This is in agreement with Siri von Reis Altschul (1972), who maintained that Tunebo territory is west of the reported distribution of *Anadenanthera* in northern South America. However, the range of distribution of *A. peregrina* in this area seems to be broader than suggested by herbarium specimens.

An attitude of awe attended preparation or use of this snuff. To prepare it, the Tunebos peeled the seeds and roasted them in the same hearth used to dry *coca* leaves. The roasted seeds were pulverized, lime of calcined shells mixed with water added, and the mixture was kneaded and made into small cylinders kept in a container made from the beak of a toucan. The seed membranes and any remaining lime water were buried and covered by a rock. All of this work was done indoors; were it conducted outdoors, it was believed that terrible storms would result. Prior to its ingestion, the small cylinders were finely pulverized, the powder poured into a small hardwood dish *(karoá)* to be inhaled through a tube *(kwisiará)* made from the leg bone of the *pajuíl* bird *(Crax alberti* Fraser or *Mitu tomentosa* Spix; Reis Altschul 1972).

The *akuá* snuff is of mythical origin. A Tunebo tale relates how a mythical ancestor, Bistoá, pursuant to commands of the Tunebo supreme being Sirá, emerged from primordial waters with the intention of creating the earth. Since there was no earth, only water, Bistoá sat on his fingers, called his four nephews, and told them that there was no earth and to go quickly in search of some because there was no place to inhabit. Soil was brought, and once this phase of creation was concluded, Sirá ordered Bistoá to inebriate himself with *akuá* to prepare the land for the arrival of tobacco, animals, and ultimately the Tunebo. Bistoá's final act of inebriation was identified with a specific feature of the landscape. On a rocky outcrop known as Tína, near Sukúta, there exists a petroglyph depicting a seated figure wearing a tunic and holding a snuff tray and tube. The Tunebo interpret this lithic engraving as an image left behind by Bistoá on his primordial inebriation (Márquez 1979).

Akuá snuff was used almost exclusively by shamans *(karekas)*. The *kareka* received their calling directly from Sirá, who instructed the future shamans on use of the snuff as a diagnostic and oracular tool. In order to effect a healing, the *kareka* snuffed the powdered *Anadenanthera* seeds, imbibed liquid tobacco, and journeyed in his ecstatic trance to a mythical space where there exists no night. There he was offered tobacco juice by winged supernatural figures who carried the shaman to the presence of Sirá. Sirá was seated holding rattles and wearing a feathered headdress like those worn by Tunebo shamans. All spirits were instructed by the snuff spirit to seek out the Tunebo and to heal them of any ailments (Márquez 1979).

To diagnose an illness for a specific individual, the *kareka* asked the following questions of the patient: How did the disease begin? Where does one hurt? Might a patient eat and is it possible to sit erect? The *kareka* and patient then sat down, and began snuffing, and chewing *coca* and tobacco, meanwhile inquiring of the supernaturals for an answer. Blowing and sucking on the patient's body might be conducted throughout the healing session (Márquez 1979).

The existing Tunebo documentation makes apparent that *yopo* snuff enabled a shaman to have access to the supernatural realm. The snuff seemed to be imbued with vitality, being referred to as the "*yopo* spirit" (cf. Wichi later in this chapter). It was used for the diagnosis and healing of individual or community diseases and epidemics and also in oracular and divinatory activities. The seeds were used in attempts to control the weather. To propitiate the rain, several *Anadenanthera* seeds were wrapped inside cloth, which was placed in a ravine, covered with a rock. When this action had served its purpose and it was desired that the rain stop, these seeds were retrieved and burned.

Under the influence of the snuff, the *karekas* were even believed capable of flight. Avian and feline imagery were frequently associated with Tunebo snuff use. The shaman stored snuff pellets in the container made of toucan beak and inhaled it via a bird bone tube (see Plate 54 for illustrations of snuffing tube types). Guillén de Arce described the use of jaguar fur as a stopper for the snail shell snuff container, and of a spoon made of jaguar bone for distributing the snuff. No other plant admixtures seemed to be added to the *akuá* snuff of the Tunebo. However, tobacco and *coca* were used in conjunction with the snuff during the all-night sessions.

The Otomac

The first notice of psychoactive inhalants by the Otomacs, nomadic hunter-gatherers of the Meta, Apure, and Orinoco rivers, was made by Joseph Gumilla (1984). He was a Jesuit missionary who, like his contemporary Juan Rivero, had traveled extensively in the Casanare plains, and on the Meta and Orinoco rivers between 1715 and 1737. This period marked the intensification of Jesuit penetration into the valley of the Orinoco and its tributaries (Gumilla 1984) and occasioned the earliest reports of visionary plant use in this region.

Gumilla (1984) considered the Otomac warring barbarians without a socioeconomic structure, given to the excessive use of inebriants:

> They have another most evil habit of intoxicating themselves through the nostrils, with certain malignant powders which they call *yupa,* which deprives them of their judgment *(que les quita totalmente el juicio),* and furious they grasp their weapons. . . . They prepare this powder from certain pods of the *yupa (unas algarrobas de yupa)* from which the name is derived, but the powder itself has the odor of strong tobacco. That which they add to it, through the ingenuity of the devil, is what causes the intoxication and the fury. After eating certain very large snails . . . they put their shells into the fire and burn them to quicklime whiter than snow itself. This lime they mix with the *yupa* in equal quantities, and after reducing the whole to the finest powder there results a mixture of diabolical strength; so great that in touching this powder with the tip of the finger, the most confirmed devotee of snuff cannot accustom himself to it, for in simply putting his finger that touched the *yupa* near to his nose, he bursts forth into a whirlwind of sneezes. The Saliva Indians . . . also use the *yupa,* but as they are people gentle, benign, and

timid they do not become maddened like our Otomacos, who, even on account of this, have been and still are formidable to the Caribs; for before a battle they would throw themselves into a frenzy with *yupa,* wound themselves, and full of blood and rage go forth to battle like rabid tigers. (English translation from Safford 1916: 553)

Analysis of Gumilla's statement reveals aspects of the snuffing complex relevant to this study. He uses the phrase *"algarrobas de yupa"* to identify the source of the snuff. *Algarroba,* or *algarrobo,* is a generic term used in Spanish to refer to diverse American leguminous trees similar to the tree known as *algarrobo* (*Ceratonia siliqua* L.) in southern Spain. In Peru, Bolivia, and northern Chile, the term usually refers to species of *Prosopis*. Gumilla was clearly referring to the pods of an *algarrobo*-like tree. The preparation of *yupa* snuff as described in this text is similar to that reported for many other groups. The *algarrobo* bears some superficial similarities to *Anadenanthera.* The addition of calcined snail shell to the ground seeds is a feature common to this area. It should be noted, in connection with the consumption of *yopo* snuff before battle, that Chiricoa men of the Colombian/Venezuelan savannas also take snuff to enrage themselves before battle (Kirchhoff 1948). According to Father Gilli, another Jesuit missionary of this region, the Otomacs used the term *curupa* to designate the snuff referred to as *yupa* by Gumilla (Humboldt and Bonpland 1971).

Approximately 70 years after Gumilla, the German explorer Alexander von Humboldt visited the Otomacs. In June 1800, during explorations of the Orinoco, he visited the mission of Uruana (La Urbana), located on the Orinoco River between the Meta and Apure rivers (Humboldt and Bonpland 1971). Otomacs inhabited this mission during the time of his visit. Humboldt observed the preparation and use of a snuff powder, and identified one of its ingredients as *Acacia niopo* (syn. *A. peregrina* var. *peregrina*):

[T]hey throw themselves into a peculiar state of intoxication, we might say of madness, by the use of the powder of *niopo.* They gather the long pods of a *mimosacea,* which we have made known as *Acacia niopo,* cut them into pieces, moisten them, and cause them to ferment. When the softened seeds begin to go black, they are kneaded like a paste, mixed with some flour of cassava and lime procured from the shell of a *helix,* and the whole mass is exposed to a very brisk fire, on a gridiron made of hard wood. The hardened paste takes the shape of small cakes. When it is to be used, it is reduced to a fine powder, and placed on a dish five or six inches wide. The Otomac holds this dish, which has a handle, in his right hand, while he inhales the *niopo* by the nose through the forked bone of a bird, the two extremities of which are applied to the nostrils. This bone, without which the Otomac believes that he could not take this kind of snuff is seven inches long: it appears to me to be the leg bone of a plover. (Humboldt and Bonpland 1971, 2: 504-505)

Humboldt's identification of the source of *niopo* as an *Acacia* species firmly establishes its identity. Humboldt stated that the pods are moistened and left to ferment; this has not been documented among any other group. Further on in his text, Humboldt attributed the strength of the snuff preparation, not to the *Anadenanthera* seeds but to the freshly calcined lime added to them (Humboldt and Bonpland 1971). These softened and kneaded seeds cooked in cake form over an open fire have been reported more recently among the Cuiva-Guahibo, as is described later (Coppens and Cato-David 1971).

The Guahibo

The Guahibo occupy the territory south of the Otomac, between the Meta and Vichada rivers. They are hunters and fishermen who use *yopo, kapi* (*Banisteriopsis* sp.) and tobacco. They are small-scale tobacco cultivators and smoke it as cigars wrapped with the soft inner leaves of corn husks (Reichel-Dolmatoff 1944). The Guahibo are divided into four subgroups: Guahibo proper, Amoruá, Sikuani, and Cuiva. We owe to Juan Rivero (1956: 152) the first description of *yopa* powder among the Guahibo:

Inebriation with *yopa* powders is never amiss amongst them, and they carry them in large snail shells that serve as containers, and this is the only equipment they take along on their wanderings; they use the snuff powders with more excess and recklessness than the other nations, and it serves them in their superstitions and prophesies.

Fifty years after Humboldt, the English botanist and explorer Richard Spruce (1970) traveled in the region, collected botanical specimens and snuffing paraphernalia, and observed the preparation of snuff powders. Spruce traced the tree from the Amazon to the Orinoco and collected its leaves, flowers, and fruits. These samples were identified by Bentham, the English botanist and expert on the Mimosaceae, as *Anadenanthera peregrina* (then *Piptadenia*). Spruce first gathered specimens from cultivated trees at the junction of the Tapajoz and the Amazon. The following year he made a collection from wild trees along the Jauauarí, a lower tributary of the Río Negro. In 1977, the seeds collected by Spruce in 1854 were submitted to chemical analysis. The only alkaloid identified was, as expected, bufotenine, a chemical marker for *Anadenanthera* species (Schultes et al. 1977). Spruce had the opportunity to see the snuff prepared in June 1854, when he met a group of Guahibo from the Meta encamped on the savannas of Maypuré:

> [O]n a visit to their camp I saw an old man grinding *Niopo* seeds and purchased of him his apparatus for making and taking the snuff. . . . The seeds being first roasted are powdered in a wooden platter. . . . It is held on the knee by a broad thin handle, which is grasped in the left hand, while the fingers of the right hold a small spatula or pestle of the hard wood of the *Palo de arco* (*Tecomae* sp.) with which the seeds are crushed.
>
> The snuff is kept in a mull made of a bit of the leg-bone of the jaguar, closed at one end with pitch. . . . It hangs around the neck. . . . For taking the snuff they use an apparatus made of the leg-bones of herons . . . put together in the shape of the letter Y. (Spruce 1970, 2: 427-428)

Spruce's description is in agreement with observations made by Reichel-Dolmatoff (1944) almost a century later. Both authors describe a simple process of roasting the seeds and grinding them into a fine powder, with an admixture of lime or ash.

This contrasts with the more complex preparation of the Cuiva of the Capanaparo River, a tributary of the Orinoco (Coppens and Cato-David 1971). After collecting the seeds, the Cuiva let them dry for several days in a sunny spot. The seeds are then compacted into a mass that is placed in a mortar and pounded with a pestle until it becomes a soft paste. The next step starts with the processing of a shell that is first broken into little pieces and heated over a fire until it becomes incandescent. The bits of shell, now turned white, are transferred to a hard wood tray and reduced to a fine powder. The mass of macerated *yopo* seeds is removed from the mortar and mixed with the fine shell powder. The mixture is kneaded and shaped into a flat disk, which is then attached to a forked stick. This is placed over a fire until it is completely dry. When they are ready to snuff, a piece of the dried cake is placed on the same dish used to grind the calcined shell, where it is ground to a fine dust. The *yopo* is then spread in a thin layer over the tray and inhaled through a Y-shaped bird bone tube. After consuming *yopo,* it is common to have nausea accompanied by strong vomiting. Some natives induce vomiting by introducing a finger or a feather into the throat (cf. the use of vomit spatulas by the Taíno). Among the Cuiva, *yopo* could be taken by an individual alone or by invitation of another person. Most *yopo* consumption is of a collective nature. Frequently, the host distributes among his guests pieces of *yopo* cakes that are taken home for later ingestion. All the males, with rare exception, take *yopo* daily. Children are introduced to *yopo* snuffing at an early age, sometimes before the onset of puberty (Coppens and Cato-David 1971).

Spruce (1970, 2: 428) goes on to describe the chewing of *Banisteriopsis caapi* bark in conjunction with snuffing *yopo:*

> The Guahibo had a bit of *caapi* hung from his neck, along with the snuff box, and as he ground his *niopo* he every now and then tore off a strip of *caapi* with his teeth and chewed it with evident satisfaction. "With a chew of *caapi* and a pinch of *niopo*," said he, in his broken Spanish, "one feels so good! No hunger—no thirst—no tired!" From the same man I learnt that *caapi* and *niopo* were used by all the nations on the upper tributaries of the Orinoco, i.e., on the Guaviare, Vichada, Meta, Sipapo, etc.

The chewing of *Banisteriopsis caapi* is also documented by Reichel-Dolmatoff (1944) in his description of a class of Guahibo protective ritual events in which the shaman serves as an intermediary between humans and the supernatural. In these rites it is essential to snuff copious amounts and to chew *caapi* in order to be in an ecstatic state from the beginning of the performance. The practice of chewing *caapi* bark and snuffing *yopo* during the course of all-night ceremonies seems to be frequent in the region. The Guahibo of the Vichada River perform multinight ritual events that include, in addition to snuffing *yopo* and chewing *caapi,* the smoking of tobacco and the drinking of *yagé* (Wassén 1965). The Pumé of the Arauca and Capanaparo rivers conduct all-night shamanic events in which they chew the stems and the root of *Banisteriopsis caapi* in conjunction with a snuff powder made from the seeds of *A. peregrina* (Gragson 1997). The Sikuani of the Meta River, Colombia, chew the roots of *B. caapi* to enhance the experience of snuffing *yopo* (Torres 1994). Research on the mono-amine oxidase (MAO)-inhibiting effects of the harmala alkaloids suggests the possibility that sustained chewing of *caapi* bark could enhance the effects of the tryptamine-containing snuffs (see Holm-stedt and Lindgren 1967a; Ott 2001a, 2001b).

Snuffing paraphernalia is very homogenous throughout Guahibo territory (Plate 55). Reichel-Dolmatoff (1944) describes utensils very much like those sent by Spruce to the Royal Botanical Gardens (Schultes et al. 1977). The equipment is directly associated with fe-line attributes. In addition to the feathered feline bone container, the shaman wears a tiger claw headdress and carries the snuffing equip-ment in a bag made of feline fur (Reichel-Dolmatoff 1944). Guahibo inhalers are Y-shaped and made out of bird bone with a slanted cut at the distal end, and two nuts serving as nosepiece. The snuff tray is round with a fanlike handle (for other snuffing kit samples, see Granier-Doyeux 1965; Wassén 1965; Wurdack 1958).

Reichel-Dolmatoff (1944) states that *yopo* is used exclusively by males. However, Coppens and Cato-David (1971) reported that Cuiva women participated in the collecting of the seed and in snuff prepara-tion, and a few took part in its consumption. Some of the women en-gaging in snuffing among the Cuiva belonged to families of great prestige.

The three groups discussed are representatives of the different as-pects of the use of *Anadenanthera peregrina* in the Colombian and Venezuelan llanos. The Tunebo, sedentary agriculturalists, contrast in some aspects of their utilization of *A. peregrina* with nomadic hunters and gatherers such as the Guahibo and the Otomacs. Among the Tunebo, *yopo* snuff is restricted to the shamans, while among the Guahibo its use is more widespread within the community. The iden-tification of the botanical source as *A. peregrina* has been clearly established for all three groups.

Right-Bank Tributaries of the Orinoco River

The territory encompassed by the right-bank tributaries of the Orinoco River in its middle and upper course is inhabited by several groups reported to utilize *Anadenanthera* preparations. The terrain here differs from the Colombian and Venezuelan savannas, being heavily forested and including mountainous areas. Two groups that occupy this region, the Piaroa and the Yanomamö, are discussed in detail.

The Piaroa

The Piaroa occupy the area in present-day southern Venezuela bounded by the Parguaza River to the north, the lower Ventuari to the south, the middle Ventuari to the east, and the Orinoco to the west (Wilbert 1958). Their seminomadic economy is based primarily on fishing, hunting, and gathering, although they also practice small-scale agriculture. The Piaroa, Sáliva speakers, refer to their snuff powder as *yopo* and employ the seeds of *A. peregrina* as one of its components (Reis Altschul 1972; Smet and Rivier 1985; Wilbert 1958).

Alain Gheerbrant (1954) visited the Piaroa in 1949 and observed their preparation and use of *yopo* snuff. He did not attempt to identify the plant source of *yopo* but otherwise provided an account of its preparation. He told of a method of obtaining the ashes for the admixture that seems unique to this group. A small bunch of unidentified herbs hung from the roof of the shaman's hut and, suspended over a flat stone, was set on fire so that its ashes fell on the stone below. According to Gheerbrant, several other substances were added to the ashes, and the resulting deep-brown mixture was roasted over a fire. Unfortunately, he failed to identify any of the ingredients. *Yopo* was snuffed from a small board with raised edges via a Y-shaped tube. The use of *yopo* in the context of night-long ceremonies is also briefly mentioned (Gheerbrant 1954).

To collect the seeds of *A. peregrina,* the Piaroa traveled to the savanna regions of the upper Ventuari and the lower and middle Parguaza rivers during the dry months of January and February. The Piaroa made extensive use of *yopo* snuff and prepared it by roasting and pulverizing the seeds, then mixing the resulting powder with ashes from the bark of a tree known as *Coco de mono* (Lecythidaceae sp.). The snuff powder was placed on a circular dish with a fanlike handle to be inhaled through a Y-shaped bird-bone tube. Piaroa snuffing paraphernalia is very similar to that known for the Guahibo (Reis Altschul 1972; Smet and Rivier 1985; Wilbert 1958, 1963).

The Piaroa were renowned for their production of potent curare used to poison blowgun darts. They utilized a species of *Strychnos* capable of killing a prey animal within fifteen minutes (Wilbert 1958). Trade of curare for *yopo* existed with the Guahibo, who did not themselves prepare the dart poison. The *yopo* manufactured by the Sikuani (a Guahibo subgroup) of the Tuparro River was highly valued by the Piaroa (Reichel-Dolmatoff 1944).

Identification of the primary plant source for Piaroa snuff as the seeds of *A. peregrina* was definitively determined by the finding of bufotenine in Piaroa snuff samples (Smet and Rivier 1985). Smet and Rivier also found traces of harmine in one Piaroa snuff sample. Holmstedt and Lindgren (1967a) detected harmine in a Piaroa snuff sample, in addition to bufotenine. The ß-carboline alkaloid harmine is not known to be a constituent of *Anadenanthera* seeds, but it is the principal alkaloid of *Banisteriopsis* species, widely used as a primary ingredient of inebriating potions (ayahuasca, *caapi, yagé*) throughout the Amazon and Orinoco basins. There is no ethnographic evidence for use of *Banisteriopsis* species as a snuff admixture; the Piaroa did not seem to be familiar with ayahuasca potions (Smet and Rivier 1985). However, in light of the well-documented Guahibo practice of chewing *Banisteriopsis* bark in conjunction with taking snuff, we cannot dismiss the possibility that the Piaroa might have added it to their snuffs. Harmine has also been detected as component of Surará and Tucano snuffs (Biocca et al. 1964; Holmstedt and Lindgren 1967a).

The Yanomamö (Waika, Sanemá, Samatari, Xiriana)

Anadenanthera peregrina has a spotty distribution in the largely densely forested area of the upper Orinoco River occupied by the Yanomamö (Chagnon 1992), who actively use a variety of psychoactive plants, including species of *Virola, Justicia,* and *Anadenanthera* (Chagnon et al. 1971). The Yanomamö use the term *ebene* in reference to any snuff powder, regardless of source plants. They often combine previously prepared snuffs and the resulting mixture is still referred to as *ebene*. The snuff is blown by one man into another's nostrils via a 1-2 m tube.

Resin or bark extract exudate of *Virola* trees, known as *yakoana* to the Yanomamö, is a primary ingredient in their snuffs. *Virola* is so common in this area, and its use as snuff source so prevalent, that it may often be denominated *ebene,* although not all snuff powders contain *Virola* resin or extract. Various species of *Virola* (Myristicaceae) are used as components of snuffs in the northwestern Amazon area of Colombia and Brazil, and in the Orinoco River basin of Venezuela. This type of snuff escaped notice until the fieldwork of the German ethnologist Theodor Koch-Grünberg in the early twentieth century. Koch-Grünberg did not identify the plant source, but he observed preparation of snuff from the bark of a tree during his stay among the Yekwana of the upper Orinoco River in 1911-1913 (Koch-Grünberg 1917-1928; Schultes 1979a). The first published reference to the use of *Virola* in snuff was made by the botanist Adolpho Ducke (1938, 1939); Alfred Métraux (1948b) documented the drinking of a *Virola* bark decoction in conjunction with snuff taking among the Omagua (see p. 82). *Virola* was not definitively identified as a snuff source until the U.S. ethnobotanist Richard Evans Schultes (1954) observed preparation of *Virola* snuff during his extensive fieldwork in the northwestern Amazon. The Puinave, Cubeo, and many Tukano groups from the Vaupés region of Colombia also employed *Virola* species in snuffs. Leaves of *Justicia* species, notably *Justicia pectoralis* var. *stenophylla* (Schultes 1967, 1979, 1990; Seitz 1967), sometimes were added to the *ebene* snuffs; often these leaves might be pulverized and snuffed without any other admixtures or with the ashes of *Elizabetha princeps* bark (Brewer-Carias and Steyermark 1976; Seitz 1967). The role of *Justicia* leaves, known as *mashahiri* to the Yanomamö, in psychoactive preparations is not clear. No alkaloids of an activity comparable to the tryptamines have been found with certainty, although they have been reported twice (Ott 1996; Schultes 1990); the presence of non-nitrogenous psychoactive compounds has been suggested (Schultes 1990). The Tototobí Waikás (Yanomamö) are reported to use resin from the trunks of *Virola theiodora* as sole ingredient of their snuffs and dart poisons (Agurell et al. 1969). The predominant alkaloids in *Virola* barks are 5-methoxy-DMT and DMT (Ott 1996).

Some Yanomamö prefer snuffs made from *Anadenanthera peregrina* (*hisioma, sisioma* in some dialects) seeds because they may be stronger than *Virola* bark snuffs (Chagnon et al. 1971); only a small amount is needed to attain desired effects with a minimum of malaise and nausea. One of Chagnon's informants commented, "*[H]isioma* is really the strongest of the snuffs. To get inebriated with *yakoana* one must inhale a lot, dose after dose into the nose. It makes you vomit all your food, then one becomes hungry" (Chagnon et al., 1971: 73). This remark is supported by the differences in alkaloid concentration between *hisioma* and *yakoana* snuffs. Analytical results reported by Chagnon and his team indicated that one sample of *hisioma* yielded 7.4 percent bufotenine, whereas two samples of *yakoana* yielded 0.15 percent and 2.0 percent 5-methoxy-DMT and its *N*-oxides respectively (Chagnon et al. 1970).

Distribution of *A. peregrina* in Yanomamö territory is disperse and spotty. Villages proximate to wild or feral populations of the tree may specialize in the trade of its seeds, which are peeled, then packed into foot-long cylinders traded over an extensive range. The Maruiá Waikás make annual trips to collect *Anadenanthera* seeds from trees growing in open pastures (Prance 1972). Schultes (1954, 1967) has stated categorically that the genus *Anadenanthera* is absent from this region, and proposed that any groves of *Anadenanthera* present are recent introductions from the adjacent savanna areas. Chagnon argued that *Anadenanthera* had wider distribution in the forest, noting that all Yanomamö groups he had visited knew of the tree and referred to it by the same name: *hisioma* or *sisioma* (Chagnon et al. 1970; see also Brewer-Carias and Steyermark 1976). The presence of *Anadenanthera* in a village on the Marauiá River has likewise been documented by Georg Seitz (1969; Wassén 1965). Spruce (1970) saw *A. peregrina* growing wild in the Jauaurí River, a tributary of the lower Río Negro. Bufotenine was detected in snuff cakes collected among Makeko-toterí Waikas of the upper Orinoco River, suggesting *Anadenanthera* as one of its components (Marini-Bettòlo et al. 1965). *Anadenanthera peregrina* has been planted in several Yanomamö villages in the upper Orinoco. Some Yanomamö groups have introduced the tree to areas where shifts in trade and warfare patterns have interrupted the seed trade. It should be noted that any villages trading for *hisioma* seeds generally have ready access to *Virola* trees (Chagnon et al. 1970, 1971).

These snuffs are used in a shamanic context, although secular use is also frequent. Shamans as a rule perform their cures in the afternoon, although not exclusively. Experienced shamans do not inhale large amounts; small pinches are all that is required to achieve inebriation. Ecstatic trances catalyzed by these snuffs may provoke frenetic dancing as a means to invoke the *hekura,* diminutive spirits that can harm enemies and dispel sickness from the community. *Ebene* is sprinkled over the ashes of cremated individuals who have died in warfare. It is also used in mourning ceremonies for the recently deceased (Chagnon et al. 1970).

THE AMAZON BASIN

Distribution of *Anadenanthera* in the Amazon basin is limited by the intolerance of this genus for tropical rain forest conditions. *Anadenanthera peregrina* var. *peregrina* is found in pockets of savanna within the jungle, but appears not to be found at all in western Amazonia (Reis Altschul 1964). Reichel-Dolmatoff (1978) has proposed that the Guaviare River is the dividing line between *Anadenanthera* and *Virola* snuff usage. We first discuss A. *peregrina* var. *peregrina*–using groups such as the Kaxúyana, Maué, and Mura. *Anadenanthera colubrina* var. *Cebil* is the species and variety native to the Southern Hemisphere, and next we discuss its use by the Cocama and Piru of the upper Ucayali River, and the Tupari of western Brazil, among others.

The Kaxúyana

Documentation of *Anadenanthera* use in the lower Amazon basin is scarce and is limited to a few native groups. Frikel (1961) and Polykrates (1960) collected suggestive evidence from the Kaxúyana, a Karib group of the Trombetas River, to postulate that its seeds were used as an ingredient of their snuff powders. The Kaxúyana refer to snuffs and to the ritual in which they are used as *morí.* The *morí* ritual is ancient and was instituted by *Uhhtarére,* a mythological shaman and intermediary between worlds. The purpose of attaining a visionary state through snuff inhalation was to establish contact with this entity (Frikel 1961).

Frikel (1961) differentiated three types of snuffs. Tobacco was the sole ingredient of the first type. The second consisted of unidentified tree bark, seeds, and nuts, while the third was a combination of the first two. However, *Anadenanthera peregrina* seeds were present in Polykrates's collection for the Danish National Museum (Wassén 1965). Flexibility characterizes indigenous drug preparation and snuffs might vary in ingredients from batch to batch. The snuffing equipment consisted of parallel snuffing tubes, a snuff tray, a bird-shaped staff, and containers for the powder. The tray itself is called *yará-kukúru,* or "image *(kukúru)* of the mythological water jaguar *(yará).*" The staff is known as *"kurúm-kukúru,* or image *(kukúru)* of a parrot-like bird *(kurúm),*" and is used during chants and dances preceding and during the *morí* ritual (Frikel 1961).

Kaxúyana snuffing paraphernalia differs from that described for the Guahibo and Piaroa. Snuff trays are not circular but rectangular, and more closely resemble pre-Columbian Andean snuff trays, although these are larger in size. One such tray has been documented by Frikel (1961; see also Wassén 1967a) and two by Polykrates (1960); all three are quite similar in form and iconography. The trays illustrated by Frikel and Polykrates (1960) have a handle consisting of paired felines (Plate 56).

The Maué

This native group inhabited the lower Tapajoz River to its confluence with the Amazon (Nimuendajú 1948a). One of the earliest accounts of snuffing among the Maué is that of Alexandre Rodrígues Ferreira. This Brazilian scholar had conducted one of the first scientific expeditions to the Amazon basin at the request of the Portuguese government, between 1783 and 1792 (Wassén 1972a). In 1786, he documented the snuff implements used by the Maué in his "Memorial about the instruments used by the savages for taking paricá-snuff" (in Wassén 1970). These included a mortar with its pestle, a small brush used to clean the mortar and to gather the snuff on the tray, a snail shell fitted at its helical vertex with the neck of a gourd serving as a snuff box, a wooden rectangular tray, and parallel bird bone snuff tubes. The snuff was taken by pouring some powder contained in the snail shell onto the snuff tray to be spread evenly with the brush. The tray was grasped by the handle with the left hand, the dish turned toward the body to inhale the powder via the parallel bird bone tubes. One of the illustrations accompanying Ferreira's manuscripts depicts a wooden snuff tray with three figures projecting from one of the narrow sides of the tray (Wassén 1970, 1972a). This is a common occurrence, as previously discussed, in archaeological snuff trays from the south central Andes; this is the only snuff tray of this type in the Amazon basin. The same illustration depicts two individuals engaged in snuffing via a long tube. It can be concluded that the two methods of snuffing, self-administered and collaborative, were practiced by the Maué. The material collected during the expedition was sent to Lisbon, and as of 1806 most of these artifacts became part of the collection of the Museu e Laboratório Antropológico da Universidade de Coimbra, Portugal (Hartmann 1982b; see also Hartmann 1982a).

The German explorers Johann B. von Spix and Carl von Martius visited the Mura and the Maué ca. 1819 and provided detailed accounts of their snuffing practices. Spix and Martius (1823-1831) and the Austrian naturalist Johann Natterer were part of a scientific expedition to Brazil organized at the behest of Austrian Emperor Franz I. The expedition lasted from 1817 to 1821. Spix and Martius returned to Europe with the rest of the expedition members, but Natterer stayed in the Americas until 1835 (Smet and Rivier 1987). During his travels in Brazil, Natterer collected three elaborately carved wooden snuff trays from the Maué, as well as two snuffing tubes, two shell containers, and two hardwood pestles. These objects are all part of the collection of the Museum für Völkerkunde of Vienna. This museum owns three additional Maué snuff trays and four snuffing tubes, acquired in 1901 as part of the Loreto collection (Becker-Donner 1953; Wassén 1965).

Natterer's diaries were destroyed by fire during civil disturbances in Vienna in October 1848. The museum's inventory was written under his direction, and it is still extant (Wassén 1965). His collection also included seeds labeled as being "of the *Paricá*-tree." Chemical analysis conducted by Smet and Rivier detected 15 milligrams of bufotenine per gram of dried seed material. According to Natterer's catalogue notes (quoted in Wassén 1965 and in Smet and Rivier 1987), the seeds were crushed, then mixed with ashes of *Cecropia* species. The resulting mix could be snuffed or administered as an enema. Natterer also recorded the use of *A. peregrina* among the Mura and the Capiruna.

Spix and Martius visited the Maué, collected one snuff tablet (Plate 57; Zerries 1964, 1980), and mentioned that by the time of their visit in 1819, snuff from *A. peregrina* seeds was less frequently used than previously. Like Natterer, Spix and Martius described simply roasting the seeds then adding *Cecropia* ashes. Such a method has been attributed to the Maué by other investigators (Stolpe 1927; Wassén 1965).

Of the extant Maué snuff trays, the great majority are decorated with snakes. Approximately 22 carefully carved wooden snuff trays from the Maué region are preserved in museum collections in Europe and South America (Hartmann 1982a, 1982b; Phelps 1976; Serrano 1941; Zerries 1988). The role of snakes as fathers or procreators of the Maué (Nimuendajú 1948a) might in part explain the great importance of ophidian imagery in their snuff tablets.

One of the snuff trays collected by Johann Natterer in Brazil (Plate 58) features a round cavity, not common in Amazonian nor any other snuff tablets. The receptacle frame was decorated with a butterfly design above and below the circular cavity. The handle is engraved with a low-relief carving of a butterfly and dragonfly joined together at the rear. The motif of the posteriorly united butterfly and dragonfly was connected by Claude Lévi-Strauss (1979) to a Tucuna tale, "The Errors of Cimidyuë." Through deceit and cunning, Cimidyuë is abandoned by her husband during a hunting expedition. She did not know the way home, and in her wanderings encountered a series of misadventures. She was held captive by a group of supernatural monkeys that in human form offered the hospitality of their hut. The next morning there was no hut and the monkeys had returned to their animal form. The lord of the monkeys was a jaguar that could also manifest as a human being, and personally held her hostage. With the help of a tortoise, Cimidyuë finally escaped her captors. She wandered in the forest, lost, until she arrived at a familiar valley where she fell asleep among the root buttresses of a large kapok tree. In the morning she was awakened by the lord of the tree, a blue butterfly, who was hungry for pineapples from the garden of Cimidyuë's father. She followed the butterfly to a river. Then she suddenly saw her father's hut on the other side but was not strong enough to reach it unaided. The butterfly uttered a magic formula that transformed Cimidyuë into a red dragonfly; with the help of the butterfly both flew together to the other side.

The structure of the story and its careful encoding of displacement and transformation essentially tells of passing from one realm to another. The resolution of the crisis occurred when Cimidyuë encountered an intermediary who allowed passage to her place of origin. The blue butterfly *(Morpho menelaus),* usually invested with evil connotations throughout the Amazon, reverses role and becomes the helpful intermediary. The allusion to this tale on a snuffing implement situates visionary plant preparations at the intersection between worlds; ecstatic agents acted as intermediaries so that human beings could contact the supernatural to cross the river, as expressed metaphorically in "The Errors of Cimidyuë."

The Mura, neighbors of the Maué who occupied the area of the lower Madeira River, shared several aspects of this snuffing complex with the Maué. According to Curt Nimuendajú (1948b), who refers to Mura and Maué snuff powders by the generic term *paricá,* the seeds of *A. peregrina* were pulverized and taken as a snuff or an enema. The snuff was blown into the nose by another via a long tube. This contrasts with the Maué's method of self-administration employing Y-shaped or parallel bird bone tubes. Wassén (1972a: 6-7) quoted a rare passage from the work of the Brazilian explorer João Barbosa Rodrígues written ca. 1870, describing a puberty rite:

> Ripe seeds of *paricá, Mimosa acacioides,* are collected and crushed in a wooden mortar. During this process, and because of the oil they contain, a kind of dough is formed and therefore one adds ashes from the bark of wild cacao, *Theobroma silvestre.* Having been kneaded well, three-inch long cakes are formed which are put on a forked pin and dried by the fire. When dried, the material is again crushed in another mortar . . . and the powder is kept in a box of snail shell. . . . The feast starts with flagellation, by two Indians whipping each other. . . . Each man flagellates the other in turn. This ceremony sometimes goes on for six days depending on the number of young men who have attained majority. All those who have been flagellated take *paricá* either as a snuff or dissolved in water as a clyster. During the dancing the old women who have prepared the *paricá* either fill a bamboo tube with powder and give it to one of the dancers who places one end of the tube in one of the nostrils of a com-

rade and blows in the other end, or gives him a syringe of rubber filled with *paricá* in cold water to administer.

Spix and Martius (1823-1831) had previously described a similar puberty rite of the Mura, which lasted several days and involved copious use of fermented drinks and the snuffing of *paricá*. Rodrígues Ferreira described a similar feast of the Maué, ca. 1786 (Wassén 1970). He labeled such events "great *Paricá* bacchanals," which took place in a house known as a *paricá* house and constructed especially for this purpose. These ceremonial drinking and snuffing bouts began with the participants flogging each other in pairs. In Rodrígues Ferreira's narrative, the performance lasted eight days, accompanied by copious use of snuff. Safford (1916) also described a flagellation ritual by native groups of the Negro River.

The Middle and Upper Amazon

Western Amazonia and northeastern Peru lay outside the natural range of *Anadenanthera* species. On the other hand, reports by scientific observers (Koch-Grünberg 1909-1910; Métraux 1948b; Reichel-Dolmatoff 1944) suggest a probable, albeit scattered, use of *Anadenanthera* snuffs and enemas. This evidence is examined in a westward direction to the drainage of the upper Amazon and its tributaries.

The Catauixí (Katawishi) of the Purús River, a right-bank tributary to the Amazon west of the city of Manaus, were known to use both *Anadenanthera* clysters and snuffs. In 1851, Spruce (1970) purchased a set of snuff-taking implements used by the Catauixí. The most unique piece is a V-shaped bird bone tube. It consists of two pieces joined together at an angle that would allow one end to be placed in the nostril and the other in the mouth of the same individual. The powder was placed in the tube and forcibly blown into the nose. Spruce (1970, 2: 429) reported that Catauixí hunters administered *paricá* clysters to themselves and their hunting dogs "to clear their vision and render them more alert!" The Piro of the upper Ucayali River also gave *Anadenanthera* to their dogs prior to hunting. The Piro are the most southerly Arawakan tribe for whom snuffing is known (Farabee 1922; Wassén 1965). The Piro also self-administered snuff by means of a V-shaped tube (Reis Altschul 1972; Steward and Métraux 1948; Wassén 1965). The source of the Piro snuff was most probably *Anadenanthera colubrina* var. *Cebil*—the Piro area lies within the range of this taxon (Reis Altschul 1972).

The Tuyuka and the Bará, Tucanoan groups of the Tiquié River, an affluent of the Vaupés, have also been reported to use *Anadenanthera* snuffs. This area lies well to the west of the range of this genus as described by Siri von Reis Altschul (1964, 1972); Uscátegui (1961) attributed *Virola* snuff to all Tucanoan groups. Reichel-Dolmatoff (1944) made brief mention of the Tuyuka in a discussion of groups utilizing *Anadenanthera*-based snuffs. The German explorer Theodor Koch-Grünberg (1909-1910) identified *A. peregrina* as the source of Tuyuka and Bará snuff powders. Thomas Whiffen (1915; see also Wassén 1965), in his pioneering work on the northwestern Amazon, stated that the Tuyuka and other groups north of the Japurá River use a snuff, which he labeled *niopo,* prepared from the dried seeds of a *Mimosa.*

La Condamine (1778), in his expedition down the Amazon in 1743, distinguished the use of two psychoactive plants by the Omagua, which he encountered at the mouth of the Napo River:

> One called by the Spaniards *floripondio,* with flowers shaped like a drooping bell, which has been described by Pere Feuillée; the other in the native vernacular called *curupa,* ground and roasted seeds, both of them purgatives. They cause inebriation lasting 24 hours, during which it is pretended that they have strange visions. The *curupa* is taken in the form of a powder, as we take tobacco, but with more apparatus. The Omaguas make use of a cane tube terminating in a fork, of Y-shaped form, each branch of which they insert into one of their nostrils. This operation, followed by a violent inspiration, causes them to make diverse grimaces. (translated from Safford 1916: 553)

The *curupa* snuff was said to come from ground seeds and to be snuffed via Y-shaped tubes. La Condamine did not elaborate on the nature of *curupa,* but this term is used to designate *Anadenanthera* preparations in other areas (Métraux 1948b; Wassén 1965). Prior to La Condamine, the use of *curupa* had been mentioned by Father Fritz in 1699-1700 in the context of religious conflicts between Spanish soldiers and missionaries with the Omagua (Fritz 1922).

Alfred Métraux (1947, 1948b) associated the *curupa* of the Omagua with *Anadenanthera* species in two of his works. He stated that the

Omagua made rubber syringes with a bone spout to administer powerful clysters of *Anadenanthera* seeds (Métraux 1947). Métraux told how Omaguan shamanic apprentices trained for a period of five or six months under the guidance of experienced shamans. Their training included fasting and use of tobacco and *curupa,* as well as a decoction of *Virola* bark. This is one of the earliest mentions of the use of *Virola* as an ingredient of psychoactive preparations.

The area of the upper Ucayali, Purús, Madeira, Guaporé, and Branco rivers of eastern Peru and western Brazil lies within the range of *Anadenanthera colubrina* var. *Cebil* (Reis Altschul 1964, 1972). The most intensive snuff use in this region is centered on the Guaporé River and its right-bank tributaries such as the Rio Branco. The snuffing of *A. colubrina* has been reported for the Arua, Macurap (Lévi-Strauss 1948), and Tupari (Caspar 1956). This is not a homogenous cultural area, and the right-bank tributaries of the Guaporé, such as the Branco and the Mequens, are bastions of Amazonian culture (Lévi-Strauss 1948).

The Arua and the Macurap of the Rio Branco used a snuff composed of crushed *angico* (*A. colubrina* var. *Cebil*), tobacco, and ashes. The powder was inhaled through long tubes terminating in a nosepiece shaped like a bird's head. Rio Branco shaman's equipment included, in addition to snuffing tubes, a snuff tray with a handle and a feathered stick (Lévi-Strauss 1948; Reis Altschul 1972). Other right-bank tribes of the Guaporé area were reported to use *A. colubrina* preparations, but the information is scanty. The Guaratägaje, the Amniapä, and the Aikaná were mentioned in passing by several authors, but no salient details were given (Snethlage 1937; Wassén 1967a; Zerries 1964).

The most detailed information regarding the use of *A. colubrina* snuffs in the Guaporé area refers to the Tupari. This Tupi-speaking group inhabited the area of the headwaters of the Machado (Gi-Paraná) River (Lévi-Strauss 1948). The Tupari prepared their snuff from roasted and powdered *A. colubrina* seeds mixed with ashes and tobacco; the snuff was known as *aimpä (aimpë).* The snuff-taking rituals usually began in the morning and lasted late into the afternoon, ordinarily taking place indoors. Snuffing equipment consisted of a temporary table made by hammering three sticks into the ground and placing a wide board atop them. A shaman's assistant would place two long snuffing tubes terminating in hollow nuts shaped like bird heads on the table, with two snuff powder containers, a brush made from tail hairs of a giant anteater, and two cigars wrapped in corn husks (Caspar 1956; Wassén 1965). Caspar (1956) witnessed a series of three snuff-taking sessions conducted for the benefit of a child who had died the previous week. These rituals included offerings of food, and bracelets and other ornaments for the ears, nose, and lips of the deceased child. The Tupari also conducted snuffing rituals to dispel rain storms (Caspar 1956).

THE SOUTHERN AMAZON BASIN PERIPHERY

This area lies within the range of *A. colubrina* var. *Cebil* (Reis Altschul 1964) and includes the Matto Grosso of southwest Brazil, the Paraguay River basin, and the Gran Chaco. The Matto Grosso and the upper Paraguay River are not at all well known in this respect. The Bororo of the upper reaches of the Paraguay River and its tributaries seem to use *A. colubrina* preparations, but we possess practically no pertinent information. They refer to *A. colubrina* as *akiri*. This word means "white down" and it is applied to this tree because its flowers are said to resemble down. The Bororo call the Pleiades *akiri-doge* (*doge* is a pluralizer). These stars are used for calendrical calculations. A possible correlation exists between the annual flowering cycle of *A. colubrina* and the annual sidereal cycle of the Pleiades (Fabian 1992).

The Gran Chaco

Evidence for the use of *A. colubrina* var. *Cebil* in the Gran Chaco is available since the early colonial period. Pedro Sotelo de Narvaez 1965, 2: 395), in his *Relación de las Provincias de Tucumán,* written ca. 1583, mentioned use of *cebil* for the Comechingon and Zanavirona of the area north of Cordoba: "These people have few rituals, almost like those from Santiago (del Estero). *Azua (chicha)* is not held in such high esteem as is done by the Peruvian Indians. By the nose they take *sebil* which is a fruit like *vilca;* it is powdered and drunk through the nose." The identification of *sebil* as a fruit like *vilca* confirms *A. colubrina* var. *Cebil* as the probable botanical source. This area is located at the southern limits of the distribution of this genus (Hunziker 1973) and is slightly south of the Chaco area.

In the early 1700s, the Jesuit priest Pedro Lozano (1941: 288) described the use of *cebil* by the Lule of the Chaco, north of Santiago del Estero:

> When water for the sown fields is desired they pray to the ancestors, to summon the rain, and these having blown with a tube into the nose the pulverized seeds of a tree known as *sevil* in such a manner that they penetrate deeply, these powders are so potent, that it deprives them of their judgment, inebriated they begin to jump and bounce in an open space screaming and howling, and singing with dissonant voices, to call the rain so they say, since it happens that sometimes it has rained during or after this enchantment, they firmly believe that by virtue of those prayers the rains have come.

The use of snuff in ritual attempts to control the weather has already been discussed in relation to the Tunebo (Márquez 1979), and the Tupari (Caspar 1956). The Abipones of the Chaco, ca. 1784, were using *cebil* bark for tanning leather. To achieve an intense state of inebriation, they would tightly close their huts and set fire to *cebil* pods and seeds, and vigorously inhale their smoke through both mouth and nose (Dobritzhoffer 1967). A similar practice of collective fumatory inhalation was attributed to the Mbayá, a Chaquean tribe of the Paraguay River. The Mbayá and Guaraní of Paraguay referred to *A. colubrina* snuffs as *kurupá* (Pagés Larraya 1959; Pardal 1937).

The Wichi (Mataco)

The practice of snuffing and smoking seeds of *A. colubrina* var. *Cebil* has continued in the Chaco up to the present. Among the Wichi, also known as Mataco, *cebil* seeds are ingested during shamanic rituals (Alvarsson 1995; Califano 1976; Dasso 1985; Dijour 1933; Métraux 1939, 1946; Palavecino 1979). The Wichi inhabit the area of the Pilcomayo and Bermejo rivers (Alvarsson 1988). This area, known as the Chaco Central (Plate 59), is culturally and ecologically a transitional zone between the Amazon, the Pampas, and the Andes. Consequently, the Wichi share cultural traits with all of these regions. Religious beliefs and shamanic practices are similar to those of Amazonia (Métraux 1946). Notable cultural differences exist between the numerous Wichi groups occupying this immense region. Wichi communities are relatively isolated from one another and each accordingly has developed specific characteristics (Califano 1995). The shamanic use of *A. colubrina* var. *Cebil* seeds, known to the Wichi as *hatáj* (*jatáj*) or *hatáj-ilé,* is one trait shared by most communities.

The profession of shaman or *jayawú* in Mataco can run in a family, but it is not strictly hereditary. When election occurs through a family member, this is indicated in the moments before her or his death (personal observation; Califano 1976). A shaman might also be selected and initiated simultaneously by a type of supernatural being *(aját)* known as *welán.* The concept of *welán* could also be understood as a specific state of consciousness in which the shaman acquires the condition of *aját* (see Califano 1995). One notable difference between election by a related moribund shaman and spiritual election is that in the first type there is a brief delay between election and subsequent initiation (Califano 1976). Mario Califano (1976), in his comprehensive study of Wichi shamanism, mentioned the drinking of an *Anadenanthera*-based potion in relation to shamanic initiation. This potion allowed the drinker, said to perceive herself or himself as purely of bone, to enter the spirit world (Califano 1976). Oral ingestion of a decoction of *Anadenanthera* seeds has been recorded for many diverse cultures. The Guahibo prepared a drink called *yaraque,* which included *yopo* powder (Reis Altschul 1972). The addition of *vilca* to fermented drinks has been amply documented in the Peruvian Andes during the early colonial period (Cobo 1964; Ondegardo 1916). Iconographic evidence suggests, as previously discussed, that the Moche of the northern Peruvian coast drank an *Anadenanthera*-based potion.

The problem of oral administration is a complex one. Psychoactive tryptamine alkaloids such as those found in *Anadenanthera colubrina* var. *Cebil* are deaminated in the gut by the enzyme MAO; therefore snuffing, smoking, and enemas are the most efficient means of administration. Bufotenine and 5-methoxy-DMT, unlike DMT, are both orally active. It is possible to render these tryptamines more active orally by adding admixture plants that contain β-carboline alkaloids (such as harmine and harmaline), and which have the effect of temporarily inhibiting activity of MAO (Ott 2001a). One such plant combination survives today in the Amazon under the names ayahuasca, *caapí,* and *yagé.* As formulated today, it consists of two basic plants: stems of the liana *Banisteriopsis caapi* (which contains harmine and harmaline) and DMT-containing leaves of the Rubiaceous shrub *Psychotria viridis* (see McKenna et al. 1986; Ott 1994) and other plants. The possibility that other pre-Columbian as well as postcontact cultures were able to prepare such a complex drug must be entertained.

After the initiation, the shaman endured a period of learning shamanic techniques and of handling ritual instruments. One key shamanic technology was preparation and ingestion of *hatáj*. *Hatáj* permitted voyages of the *o-'nusék* (soul, spirit), which was thus capable of being separated from the body, a technique taught during the initiatory process (Califano 1976; see also Arenas 1992). The ingestion of *hatáj* allowed a prospective shaman to enter a state conducive to the learning process. This might include spirit abduction, the spirit treating the shaman as he would then treat his future patients, and a period of solitude during which a rigorous fast was observed (Métraux 1946). The ingestion of the seeds of *A. colubrina* was invested with sacred connotations, since these were seen as a doorway leading to shamanic journeying. Each seed purportedly possessed in its interior a supernatural entity that might transfer its potency or life force to a shaman. Ingestion of the seeds was generally reserved for serious, indeed grave, occasions.

A Wichi tale told of the origins of the *hatáj* tree in the context of a cataclysmic fire that caused the destruction of the world, followed by its subsequent regeneration. Only three beings survived the fire: Tokjwáj, the chief of all shamans and the initiator of healing practices (Califano 1976), and Chuña and Icanchu, his two avian familiars. All escaped the fire by running to the hills and seeking refuge in a cave. After the fires had subsided Tokjwáj decided to stay, but his two companions wished to return to their places of origin. Tokjwáj told them that it would be very difficult to find the place where they had lived before the fire, but, were they to follow his instructions, they should be able to locate it. After much traveling, they at length found the place where they had lived before the fire. All the trees had been burned and hence there was neither food nor shade. Icanchu started digging, but all he could find was charcoal. He began to dance and beat on a piece of charcoal as if it were a drum. He danced and played all day, and soon observed that a shoot was sprouting from the scorched earth. He continued dancing and playing his charcoal drum, until the shoot became a larger branch. Icanchu kept on playing and dancing until the tree grew large and strong. He soon noticed that every branch was in fact a different tree. Icanchu began to throw rocks at the tree to break its branches, and as the branches sundered and fell to earth different trees sprouted from each of them. After every branch had fallen, the *hatáj* tree grew from the center. In this way the regeneration of the world was achieved (Barabas and Bartolomé 1979).

Among the Wichi of the area of General Mosconi in the western Chaco Central, *cebil* seeds are collected once yearly, during the month of August, then prepared as needed. The preparation follows a very simple procedure: the roasted seeds are ground in a mortar until they become a coarse powder. The shaman might snuff this powder, or mix it with tobacco and smoke it in a pipe or as a cigar. Califano (1976) stated that pipes were most frequently used during lengthy nocturnal sessions, when several *jayawú* get ready to deal with a difficult case. It should also be noted in reference to admixture plants that Wichi shamans combine chewing of *coca* leaves with snuffing or smoking. No clear references to dosage are found in the literature on Wichi shamanism. Personal observations indicate that 8 to 10 seeds are used when mixed with tobacco and smoked as a small cigar. This seems to be strong enough, inasmuch as the shaman generally smokes only half of the cigar. The effects last for approximately two hours, and the shaman might smoke a second time during the same session. There are other uses of *cebil* by the Wichi. The bark, which has a high tannin content, is used as a dye for leather and fibers. A decoction of the bark is also used to treat gastric ailments (Alvarsson 1995; Koschitzky 1992; see also Mell 1930). The Wichi also wash their head with a decoction of leaves and pods to treat headaches.

Three broad categories of Wichi shamanic activity can be distinguished: (1) in curing the sick individual; (2) for the benefit and protection of the community (weather control, to forestall or dispel famines, epidemics, supernatural dangers); and (3) in oracular or divinatory activities (Califano 1976; Dasso 1985; Métraux 1946). Disease is allegedly caused by the magical intrusion of an object or animal into a person, or by loss of the soul. Soul loss as a cause of illness is seen by Métraux (1946) as one of the Andean traits present in the Chaco. Pathogenic substances can supposedly be introduced by spirits acting independently or through the will of a shaman. The ingestion of *hatáj* gives a shaman the capacity to visualize and remove these intrusive pathogenic objects. In addition, it also allows the separation of the *o-'nusék* (soul) and the acquisition of animal characteristics during the shamanic journey, thereby facilitating retrieval of a lost soul. Animal transformation, usually into a bird or a jaguar (Califano 1976; Métraux 1946), is a characteristic shared with Amazonian shamanism. Califano (1976) related how, under the influence of the snuff, a shaman vigorously played a flute made from the leg bone of a *yulo* bird *(Tantalus cristatus)*. His soul *(o-'nusék)* transformed into a bird, then separated from his body to accomplish his goal. When travels of the *o-'nusék* are not aided by the bird bone flute, the shaman might beat his chest with the wings of a hawk. The wings extract the *o-'nusék* from his body and fling it into the air to initiate its travels (Califano 1976). Curing sessions always take place at night and could last several nights depending on the complexity of the situation. Private sessions among several shamans might take place, especially when dealing with issues of concern to the whole community (see also Palavecino 1979). Wichi shamanism represents the last vestiges of ancient south central Andean and Amazonian *Anadenanthera* use.

The preceding sections have provided a historical and cultural study of the use of *Anadenanthera,* not only as shamanic inebriant, but also as a contributor to the development of South American native ideologies. Use of its roasted seeds as an ingredient in snuffs, enemas, fumatories, and potions for several millennia attest to its cultural significance and efficacy. To achieve a more comprehensive understanding of this genus and of its effects on human affairs, the next two chapters discuss chemical and pharmacological aspects. These chapters include extensive discussion of the active constituents of visionary preparations derived from its seeds.

APPENDIX: INDIGENOUS USE OF ANADENANTHERA IN THE ORINOCO-AMAZON BASIN AND ITS SOUTHERN PERIPHERY

Native group	Location	Linguistic affiliation	Species	Native name	Use	Reference
Abipones	Chaco, Argentina	Guaicurú	colubrina	Cebil	Smoke inhalation	Dobritzhoffer 1967
Achagua	E. Colombia, W. Venezuela-Meta River	Northern Maipuran (Arawak)	peregrina	Yopa	Snuffing	Hernández de Alba 1948a; Rivero 1956
Airico	Meta Prov. (E. Colombia)	Betoya	peregrina	Yopa, yopo	Snuffing	Hernández de Alba 1948b; Rivero 1956
Amniapä	Branco and Mequens rivers, W. Brazil	Tupí	colubrina		Snuffing	Lévi-Strauss 1948; Wassén 1967a
Amorúa	Meta and Inírida rivers	Guahiban	peregrina	Yopo	Snuffing	Reichel-Dolmatoff 1978; Uscátegui 1961
Arua	Rio Branco basin, Bolivia	Tupí	colubrina	Angico	Snuffing	Lévi-Strauss 1948
Baniva	South of Vichada River	Northern Maipuran (Arawak)	peregrina		Snuffing	Reichel-Dolmatoff 1975
Bará	Tiquié River	Tucanoan	peregrina		Snuffing	Koch-Grünberg 1909-1910
Bororo	Upper Paraguay River, Matto Grosso, Brazil	Bororo (Macro-Ge)	colubrina	Akiri	Snuffing?	Fabian 1992

90

Caripuná	Purús River	Panoan	*colubrina*		Snuffing, enema	Smet 1985; Métraux 1948a; Wassén 1965
Catauixís (Katawixi)	Purús River	Katukinan	*peregrina*	*Niopo*	Snuffing, enema	Smet 1985; Spruce 1970
Chama	Juruá-Purús rivers	Panoan	*colubrina*		Snuffing	Reis Altschul 1972
Chiricoa	Colombian-Venezuelan Llanos	Guahiban	*peregrina*		Snuffing	Kirchhoff 1948
Chiriguano	W. Bolivia	Tupí-Guaraní	*colubrina*	*Kurupai*	Snuffing	Reis Altschul 1972
Cocama	Ucayali and Huallaga rivers	Tupí-Guaraní	*colubrina*	*Curupá*	Snuffing, enema	Métraux 1948b
Comech-ingones	Córdona, Argentina (sixteenth century)	Comech-ingon	*colubrina*	*Sebil*	Snuffing	Cooper 1949; Sotelo de Narvaez 1965
Cuiva-Guajibo	Meta, Apure, and Inírida rivers	Guahiban	*peregrina*	*Yopo*	Snuffing	Coppens and Cato-David 1971; Uscátegui 1961
Guahibo	Llanos Orientales, Colombia; Orinoco basin	Guahiban	*peregrina*	*Yopo*	Snuffing	Reichel-Dolmatoff 1944; Spruce 1970
Guaraní	S.E. Brazil	Tupí-Guaraní	*colubrina*	*Kurupá*	Snuffing	Pardal 1937; Serrano 1941; Reis Altschul 1972
Guaräta-gaje	Branco and Mequens rivers, W. Brazil	Tupí	*colubrina*		Snuffing	Lévi-Strauss 1948; Wassén 1967a
Guayabero	Meta and Inírida rivers	Guahiban	*peregrina*		Snuffing	Reichel-Dolmatoff 1978; Uscátegui 1961

91

Group	Location	Language	Species	Native name	Use	References
Guayupe	Guaviare River	Arawakan	*peregrina*	*Yopa*	Snuffing, smoking	Aguado 1956
Igneri	Trinidad	Arawakan	*peregrina*	*Yopa*	Snuffing	Reichel-Dolmatoff 1975
Jirara	Meta Prov. (E. Colombia)	Betoya	*peregrina*	*Yopo*	Snuffing	Hernández de Alba 1948b; Rivero 1956
Kaxúyana (Cashuena)	Cashorro River, tributary of middle Trombetas, Brazil	Carib	*peregrina*	*Morí*	Snuffing	Frikel 1961; Polykrates 1960
Kuripacos	Meta and Inírida rivers	Northern Maipuran	*peregrina*		Snuffing	Uscátegui 1961
Lule	Chaco	Lule-Vilela	*colubrina*	*Sevil*	Snuffing, smoking	Lozano 1941; Métraux 1946; Wassén 1965
Macurap	Rio Branco basin, Bolivia	Tupari (Tupí)	*colubrina*	*Angico*	Snuffing	Lévi-Strauss 1948; Reis Altschul 1972
Maué	Tapajóz River	Tupí	*peregrina*	*Paricá*	Snuffing, enema	Smet and Rivier 1987; Spix and Martius 1823-1831
Mbayá	Paraguay River	Guaicurú	*colubrina*	*Curupá, curupay*	Snuffing, smoking	Pagés Larraya 1959
Mundurucú	Lower Madeira and Tapajóz rivers, Brazil	Mundurukú (Tupí)	*peregrina*	*Paricá*	Snuffing	Reis Altschul 1972; Montell 1926
Mura	Lower Madeira River	Mura	*peregrina*	*Paricá*	Snuffing, enema, smoking	Smet 1985; Nimuendajú 1948b
Omagua	Mouth of the Napo	Tupí-Guaraní	*peregrina* (?)	*Curupá*	Snuffing, enema	Métraux 1948b; La Condamine 1778

Otomac	Venezuelan Llanos (between Orinoco, Apure, and Meta rivers)	Otomac	*peregrina*	*Curuba, ñopo*	Snuffing	Gumilla 1984; Humboldt and Bonpland 1971
Palenque	Lower Orinoco basin, S.W. of Cumaná	Carib	*peregrina*	*Yopa*	Snuffing	Hernández de Alba 1948a
Paravilhana	Rio Branco, N.E. Brazil	Carib	*peregrina*		Snuffing	Uhle 1898; Wassén 1967a
Piapoco	Meta and Inírida rivers	Northern Maipuran	*peregrina*	*Yopo*	Snuffing	Cooper 1949; Uscátegui 1961
Piaroa	S. Venezuela (Guiana highlands)	Sálivan	*peregrina*	*Yopo*	Snuffing	Smet and Rivier 1985; Wilbert 1958, 1963
Pijao	Upper Magdalena River, S. Colombia	?	*peregrina*	*Jopa*	Snuffing?	Reichel-Dolmatoff 1978
Piritu	Lower Orinoco basin, S.W. of Cumaná	Carib	*peregrina*	*Yopa*	Snuffing	Hernández de Alba 1948a
Piro	Upper Ucayali River	Southern Maipuran	*colubrina*	*Yopo*	Snuffing	Cooper 1949; Steward and Métraux 1948
Puinave	Meta and Inírida rivers	Arawak	*peregrina*	*Yopo, noopa*	Snuffing	Uscátegui 1961; Wurdack 1958
Pumé	Arauca, Capanaparo, and Riecito rivers, Venezuela	Yaruro (Macro-Chibchan)	*peregrina*		Snuffing	Gragson 1997
Sáliva	Meta and Inírida rivers	Sálivan	*peregrina*	*Yupa*	Snuffing	Gumilla 1984; Rivero 1956; Uscátegui 1961

Group	Location	Language/Family	Species	Name	Use	References
Shiriana	Upper Orinoco	Macro-Chibchan family	*peregrina*	*Yopo*	Snuffing	Reis Altschul 1972; Wurdack 1958
Sikuani	Meta and Inírida rivers	Guahibo	*peregrina*	*Yopo*	Snuffing	Uscátegui 1961; Reis Altschul 1972
Tucuna	Left tributaries of the Solimões	?	*peregrina*		Snuffing	Wassén 1965
Tunebo	Arauca River (E. Colombia)	Chibcha	*peregrina*	*Akuá*	Snuffing	Márquez 1979; Rivero 1956
Tupari	Rio Branco and Guaporé, W. Brazil	Tupari (Tupí)	*colubrina*	*Aimpë, aimpä*	Snuffing	Caspar 1956; Wassén 1965
Tuyuka	North of Japurá River, Tiquié River	Eastern Tucanoan	*peregrina*		Snuffing	Koch-Grünberg 1909; Reichel-Dolmatoff 1944
Wichi (Mataco)	Chaco, Argentina/Bolivia	Mataco-Maká	*colubrina*	*Jatáj, hataj*	Snuffing, smoking	Alvarsson 1995; Califano 1976; Métraux 1946
Yanomamö	Upper Orinoco, S. Venezuela, N. Brazil	Yanomam	*peregrina*	*Hisioma, sisioma*	Snuffing	Chagnon et al. 1970, 1971; Prance 1972
Yaruro	Capanaparo and Cinaruco, Orinoco tributaries	Yaruro	*peregrina*	*Curuba, yopo*	Snuffing	Cooper 1949; Reis Altschul 1972
Yecuaná	Upper Ventuari River	Carib	*peregrina*	*Acuja*	Snuffing	Koch-Grünberg 1917-1928; Wassén 1965
Zanavirona	Córdona, Argentina (sixteenth century)	Zanavirona	*colubrina*	*Sebil*	Snuffing	Cooper 1949; Sotelo de Narvaez 1965

Chapter 4

The Chemistry of the Genus
Anadenanthera

CHEMICAL MAKEUP AND COMMERCIAL USES
OF ANADENANTHERA

Our knowledge of *Anadenanthera* chemistry is extensive, reflective of nearly a century of contemporary economic interest and some 200 years of scientific interest. Of course, New World human involvement with *Anadenanthera* and the closely allied genus *Piptadenia* is at least 4000 years old. *Anadenanthera* species, both wild and cultivated, are sources of timber for milling lumber, of dyestuffs for the textile industry, of tannins for leather curing, and of pulp for paper production. In addition, *Anadenanthera* and related species of *Piptadenia* have served as sources of an adhesive and medicinal agent known as *angico* gum. Various medicinal properties ascribed to *angico* gum include the treatment of respiratory infections such as pneumonia and bronchitis (Le Cointe 1947), use as an abortifacient (Hieronymus 1882), and use as snuff to cure constipation and headaches (Hoehne 1939). However, one of the most interesting aspects of the genus has been its role in the manufacture of various drug preparations used in traditional healing practices throughout South America and the Caribbean.

A comprehensive review of the chemistry of any genus must take into consideration the interdisciplinary nature of the study. For example, any attempt to correlate the reported chemistry of certain genera and species must account for botanical synonymy. Benson (1959: 664) defined synonymy as follows: "A name which is not used because one applied earlier designates the same plant or because the same name was used earlier for a different plant." Synonymy therefore refers to the series of names applied to a single taxon. Occasional discarding of names occurs when botanists revise generic taxonomic concepts and/or regroup or separate previously recognized taxa. Although the genus *Piptadenia* Bentham was established in 1841, numerous additions and revisions have occurred since then. The four species of *Anadenanthera* Speg., with which this monograph is mainly concerned, were once part of the genus *Piptadenia* Benth. In this chapter, botanical names cited in the chemical literature were retained in order to afford historical continuity. Synonymy with one of the four species of *Anadenanthera* is indicated in brackets (see also Appendix to Chapter 1).

The use of natural products in commerce was still quite prevalent at the beginning of the twentieth century. Practiced for centuries, the art and science of tanning and dyeing of leather led to extensive research in all corners of the world for sources of tanning agents. The quest for new sources of tannins from tropical forests grew in the early to mid-twentieth century as northern, temperate forests were extensively logged. Several South American species of the genus *Piptadenia* were among the tropical trees that were investigated as sources of tannins and dyes. Among these species were *Piptadenia rigida, P. peregrina, P. macrocarpa,* and *P. speciosa,* known generically as *angicos.* Generally, the bark served as the organ richest in tannin; however, with the leguminous trees, seed pods could also be used. A mid-twentieth-century study from Brazil reported a tannin content from *P. rigida* bark of 15.0 percent (Primo 1945).

In an extensive study of the trees of Argentina, Prado and Ricci (1956) reported the percentage of tannins in the bark of *P. rigida* to be 16.85 percent and that of *P. macrocarpa* to be 15.38 percent. The seed pods of *P. macrocarpa* contained a lesser amount, 3.0 percent, the heartwood of the same species 1.8 percent.

Trease and Evans (1971: 146) gave the following definition of tannin: "The term tannin was first applied in 1796 to denote substances present in plant extracts which were able to combine with protein of animal hides, prevent their putrefaction, and convert them into leather." The quantitative test for tannins in water-soluble extracts of plants consists of absorption on "standard hide powder," which is then weighed. Tannins are polymeric substances with a molecular weight between 1000 and 5000 mass units. Two types of "true" tannins are known, those containing linked monomers and dimers of either gallic acid or ellagic acid, known as "hydrolyzable tannins," and "condensed tannins" consisting of catechins and flavan-3,4-diols. Using the powdered leather method in a study of tropical tannins, Doat (1978) suggested that the tannins of tropical woods were of the condensed tannin class, that is, "of a catechic nature."

Often dyestuffs for leather were also obtained from the same plant sources as tannins, as reported by Mell (1930: 754). Mell's work is unusual for its day, since it contained a rather thorough description of both habit and habitat of *Piptadenia peregrina*. What follows are excerpts from this study:

> The outer corky layer [of the bark], which is designed by nature to serve as a nonconductor of heat and moisture, is exceedingly rough having very conspicuous, short, irregular ridges or persistent conical projections. The external appearance varies from a dark-grayish brown to a dark reddish shade depending upon the degree of exposure to the direct rays of the sun or to the drying wind. (Mell 1930: 754)

Mell further states:

> Few other kinds of tropical trees develop such a thick, coarse bark as the species of *Piptadenia* under review, which is known to grow pretty generally throughout the West Indian Islands and in many parts of the mainland from Guatemala southward to Brazil. . . . The bark of this species [*P. peregrina*] is highly esteemed for tanning and dyeing leather wherever the tree grows. . . . Moreover, the dyeing qualities are claimed to be superior to that of mangrove bark and of the wood of *quebracho*. (Mell 1930: 754)

Perhaps as an echo of the past, Mell (1930: 754) states, "The fact is that the *Piptadenia* species are so closely related to the species of other genera of the family that it is often quite difficult to say just where they belong."

Tannins were also used in the preparation of medicines, most notably quinine tannate as a non-bitter-tasting preparation of the antimalarial drug quinine. Wassicky (1944: 266) of Sao Paulo reported, "Quinine tannate is not bitter but tasteless or nearly so, depending on the kind of tannin used. . . . Tannins from the barks of the Brazilian tree(s) . . . *Piptadenia speciosa* . . . were as satisfactory as imported tannin."

Prior to the advent of the modern chemical age, various members of the Leguminosae were used throughout the world as sources of mucilages and adhesives. The best known of these adhesive preparations is gum arabic, extracted from *Acacia senegal* Willd. Gum arabic has been known since the seventeenth century B.C., first described by Theophrastus (Trease and Evans 1971) as a product of upper Egypt. Five types of the closely related *angico* gum are known from twentieth-century South America. These types and their properties and uses were described by Rangel (1943: 16):

> *Angico branco* [white *angico*]—*Piptadenia colubrina* Benth. or *Acacia colubrina* M.—also known as *cambui.*
> *Angico do campo* [wild *angico*]—*Piptadenia macrocarpa* Benth. Or *Acacia grata* Willd.—also called *arapiraca* or *curupái.*
> *Angico Roxo* [red *angico*]—*Piptadenia cebil* Griseb.
> *Angico verdadeiro* [genuine *angico*]—*Piptadenia rigida* Benth. Or *Acacia angico* M.—also known as *angico amarelho* and **paricá.** (Emphasis ours).
> *Angico vermelho* [red *angico*]—This also refers to the species *P. rigida* Benth.

Angico gums were also used as medicines for the treatment of respiratory illnesses such as bronchitis. The chemistry of *angico* gum was studied by Rosenthal (1955). Figure 4.1 shows the monosaccharides derived from the acidic hydrolysate of the gum.

Other economic uses for several species of *Piptadenia* and *Anadenanthera* have been suggested and some have been implemented with limited success. The Zona da Matas region of Minas Gerais State, Brazil, comprises an area of some 55,000 square kilometers. Although, as its name suggests, it was originally covered with forests, as of 1972, only 10 percent of the region was still forested (Gomide et al. 1972). During the nineteenth century, much of the forest was removed in order to establish coffee plantations. The steep slopes of this mountainous region make it unsuitable for general agricultural use, and much of the area has since undergone extensive erosion. The government of Brazil has commissioned studies of the possibility of making the region a forest zone once again. Any such reforestation

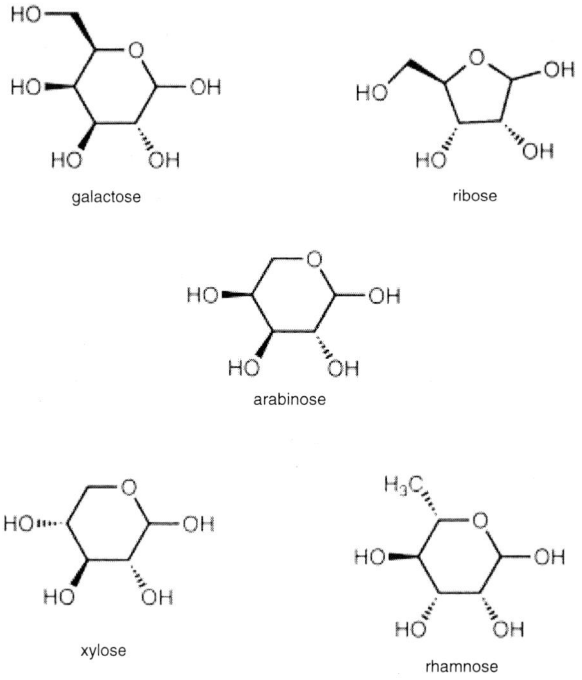

FIGURE 4.1. Monosaccharides derived from saponification of *angico* gum. *Source:* After Rosenthal 1955.

project must take into account the potential profitability of such an undertaking.

Of the eight major species that originally made up the forests of the Zona da Matas, three are of interest here: the previously mentioned *angico vermelho (Piptadenia rigida), angico branco (Anadenanthera colubrina),* and the related species *jacare (Piptadenia communis). Angico branco* is the only one of these three that has been used commercially in pulp production for the manufacture of paper. Study of the possible use of these species in the production of paper pulp demonstrated that *angico vermelho* produced a pulp yield that was comparable to the control species *(Eucalyptus saligna),* and *jacare* produced the highest yield (Gomide et al. 1972). Characteristics such as flexibility, intrinsic fiber strength, bursting strength, density, tensile strength, and tear factor indicated that while the species in question could be used to prepare paper pulp, their overall quality was not as good as that of *Eucalyptus saligna,* although *jacare,* which produced a good yield (of growth) per hectare was suitable for the production of pulp where low density was desired. A related study (Marques de Melo et al. 1971) determined the cellulose, lignin, pentosan, and ash content that would be required to use various tropical trees in the production of paper pulp.

Species of *Piptadenia* and *Anadenanthera* were used throughout the twentieth century for lumber and other wood products. An early study by Record and Mell (1924) described the useful properties of *Piptadenia rigida* and of *curupáy,* an Argentine species then of unknown identity. Describing the general properties of the wood of *P. rigida,* these authors stated:

> Color rather pale reddish-brown; fairly lustrous; mahogany-like. Sapwood thick, pinkish gray; distinct but not very sharply defined. Odor and taste absent or not distinctive. Hard and heavy. Specific gravity (air dry) 0.95. Weight about 59 pounds per cubic foot. . . . Wood fairly easy to work, finishes smoothly, takes a high polish, appears durable. (Record and Mell 1924: 221)

Of *curupáy:*

> Its principal source seems to be the lowland forests of Paraguay. . . . it is said to be a large tree and fairly abundant. . . . It also occurs in parts of southern Brazil. The timber enters the market in the form of squared logs, and it is used for all sorts of heavy durable construction. . . . It is too hard, however, for furniture and general carpentry, though of beautiful figure and color and taking a high polish. (Record and Mell 1924: 221)

The wood of this species was easily distinguished from that of *P. rigida* by a deeper red color and black markings and a greasy feel.

Later, Tortorelli (1948) conducted a thorough study of the xylotechnology and forestry aspects of four species of *Piptadenia* (*P. macrocarpa* Benth. [*Anadenanthera colubrina* (Vell.) Brenan var. *Cebil*], *P. excelsa* [Gris.] Lillo, *P. rigida* Benth., and *P. paraguayensis* [Benth.] Lindm.), which were considered to be the principal species of the genus growing in northern Argentina. This work described the macroscopic properties and wood anatomy (both gross and minute), as well as the uses of the wood, and various timber and forest characteristics such as the merchantable volumes in cubic meters *per* hectare, average diameter, and percentage of diseased trees. In addition, this study included a botanical key to the four species as well as the range, habit, and habitat of the species. Tortorelli here applied the names *cebil colorado* and *curupay* to signify *A. colubrina,* and *Horco Cebil* to designate *P. excelsa.* Tortorelli (1948: 1) emphasized the importance of the genus to the Argentine economy: "[T]he woods of the species which make up the genus are very valuable and also because the tree can be reproduced easily, either naturally or artificially." An interesting use of the wood was said to be in the cooperage industry: "[W]ine bottled with shavings and with chips of Cebil Colorado for two years had a darker color than the control specimen. . . . No differences were noticed in the odor; the taste was slightly bitter" (Tortorelli 1948: 10). Tortorelli reported that in 1946, five tons of wood of *cebil colorado* were removed from public forests and 962 tons from private forests in the Misiones region.

Ten years later, Brazier (1958) updated this study with the timber anatomy of the species of the newly created genus *Anadenanthera* Brenan (see Chapter 1). This study was undertaken to determine whether the genera established by Brenan could be distinguished on the basis of their wood anatomy. Brazier (1958: 49) concluded that although the color, texture, and weight of the woods of species of *Anadenanthera* were similar to those of *Piptadenia rigida,* anatomically the timbers of the two genera were "readily distinguishable on ray width, the rays in *P. rigida* being mainly bi- or occasionally triseriate whereas in *Anadenanthera* they are typically four and occasionally more cells wide."

As recently as 1976, active logging of *Anadenanthera colubrina* was reported in Argentina. The company Celulosa Argentina published a short account (*Libro del árbol* 1976) of the characteristics and uses of the logged species. Uses included naval construction (canoes and barges) since the angles and curvatures of the tree were so well suited to the formation of hulls and braces. General construction purposes included fence posts, telephone poles, piles and piers, window and door frames, and as floors and platforms of railway cars.

Lumber from *A. colubrina* has also been exported from Argentina. It is used in Japan as a fancy sliced veneer because of its light color and distinctive black stripes. Variations in wood color are artificially produced by irradiation of the timber with ultraviolet light. This darkens the wood considerably and care must be taken to limit the exposure to ultraviolet rays since the longer the irradiation time, the less is its decorative value. In an attempt to provide a quantitative measure of this ultraviolet-irradiated darkening process, Miyauchi et al. (1976) reported the results of a chemical analysis of the heartwood of *Piptadenia macrocarpa (A. colubrina)*. Figure 4.2 gives the chemical structures of the compounds obtained from chromatography of both a hexane and an ether extract. It was concluded that the photo-induced

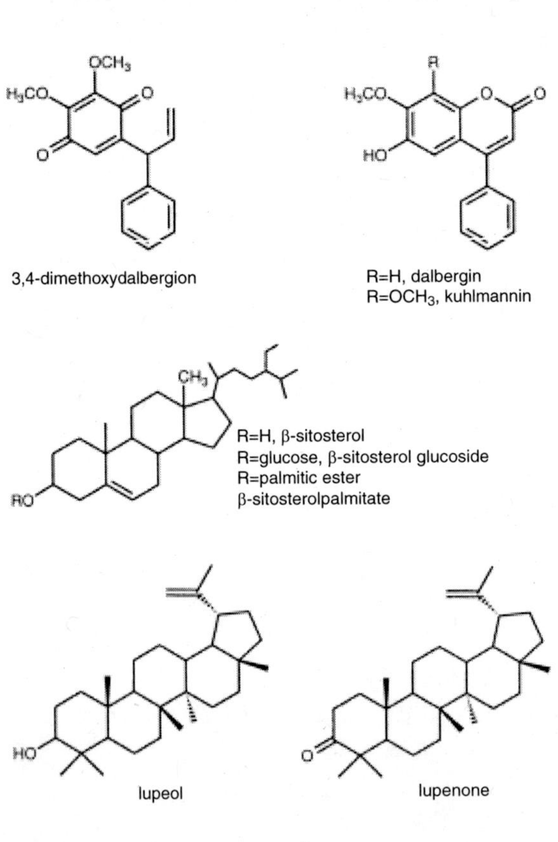

3,4-dimethoxydalbergion

R=H, dalbergin
R=OCH₃, kuhlmannin

R=H, β-sitosterol
R=glucose, β-sitosterol glucoside
R=palmitic ester
β-sitosterolpalmitate

lupeol   lupenone

FIGURE 4.2. Neoflavanoids, steroids, and triterpenoids from *Anadenanthera*. *Source:* After Miyauchi et al. 1976.

color change was strongly influenced by these wood extractives (Miyauchi et al. 1976).

A number of other nonalkaloidal constituents have been reported to occur in species of *Anadenanthera*. Paris and colleagues (1967) isolated four C-flavanosides from the leaves of *P. peregrina* Benth. (Figure 4.3). These were the β-D-glucopyranosyl derivatives of 2-(mono- and di-hydroxy-phenyl)-5,7-dihydroxy-4*H*-1-benzopyran-4-one. Orientin and vitexin differ from homoorientin and homovitexin by the position of the carbon-carbon linkage of the sugar moiety to the aglycone, the former at carbon 8, the latter at carbon 6. Vitexin was the first C-flavanone to be isolated from natural sources. Of little use in chemotaxonomy or chemical systematics (the use of chemical constituents as taxonomic characters), convergent formation of these

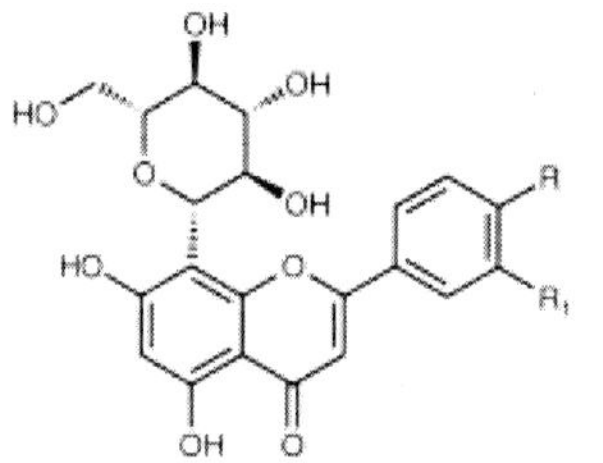

R=R₁=OH orientin, 2-(3,4-dihydroxyphenyl)-8-β-
D-glucopyranosyl-5,7-dihydroxy-4H-1-benzopyran-4-one

R=OH, R₁=H vitexin

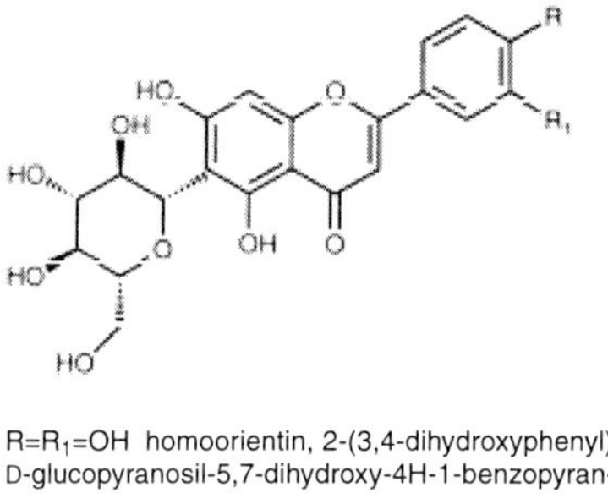

R=R₁=OH homoorientin, 2-(3,4-dihydroxyphenyl)-6-β-
D-glucopyranosil-5,7-dihydroxy-4H-1-benzopyran-4-one

R=OH, R₁=H homovitexine

FIGURE 4.3. C-flavanosides found in *Anadenanthera*. *Source:* After Paris et al. 1967.

flavanoid C-glycosides is indicated by their detection in at least 18 unrelated families scattered throughout the plant kingdom, including ferns and monocotyledons (Trease and Evans 1971). Another such study (Plouvier 1962) attempted to relate the distribution of the cyclitols L-inositol, D-pinitol, L-quebrachitol, L-bornesitol, and D-ononitol to the chemotaxonomy of 27 families of the Leguminosae, including species of *Piptadenia.*

Krauss and Reinbothe (1973) published a major work aimed at establishing the connection of chemical markers to botanical taxonomy in one leguminous family, the Mimosaceae. They studied the occurrence of 20 rare amino acids (also called nonprotein amino acids) in 104 species of 40 genera of this family. Five of these amino acids (Figure 4.4) were detected in several species of *Anadenanthera* and

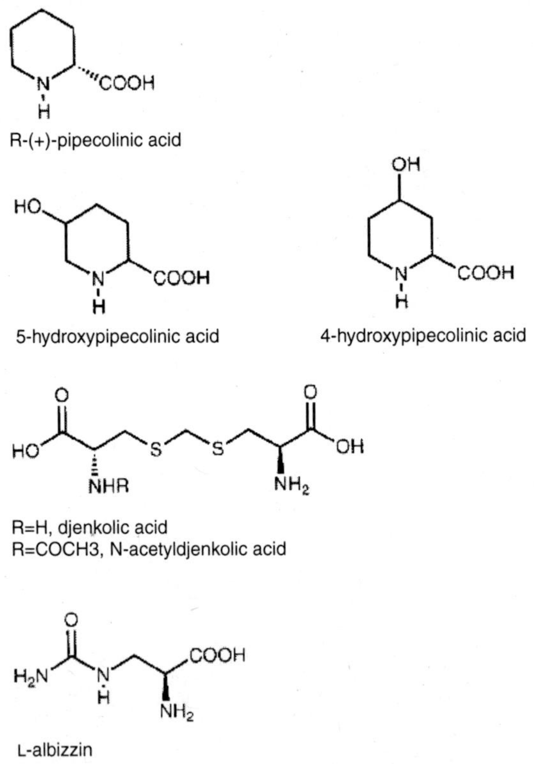

R-(+)-pipecolinic acid

5-hydroxypipecolinic acid

4-hydroxypipecolinic acid

R=H, djenkolic acid
R=COCH3, N-acetyldjenkolic acid

L-albizzin

FIGURE 4.4. Rare amino acids from *Anadenanthera. Source:* After Krauss and Reinbothe 1973.

Piptadenia. They used the botanical classifications published by Hutchinson (1964) and Bentham (1874-1875) as the basis for comparison of their results with the (then) known taxonomy. They placed *A. macrocarpa* in the section Mimosae and *Piptadenia macrocarpa* and *P. excelsa* in section Adenantherae. In this study, both species of *Piptadenia* differ from *Anadenanthera* based upon the occurrence of the sulfur-containing compounds djenkolic acid and acetyl-djenkolic acid, and pipecolic acid and 5-hydroxypipecolic acid in the latter, and by the occurrence of larger amounts of 4-hydroxypipecolic acid in the former. However, both *A. macrocarpa* and *P. macrocarpa* differ from *P. excelsa* by the presence of a large quantity of *an unknown amino acid.*

In the same year, Reis Altschul (1964) published a revision of the genus *Anadenanthera* Brenan in which she placed *P. macrocarpa* Benth. and *A. macrocarpa* (Benth.) Brenan in synonomy with the newly created taxon *Anadenanthera colubrina* (Vell.) Brenan var. *Cebil.* One is then left with the dilemma of how to explain apparent chemical differences in the same species. Even so, studies such as the one by Krauss and Reinbothe (1973) are very useful because they serve to enlarge the knowledge of the natural occurrence of diverse chemical substances. However, Trease and Evans (1971: 242) point out, "As more information becomes available it is increasingly evident that there is no simple application of comparative phytochemistry to taxonomy and most modern authors are extremely cautious in their interpretations of data."

The largest and most thoroughly studied group of chemical compounds found in species of *Anadenanthera* and *Piptadenia* are the alkaloids, nitrogen-containing substances that have basic (as distinguished from acidic) properties (hence the name *alkaloid*—alkali-like). The term alkaloid is of broad meaning and refers to chemical compounds containing one or more nitrogen atoms either in a heterocyclic ring or on an isolated side chain (Trease and Evans 1971). Since 1967, over 1100 studies have been published dealing with various aspects of the major alkaloids of *Anadenanthera.* The largest number of these concern two areas of study: chemistry and pharmacology. These attest to a single fascinating aspect of these chemicals: their ability to produce intriguing and profound effects in a variety of test animals, including human beings. Although it is true that many alkaloids are known to exert powerful pharmacological effects, sometimes in very small doses (strychnine, morphine, atropine, histrionico-toxin, for example), up to and including death, the *Anadenanthera* al-kaloids belong to that peculiar pharmacological niche known as hallucinogens. There have been many attempts to capture the nature of the effects of these materials with a single descriptive word (e.g., psychedelic, psychotomimetic, psychodesleptic, entheogenic). A dis-cussion of this is beyond the scope of this work. The reader is referred to the works of Hoffer and Osmond (1967), Brimblecombe and Pinder (1975), Schultes and Hofmann (1980), and Ott (1994, 1996). The preface from Hoffer and Osmond (1967: v) succinctly captures the nature of research with the hallucinogens:

> The use of hallucinogens has been described as one of the major advances of this century. There is little doubt that they have had a massive impact upon psychiatry and may produce marked changes in our society. The violent reaction for and against the hallucinogens suggests that, even if these compounds are not universally understood and approved of, they will neither be for-gotten nor neglected.

The first systematic combined chemical and pharmacological study of *yopo* snuff (presumably from *A. peregrina* Benth. collected in Co-lombia) was that of Henker and Huston (1950). They utilized simple precipitation and colorimetric tests to ascertain the nature of the ac-tive principles contained in a hot aqueous extract of the snuff. Phar-macological examination, both in vitro and in vivo, was fairly sophis-ticated for its day, demonstrating an inhibition of the ciliary action of frog esophagus tissue and a depression of heart rate upon injection into a pithed frog. Central nervous system depression was observed after intraperitoneal injection of a sublethal dose into rats; a marked analgesic effect was noted. These researchers concluded that the ac-tive principles were apparently not alkaloidal, but could be saponins.

A rather curious study of *yopo* was published in Italy several years later by Stagno d'Alcontres and Cuzzocrea (1956-1957). Utilizing both aqueous and alcoholic extracts of *A. peregrina* snuff from Vene-zuela, these workers used precipitation tests and colorimetric reac-tions to follow the course of their extractions. They employed a now-classic alkaloidal enrichment procedure, which involved partitioning of the concentrated crude alcoholic extract between aqueous dilute hydrochloric acid and chloroform followed by precipitation of the alkaloids from the aqueous layer with alkali and re-extraction with chloroform. Using paper chromatography, ultraviolet spectroscopy, and electrophoresis techniques, they tentatively reported that the active principles were the dimeric strychnine-related alkaloids C-calebassine, C-curarine, C-calebassinine, and C-alkaloid D. The presence of these compounds has never been verified by other investigators. However, consideration must be given to these workers since less than a gram of material was available for study.

However, two years earlier, Stromberg (1954), working at the National Heart Institute, Bethesda, Maryland, had reported the first isolation of bufotenine (5-hydroxy-*N,N*-dimethyltryptamine; Figure 4.5) from the seeds of *A. peregrina* Benth. collected in Puerto Rico. From nearly 900 g of ground material, Stromberg isolated 4 g of crystalline bufotenine free base, representing 0.44 percent yield. Positive identification of the compound was made by ultraviolet and infrared spectrometry and by comparison of the melting points of derivatives such as picrate and methiodide with those of an authentic, synthetically prepared sample. The synthetic sample was provided by Dr. M. E. Speeter of Upjohn, using technology that he had recently published (Speeter and Anthony 1954).

The following year, Fish, Johnson, and Horning (1955) confirmed the finding of bufotenine in seeds of *A. peregrina* (L.) Benth. from the same material analyzed by Stromberg. In addition, the alkaloidal constituents of two other species and several other collections of *A. peregrina* from Puerto Rico and Brazil were examined for the first time. These were samples of *P. macrocarpa* Benth. *(A. colubrina)* from Brazil and Florida and *P. paniculata* Benth. from Brazil. Leaves, bark, seeds, and pods were extracted. This study was important for several reasons: First, additional chemical compounds were isolated and identified, including the first isolation of *N,N*-dimethyltryptamine (DMT), its *N*-oxide, and bufotenine *N*-oxide (Figure 4.5). Second, this study established a connection between the suggested source of the snuff and the snuff itself. These investigators compared the chemical findings of their "synthetically" prepared snuff, using the descriptions of Humboldt and Bonpland (1971) and Spruce (1970), to a snuff contained in a Piaroa snuff box from the Smithsonian Institution. Third, the distribution of the alkaloids between different plant organs was not the same. Only DMT was found in the pods, while bufotenine, its *N*-oxide, and DMT *N*-oxide were confined to the

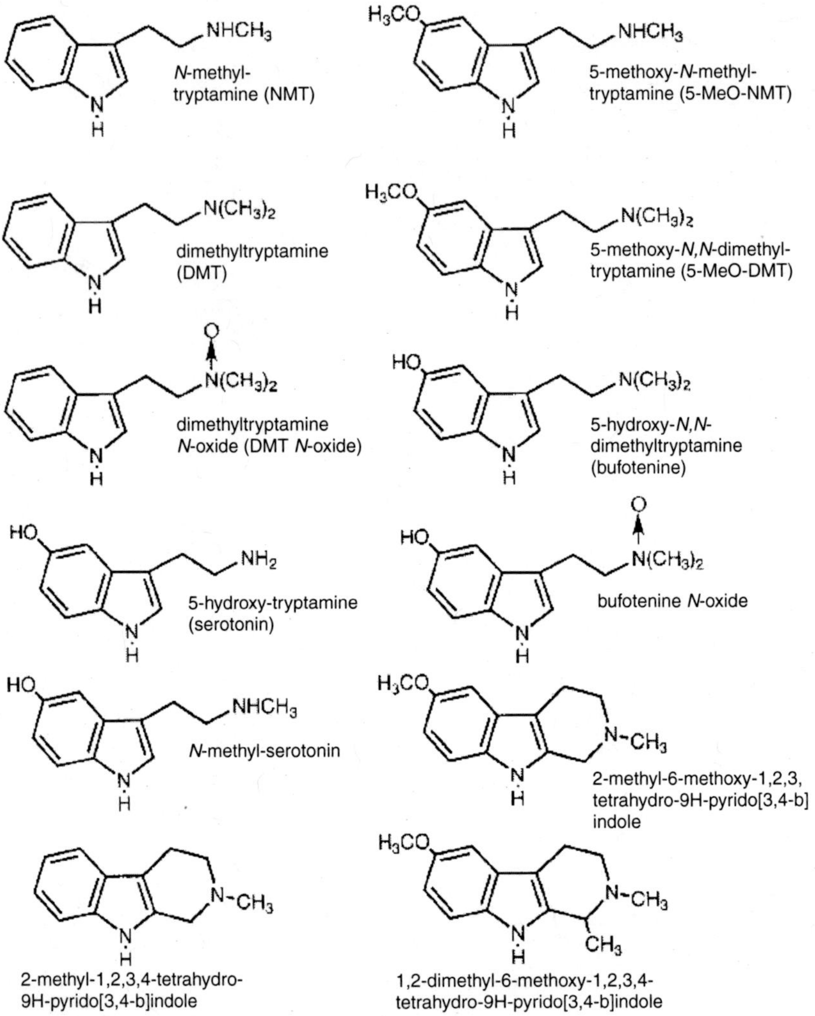

FIGURE 4.5. Indole alkaloids reported to occur in *Anadenanthera* species.

seeds. Last, these authors speculated on questions of comparative biochemistry and metabolic pathways and stated:

> The presence of bufotenine in such varied sources as *Piptadenia* seeds, toads, certain mushrooms and human urine indicates a

ubiquitous nature. This compound is evidently associated with serotonin as a product of tryptophan metabolism, but its metabolic route of synthesis and its function are unknown. (Fish, Johnson, and Horning 1955: 5893)

Stimulated by the finding of DMT *N*-oxide in nature, Fish et al. (1956) studied the tertiary amine oxide rearrangement as a model for biological *N*-dealkylation.

Before the close of the decade, bufotenine was isolated in 2.1 percent yield from the extraction of more than 2 kg of seeds of *A. colubrina* (Vell.) Benth. from Rio de Janeiro, Brazil (Pachter et al. 1959). This study incidentally also suggested the identity of DMT with the previously isolated alkaloid "nigerine" found in the Brazilian preparation known as *vinho da jurema* (wine of *jurema*). The source of this drink was identified as *Mimosa hostilis* Benth. (Gonçalves de Lima 1946). DMT had also been isolated from the species *Prestonia amazonica* (Hochstein and Paradies 1957; for additional plant sources of DMT, see Raffauf 1970; Ott 1996; Shulgin and Shulgin 1997).

The 1960s witnessed a global flurry of scientific inquiry into the many aspects of the visionary *Anadenanthera* snuffs, including archaeological, anthropological, pharmacological, psychiatric, and chemical. Other investigators verified the presence of these alkaloids in *Piptadenia-Anadenanthera* species. Giesbrecht (1960) isolated bufotenine from the seeds of *Piptadenia falcata* (*A. peregrina* var. *falcata*) Benth. The number of alkaloids present in *A. peregrina* Benth. was expanded when Legler and Tschesche (1963) reported the isolation of 5-methoxy-*N,N*-dimethyltryptamine (0.64 percent yield), 5-methoxy-*N*-monomethyltryptamine (0.4 percent), and *N*-methyltryptamine (0.4 percent yield) along with *N,N*-dimethyltryptamine and bufotenine from the bark of material collected in Brazil. This study was unusual because of its quantitative nature and attention to detail. These authors also commented on the possible biochemical pathways by which such compounds could arise and suggested that perhaps specific enzyme systems existed in plants that could convert the monomethyl derivatives into dimethyl compounds. The compound 5-methoxy-DMT had previously been isolated from the Brazilian tree *Dictyloma incanescens* D.C. (Pachter et al. 1959) and 5-methoxy-*N*-monomethyltryptamine had been obtained from a member of the Gramineae or grass family, *Phalaris arundinacea* L. (Wilkinson 1958).

Iacobucci and Ruveda (1964) examined five species of *Piptadenia* native to Argentina. They used paper chromatography to follow the course of their extractions and ultraviolet and infrared spectroscopy as well as melting points and mixed melting points to identify the alkaloids found. In this study, *P. macrocarpa* Benth. (*A. colubrina* var. *Cebil*) was found to be the richest in total alkaloid content and in the number of compounds present in different parts of the plant. Bufotenine and *N,N*-dimethyltryptamine were found both in seeds and seed pods; bufotenine *N*-oxide was found in the seeds. The bark yielded 0.1 percent 5-methoxy-*N*-monomethyltryptamine. This was the only compound for which these authors reported an actual isolated yield. The concentration of bufotenine must have been fairly high, however, as it was isolated as the crystalline free base directly from the basic extract. This paper was of further importance because for the first time, a species of *Piptadenia* not considered in synonymy with the four species of the genus *Anadenanthera* was found to contain alkaloids (Figure 4.6).

From the seeds of *P. excelsa* (Gris.) Lillo *(horco cebil),* bufotenine and its *N*-oxide were detected by paper chromatography and bufotenine was actually isolated. Although no yield was given, the amount of bufotenine found was "much lower than from the seeds of *P. macrocarpa*" (Iacobucci and Ruveda 1964: 217). *N,N*-dimethyltryptamine was detected in the seed pods of *P. excelsa.* A quaternary alkaloid of undetermined structure had been reported from the bark of this species by Stucker and Paya (1938). The three other species, *P. paraguayensis* (Benth.) Lindm., *P. rigida* (Benth.) (syn. *angico vermelho*), and *P. viridiflora* (Kunth.) Benth., were found to be alkaloid negative, although paper chromatography revealed a single compound that gave a positive "test" (no reagents were specified) for a nonindolic alkaloid being present in the bark of *P. paraguayensis.* These authors also commented on the "isomorphic" nature of crystalline bufotenine free base, that is, different crystalline forms having different melting points. The original isolated material crystallized from ethyl acetate and had the melting point 123-124°C. A synthetic sample of bufotenine had a melting point of 146-147°C. When the natural isolated material was again recrystallized with seeding of the synthetic material, the melting point was raised to 146-147°C. The higher-melting ("more stable") form could not be reconverted to the lower-melting form.

Marini-Bettòlo and co-workers (1964) conducted a chemical analysis of *epéna (ebene)* snuff from the Yanomamö of the upper Rio Orinoco, Brazil. Using column chromatography on alumina, these workers isolated 1.0 percent bufotenine, 0.13 percent *N,N*-dimethyltryptamine, and smaller quantities of their respective *N*-oxides from a dilute acetic acid extraction of a 33 g snuff sample. The source of the snuff was not identified but was said to be from a tree, a member of the leguminosae (Marini-Bettòlo et al. 1964). In the same issue of the journal *Annali di Chimica,* the same workers (Biocca et al. 1964) reported the results of a study of a liana used as the source of *paricá* snuff obtained from shamans of a Tukanoan tribe of the Vaupés River region of the Amazon. On the basis of chromatographic evidence, melting points, and ultraviolet spectroscopy, the structures of the isolated alkaloids were determined to be harmine, harmaline (dihydroharmine), and tetrahydroharmine. The liana was identified as belonging to the family Malpighiaceae, probably the genus *Banisteriopsis.*

The next year, Holmstedt (1965) published a significant study of *epéna* snuff collected four years earlier by George J. Seitz from the Waika (Yanomamö) tribe of the Negro River region of northwestern Brazil. This research included the use of analytical and preparative paper chromatography, silica gel thin-layer chromatography, and both activation and fluorescence spectrophotofluorometry. In addition, a pharmacological assay (Vane 1959; Barlow and Khan 1959a, 1959b) was used as an aid to structure determination. The ability of a compound to cause contraction of a rat gastric fundus strip preparation was used as a measure of serotonin-like (5-hydroxy-tryptamine) activity. In this assay, activity of bufotenine relative to 5-methoxy-DMT could be determined when the log of the concentration of respective drug was plotted against the amount of contraction of the strip. Isolation steps were followed with the use of colorimetric tests with Erlich's reagent (4-dimethylaminobenzaldehyde).

Since complete separation of the individual alkaloidal components could not be achieved by either paper or thin-layer chromatography, the (then) relatively sophisticated analytical technique of gas chromatography was utilized. The primary column used was a 6 foot × 4 mm glass column containing a mixture of 7 percent F-60 and 1 percent EGSS-Z (silicone-based mobile phases) supported on Gas Chrome P. The instruments used were a Barber-Colman Model 10 and an EIR Model AU-8, operating at 216°C and 19 psi with an argon ionization

detection system. Substances in the snuff were identified by their retention times relative to known, synthetic standards and to an internal
standard (anthracene). Since phenolic alkaloids (such as bufotenine)
produce broad elution peaks with long retention times, derivatization
with hexamethyldisilazane produced easily eluted trimethylsilyloxy
derivatives.

In contrast to other reported analyses of *epéna*, the results of this
study showed the major alkaloidal component to be 5-methoxy-*N,N*-
dimethyltryptamine with smaller amounts of *N,N*-dimethyltrypta-
mine and traces of bufotenine also present. This shift in the relative
amounts of alkaloids detected led Holmstedt (1965: 298) to conclude
that "there is no reason whatsoever to believe that the seeds of
Piptadenia peregrina are contained in the powder investigated by the
present author." Seitz had witnessed the preparation of the actual
snuff "from the phloem of the bark of a tree called *epena-kesi* . . .
mixed with the ashes of a species of *Acacia* . . . and the dried powder
of a herbaceous plant called *maschi-hirī*" (Holmstedt 1965: 297). Examination of the wood anatomy (the botanical specimen examined
contained neither flowers nor leaves) of an actual specimen of the primary ingredient led to the conclusion that it was a member of the genus *Virola* of the family Myristicaceae. Holmstedt (1965: 296) concluded, "In spite of careful investigations . . . the botanical origin of
many of the snuffs used among South American Indians is still enig-
matic." Commenting on the work of Reis Altschul (1964), they
added, "An important result of these studies is the fact that in many
places where the habit [of snuff taking] exists the species *Piptadenia*
is not known to occur" (Holmstedt 1965: 296).

Thus was born a controversy as to the sources of the snuff known
as *epéna* that illustrates the nature of scientific inquiry: the more a
subject is investigated, the more complicated it becomes. Each variable introduced into consideration greatly complicates the achieve-
ment of a complete, comprehensible picture. We have already seen the
problems associated with merely a single variable in this tale—the problem of botanical synonymy. As botanical families and genera are re-
arranged and new taxa are formed, one must pay close attention to
obsolete nomenclature, including citations of the published botanical
authority. Also, since most chemists do not have training in botany,
many chemical studies of natural products cannot be traced to vouch-
ered authenticated botanical materials. When one adds to this other

variables such as indigenous names, where the same name may often be applied to different plants or preparations and the admixture of more than one plant to some preparations, along with information from other disciplines such as anthropology and archaeology, and takes into consideration that such investigations have been conducted over several centuries and often under difficult conditions, one can begin to appreciate the complexity of the study of these snuffs.

Holmstedt's (1965) work is important for two reasons: (1) for the first time, the highly sensitive technique of gas chromatography had been applied to analyses of psychoactive snuffs, thus lowering the amount of material required for a successful study; and (2) the discovery of bufotenine in a snuff apparently not derived from species of *Anadenanthera* or *Piptadenia*. Prior to this time, presence of bufotenine in analyzed snuff preparations was sufficient evidence to assume the source of the snuff to be species of these two genera. However, because bufotenine had been found only in trace amounts in this study, and its detection was based solely on gas chromatographic retention times and colorimetric reactions, some doubt remains as to its identity. Since the snuff sample was four years old at the time of analysis, a possible explanation is that the traces of bufotenine arose as an artifact of the hydrolysis, over time, of the major constituent, 5-methoxy-*N,N*-dimethyltryptamine. This statement must be considered as speculation only, however, and the presence of bufotenine taken as fact. After 1965, research on alkaloids of South American snuffs would have to be conducted with yet more careful consideration of the actual plant sources involved.

The same year, Marini-Bettòlo et al. (1965) published a review of naturally occurring visionary alkaloids. He affirmed the identity of one of the variations of the *ebene* snuff of the Yanomamö of the upper Orinoco River as derived from *Piptadenia peregrina* (L.) Benth. *(A. peregrina),* a preparation containing the by-now familiar compounds, bufotenine, *N,N*-dimethyltryptamine, and their respective *N*-oxides. If things were not confusing enough, however, these authors (mistakenly?) identified the source of *paricá* snuff as *Banisteriopsis caapi* Spruce, containing the carboline alkaloids harmine, harmaline, and traces of tetrahydroharmine. This was hardly a mistake. The previous year, Bernauer (1964), working with a sample of *ebene* snuff obtained from Becher (1960) and attributed to the Surará Indians of northwestern Brazil, isolated harmine (0.38 percent) and the (+)-enantiomer of 1,2,3,4-tetra-hydroharmine (.08 percent). He used both column chromatography on alumina (in the case of the former compound) and Kugelrohr distillation (in the case of the latter alkaloid) under high vacuum to purify these compounds. The identity of these two alkaloids was confirmed by the use of ultraviolet, infrared, and nuclear magnetic resonance (NMR) spectroscopy as well as by mixed melting point. The direction (but not the magnitude) of the rotation of polarized light of the isolated tetrahydroharmine was determined at wavelengths between 480 and 700 μm. A third alkaloid of unknown structure was also isolated in trace amounts. Bernauer did not find harmaline in this sample and suggested that perhaps it arose by simple oxidation as an artifact either of preparation of the snuff or of the isolation procedure. The actual plant source of this snuff was not identified but was presumed to be *Banisteriopsis caapi* Spruce (previously known as *Banisteria caapi* Spr.).

In a previously mentioned study (Paris et al. 1967) of the chemical constituents of *P. peregrina (A. peregrina)* from Haiti and the African species *P. africana* Hook., the presence of bufotenine, its *N*-oxide, and DMT were reported in the seeds of the former species, as well as other nonalkaloidal constituents in the leaves, pods, and bark. *Piptadenia africana,* on the other hand, was devoid of alkaloids.

The year 1967 marked a zenith in research endeavors on naturally occurring psychoactive substances, or so it seemed because of the publication of the proceedings of a remarkable symposium, Ethnopharmacologic Search for Psychoactive Drugs, held in San Francisco, California, January 28-30, 1967 (Efron et al. 1967). The conference was held because of the tremendous volume of research being conducted by groups all over the world on the various aspects of these plant hallucinogens. This book still serves as a most important source of multidisciplinary information about psychoactive plants.

Holmstedt and Lindgren (1967a) reported the results of novel snuff research and reviewed the information published up until that time. They also unveiled a new and powerful technological breakthrough in the analyses of natural products: the use of combined gas-liquid chromatography and mass spectrometry. Although gas chromatography alone had been previously used (Holmstedt 1965) in analysis of snuff alkaloids, it suffered from the same drawback as other methods of chromatographic analyses, that is, it was inherently indirect since it only measured retention times relative to known, synthetic standards. Its combination with mass spectrometry, pioneered by Holmes and Morell (1957) and Rhyage (1964), provided two advantages not hitherto known: for the first time, positive identification of the structures of chemical compounds could be attained by virtue of their mass spectra, with no need for actual isolation of individual components, and even smaller quantities of plant materials were required for successful analyses, including samples from museums and herbaria.

Holmstedt and Lindgren (1967a) compared the results of their analyses of six new snuff samples with those of six others reported previously. Snuffs analyzed were from collections dated between 1948 and 1965. Four were samples called *paricá,* seven *epéna,* and one *yopo.* In addition, material from 11 different collections of six snuff plant species was included in an attempt to relate the snuffs to their botanical sources. An interesting picture emerged when comparing alkaloids found in a snuff sample relative to its respective plant source. Two samples of *paricá* contained only bufotenine, while a third contained DMT, 5-methoxy-DMT, and even harmine in addition to bufotenine. The fourth sample contained only harmine, harmaline (dihydroharmine), and tetrahydroharmine. The results from this last sample were from the previously mentioned study of Marini-Bettòlo et al. (1965). Two samples of *epéna* contained bufotenine, DMT, and their respective *N*-oxides, two other samples contained harmine and tetrahydroharmine, and three others contained only mixtures of DMT, 5-methoxy-DMT, 5-methoxy-*N*-monomethyltryptamine, and monomethyltryptamine. The single sample of *yopo* contained DMT, bufotenine, and 5-methoxy-DMT. All samples were from either Venezuela, Colombia, or Brazil. The only real constant was that all alkaloids found were indoles.

In addition, material from five collections of *Piptadenia peregrina* Benth., two collections of *P. macrocarpa* Benth., and one each of *P. colubrina* Benth., *P. excelsa* (Gris.) Lillo, *Mimosa hostilis* Benth., and *Virola calophylla* War. were examined. All collections of the seeds of *Piptadenia* but one contained bufotenine in varying mixtures with DMT and its *N*-oxide and bufotenine *N*-oxide. Bark and pod samples from collections of *Piptadenia* contained DMT, monomethyltryptamine, 5-methoxy-DMT, and 5-methoxy-*N*-monomethyltryptamine, but not bufotenine. The same alkaloids, with the exception of the latter, were found in the sample of *V. calophylla* bark, and the sample of

M. hostilis root contained only DMT. Bufotenine was not found in these two species. The single collection of seeds of *P. peregrina* Benth. obtained by F. Caspar (1956) from the Tupari Indians of Rio Branco, Brazil, were shown to contain only DMT and 5-methoxy-DMT. Although no quantitative figures were reported, a gas chromatographic trace of the analysis of this collection suggested that 5-methoxy-DMT represented 96 percent and DMT 4 percent of the alkaloid fraction. This was at the time the only analysis published of seeds of any collection of *Piptadenia* or *Anadenanthera* species in which bufotenine was not found.

Several conclusions can be drawn from these results. First, in some cases the same indigenous name applies to snuffs prepared from different plant sources (see Chagnon et al. 1970, 1971). Excepting a single report (Holmstedt 1965), the presence of bufotenine in a snuff is enough evidence to identify at least one ingredient of the snuff as *Anadenanthera* or *Piptadenia*. A relatively high concentration of 5-methoxy-DMT or the absence of bufotenine in a snuff points to one or another species of *Virola* as its source. Second, certain snuffs are prepared from mixtures of more than one plant. That would seem to be the case with snuffs that are found to contain both tryptamines and the ayahuasca β-carbolines. As of the close of 1967, tryptamines and β-carbolines had not yet been isolated from the same plant. Third, the finding of harmine suggested species of *Banisteriopsis* either as sole ingredient or as admixture in indigenous snuffs, since harmine or other 7-methoxy-β-carbolines had not been found in species of *Piptadenia, Anadenanthera,* or *Virola*.

In 1967, the finding of two reduced β-carboline alkaloids, 2-methyl- and 1,2-dimethyl-6-methoxy-1,2,3,4-tetrahydro-β-carboline (Figure 4.5), in extracts of a specimen of *A. peregrina* (L.) Speg. collected in Boa Vista, Brazil, during the *Alpha Helix* Expedition, Phase C was reported (Agurell et al. 1968). Isolated percentages of these alkaloids were not reported, but their structures were confirmed by comparison of their mass spectra with those of synthetically prepared standards.

The research vessel *Alpha Helix* was a National Oceanographic Facility of the University-National Oceanographic Laboratory System for experimental biology, which was launched June 29, 1965. The ship was owned and operated by the Scripps Institution of Oceanography, University of California, San Diego, from February

1966 to August 1980. It housed three well-equipped laboratories, a walk-in freezer, a darkroom, machine shop, and other facilities. *Alpha Helix* was used to conduct two missions of research in the Brazilian Amazon basin. The first, from February through December 1967, was near the Negro and Branco rivers and involved broad studies of animal and plant life in the region. The second Amazonian mission occurred between July and August 1976 and was devoted exclusively to the study of six native groups living along tributaries of the upper Amazon River (Scripps n.d.).

In 1969, Agurell published a detailed account of the results of chemical analyses of material collected during the *Alpha Helix* Expedition on the Amazon and Rio Negro rivers (Agurell et al. 1969). Two collections of snuffs (*epéna* and *nyakwana*) and seven collections of five species of *Virola* Warburg were analyzed for the presence of 14 different tryptamine and β-carboline alkaloids. In addition, quantitative results were reported for material from the same collection of *A. peregrina* (L.) Speg. previously examined qualitatively (Agurell et al. 1968). Unfortunately, this material had been preserved in alcohol prior to analysis, and only the bark and leaves were analyzed.

As expected, the collections of *Virola* contained 5-methoxy-DMT as the major alkaloid in bark, leaves, and flowering shoots. The *nyakwana* snuff contained an extraordinarily high concentration of this alkaloid, nearly 10 percent. No 5-hydroxytryptamines (neither bufotenine nor serotonin) were found in the snuff or *Virola* collections. The bark of *A. peregrina* was said to contain "a high amount of 5-methoxy-DMT," although the reported percentage was 0.025 percent. In addition, the bark of this collection was found to contain 5-methoxy-*N*-monomethyltryptamine (0.015 percent), 1,2-dimethyl-6-methoxy-1,2,3,4-tetrahydro-β-carboline (0.001 percent), 2-methyl-6-methoxy-1,2,3,4-tetrahydro-β-carboline (0.001 percent), DMT (0.0005 percent), and traces of *N*-methyl-tryptamine. The leaves contained 5-methoxy-DMT and DMT in equal amounts (0.0075 percent) and traces of *N*-methyltryptamine. Concentrations of these alkaloids were determined by integration of the area under their respective gas chromatographic curves relative to an internal standard of DMT. Positive identification of structures was made by mass spectral analyses.

No tryptamine *N*-oxides were found in any collection from this study. Since it was known (Ghosal and Mukherjee 1966) that 5-methoxy-DMT *N*-oxide could rearrange to 2-methyl-6-methoxy-

1,2,3,4-tetrahydro-β-carboline under certain conditions, the possibility that the latter could arise as an artifact of the extraction procedure was discounted by experiments by the authors. That the position of substitution of the methoxy group of the tetrahydro-β-carbolines was at the indole 6 carbon instead of at position 7 as in the harmine-derived *Banisteriopsis* alkaloids was determined by examination of the ultraviolet and fluorescence spectra of a number of variously substituted methoxy- and benzyloxy-indoles.

In 1971, Chagnon and co-workers reported ethnobotanical, chemical, and ethnographic findings concerning the snuffs used by the Yanomamö Indians of southern Venezuela and northern Brazil. This detailed study concerned two snuff preparations known by the names *yakoana (nyakwana)* and *hisioma*. Chemical analysis clearly differentiated these snuffs. The former was attributed to bark and bark resin of *Virola* species along with a number of plant admixtures, and the latter simply to seeds of *A. peregrina*. Various collections of *yakoana* snuff contained from 0.15 percent to 2.00 percent of equal mixtures of 5-methoxy-DMT and its respective *N*-oxide; the *hisioma* seeds contained only bufotenine in the highest quantity reported up until that time, 7.4 percent. Although an actual sample of the Yanomamö-prepared *hisioma* snuff was not available for analysis, these authors stated that "consideration of the mode of preparation of the snuff . . . suggest that little change in the nature or content of the alkaloidal constituents results from the preparation process itself" (Chagnon et al. 1971: 73).

In an investigation of chemotaxonomic relationship in *Piptadenia,* the alkaloidal fraction of the seeds from five Brazilian species of the genus was studied using paper electrophoresis and isolation techniques (Yamasato et al. 1972). Bufotenine and DMT were found in *P. colubrina* and *P. peregrina*. In addition, these two compounds were also found in two more species of *Piptadenia* not considered synonymous with any of the four varieties of *Anadenanthera: P. contorta* Benth. and *P. moniliformis* Benth. Although a sample of *P. leprostachya (P. leptostachya?)* did not contain the two tryptamines, a crystalline alkaloid was isolated in 0.03 percent yield from it. This compound was identified as theobromine, a purine alkaloid also known as 5-desmethyl caffeine, by NMR, ultraviolet, and mass spectroscopy. This was the first report of this alkaloid in the Leguminosae. (The main source of theobromine is the cocoa bean, *Theobroma ca-*

cao [Ott 1985].) It is also found in the Paraguayan tea maté, made from the leaves of *Ilex paraguariensis,* and *cassina,* a tea produced from *Ilex cassine* (Trease and Evans 1971; Tyler et al. 1981). Two unidentified indoles were also found: one was present in all five species, the other only in *P. colubrina* and *P. peregrina.*

Budowski and colleagues (1974) examined several samples of *yopo* snuff collected from the Pixaasi-Teri (Yanomamö) tribe of the Mavaca River region of the upper Orinoco. One of the samples was found to be alkaloid free, another contained only bufotenine (2.7 percent), and the third contained only 5-methoxy-DMT (1.4 percent). These authors concluded:

> It is important to underline the fact that the origin of the drug is not always sufficient to establish where the *yopo* was prepared. In effect *yopo* constitutes—as does curare—the object of trade and exchange among Indian tribes in the Amazon-Orinoco basins. (Budowski et al. 1974: 578)

Grossa and co-workers (1975) examined a sample of *epéna* snuff obtained from the Bisashi-teri of the Rio Ocamo region. They witnessed the actual preparation of the snuff from bark of a *Virola* species. A single alkaloid, 5-methoxy-DMT, was isolated in 1.2 percent yield. These authors suggested that in order to avoid confusion, a simple nomenclatural device be adopted—that all snuff drugs made from seeds be called *yopo* and all those from bark *epéna.*

Schultes and collegues (1977) conducted a phytochemical examination of seeds from *A. peregrina* originally collected by Richard Spruce in 1854. The material was obtained from the Economic Botany Museum at Kew, England, where it had been for 120 years. This study also reported analytical results for the plant organs of ten additional contemporary collections of *A. peregrina* as well as two additional snuff samples. The work involved classical alkaloid extraction and enrichment procedures and instrumental analyses by gas chromatography, gas chromatography/mass spectrometry, and the newest (then) technology in trace component analyses, mass fragmentometry (Elkin et al. 1973). These investigators conducted a thorough quantitative examination of the collection of *A. peregrina* marked, "Schultes 26363, San Juan, Puerto Rico, March 1972." Seven parts of the plant were analyzed for the presence of indole alkaloids. Seeds were shown to contain DMT (0.16 percent), 5-methoxy-DMT (0.04

percent), and bufotenine (0.013 percent). Seedlings showed DMT traces (i.e., <0.01 percent), 5-methoxy-DMT (0.024 percent), and bufotenine (traces). Pods contained DMT (traces), 5-methoxy-DMT (0.012 percent), and bufotenine (traces). The leaf analysis demonstrated the presence of DMT (0.013 percent) and 5-methoxy-DMT (0.094 percent). Ground twigs contained DMT (traces), 5-methoxy-DMT (0.04 percent), and bufotenine (traces). Bark showed DMT (0.02 percent) and 5-methoxy-DMT (0.4 percent). The analysis of root material demonstrated the presence of DMT (0.014 percent), 5-methoxy-DMT (0.68 percent), and bufotenine (traces).

Another collection of seeds from the same grove of *A. peregrina* collected three years later and marked, "Schultes, von R. Altschul, B. Holmstedt, San Juan, Puerto Rico, March 1975," although not analyzed quantitatively, was shown to contain bufotenine as 80 percent of the alkaloidal fraction with minor amounts of DMT and 5-methoxy-DMT. An alkaloid new for this species was also detected in trace amounts, 2-methyl-1,2,3,4-tetrahydro-ß-carboline, a "cyclized" tryptamine lacking either a methoxy- or hydroxy-substituent. This compound had previously been reported (Agurell et al. 1969) as a constituent of *Virola theiodora* Warb. and constituted the third β-carboline alkaloid found in *Anadenanthera*. This same collection was reanalyzed two years later to determine the effect of time on alkaloid content, something that had not hitherto been done for this species. It was found to contain only bufotenine; all other alkaloids had decomposed and vanished. Four other various collections of seeds presumably of *Anadenanthera* species were shown to contain only DMT (all less than 0.05 percent), and one also had traces of 5-methoxy-DMT. Seeds and seedlings of three other collections of *Piptadenia peregrina* as well as samples of two snuff powders from Brazil and Colombia of unknown plant origin likewise contained only DMT and 5-methoxy-DMT in trace amounts.

Several troubling aspects of this work again point to the difficulty of establishing absolute consistency in the study of the chemical makeup of natural products, even of the same genus or species. Hitherto, only one collection of seeds of *A. peregrina* (or *A. colubrina*) had failed to yield bufotenine, even as a trace constituent (Holmstedt and Lindgren 1967c). However, in Schultes et al. (1977) we have the analyses of six collections of seeds of the former species that were shown not to contain bufotenine. Even more interesting, collections of seeds from the same grove of trees, the analyses of which were only three years apart, show completely opposite results. In seeds from Schultes collection number 26363, San Juan, Puerto Rico, 1972, DMT predominated, whereas seeds from the 1975 collection (Schultes, Reis Altschul, and Holmstedt, San Juan, Puerto Rico, 1975) contained bufotenine as the main alkaloidal component (Schultes et al. 1977). Differences in alkaloid content within the same species are not uncommon, however. Considerable seasonal variation in the occurrence of alkaloids in the leaves of a related arborescent legume, *Acacia baileyana* F. v M., have been reported (Repke et al. 1973). Analysis of material collected in the spring contained mostly tetrahydroharman, while that from the fall of the same year contained only tryptamine. All material analyzed came from the same tree.

Nearly a decade elapsed before publication of any further chemical investigations of these snuffs. Bongiorno de Pfirter and Mandrile (1983) published a rather complete review of the many aspects of the species *A. peregrina* (L.) Speg., including history, botanical description, geographical distribution, chemistry, and pharmacology of the plant. They concluded that its historical importance and use, especially in the Amazon, had been unjustly underemphasized, and that it probably was the principal source of shamanic snuffs used in the region, an opinion shared by Chagnon in his studies on Yanomamö use of psychoactive plants (Chagnon et al. 1971; compare Schultes 1967).

Rendón (1984) studied the alkaloidal composition of seeds obtained from *P. macrocarpa* Benth. (*A. colubrina* var. *Cebil*) collected in Alto Beni, La Paz, Bolivia, known as *villca* or *curupáu*. Nearly half a kilogram of seeds was exhaustively extracted with boiling ethanol in a Soxhlet apparatus for 80 hours. Using column chromatography on alumina and silica gel, 0.5 percent bufotenine was isolated as the crystalline free base. Its identity was confirmed by infrared spectroscopy. The actual infrared spectrum was included in this paper. A more polar, unidentified alkaloid was also detected.

In an outgrowth of the study of the various aspects of archaeological snuffs from northern Chile (Torres et al. 1991), Torres and Repke (1996) investigated contemporary use of *A. colubrina* var. *Cebil* seeds among Wichi (Mataco) shamans of the Gran Chaco region of Argentina (Plate 59), and reported the presence of three indole alkaloids in seeds, bark, and pods of several collections of this species. Bark and pods contained minor quantities of DMT and bufotenine.

Seeds from three collections, however, were shown to contain 3.51 percent, 4.41 percent, and 12.4 percent bufotenine, along with minor amounts of DMT and *N*-methyl-serotonin. From personal observations of both the preparation and use of the seeds both as snuff and smoked cigar (mixed with tobacco), it was calculated that a single cigar might contain as much as 196 mg bufotenine. It was also concluded that bufotenine was solely responsible for the activity of the smoked seeds, since the ratio of bufotenine to DMT in the high-bufotenine collection was 200 to 1, and that the concentration of DMT (0.06 percent) was believed too low to be pharmacologically significant.

Several studies of the chemical composition of snuff powder samples from archaeological sites and museum specimens have been published. In an endnote to Núñez (1969: 94), Björn Luning commented on the importance of such investigations:

> Archaeological Indian snuffs which are found in certain dry regions of South America as well as other archaeological finds may be of diagnostic value in revealing trade ways and migrations. The origin and source are good characteristics of the many kinds of snuffs known and an analysis of these may be feasible and of great importance.

The first such undertaking was reported by Fish, Johnson, and Horning (1955) as part of a larger study of *Piptadenia* chemistry (see Appendix). These workers compared the results of analyses of "laboratory snuff" prepared from seeds of Puerto Rican *A. peregrina* with an authentic sample found in a contemporary Piaroa snuff box obtained from the Smithsonian Institution under catalog no. 387781. Using paper chromatography and visualization with Erhlich's reagent, both snuffs were found to contain bufotenine and the same unidentified indoles. The evidence indicated that the origin of the Piaroa snuff was *Anadenanthera,* although the actual species could not be identified.

The previously mentioned work of Núñez (1969) contains an endnote written by S. Henry Wassén concerning chemical analysis of three samples of snuff from snuffing kits in the collection of the Iquique Archaeological Museum. Originally excavated by the Danish pharmacist Ancker Nielsen from a site in northern Chile, these samples had been dated ca. A.D. 700-1000. Using thin-layer chromatography, results for the presence of indoles were negative for the 20 to 850 mg samples. Some problems associated with such analyses were outlined. The collection, handling, and storage of the samples, elimination of possible sources of contamination that could lead to erroneous results, and the inherent instability and subsequent deterioration of alkaloids and other chemical markers, as well as the need for exquisitely sensitive analytical methods, were found to be important for successful analyses. Paleobotanical methods such as microscopic examination of plant cells in the snuffs were suggested for identification of the plant sources.

Holmstedt and Lindgren (1972) examined eight samples of snuff powder of unknown provenance as well as several collections of leaves, carbon 14 dated to A.D. 375 from collections deposited in the Ethnographic Museum, Gothenburg, Sweden. Thin-layer chromatography, gas chromatography, and gas chromatography/mass spectrometry all gave negative results for all snuff samples. Commenting on their analysis, these authors stated that "it is not surprising that the greater surface area of the powders after such a long time should have caused the destruction of any alkaloids present" (Holmstedt and Lindgren, 1972: 142). The thousand-year-old leaves, however, were found to contain 1.0-1.8 percent caffeine and were identified as *Ilex guayusa* Loes. of the Aquifoliaceae.

Schultes and colleagues (1977) analyzed 120-year-old seeds of *A. peregrina* (L.) Speg. originally collected by Spruce (1970) in 1854 and deposited in the Royal Botanic Gardens at Kew as "Spruce 119." A single alkaloid—bufotenine—was detected in 0.6 percent yield. Comparing the analyses of fresh material to those of the same material after two years in storage, they demonstrated that all alkaloids originally present in the fresh material, except bufotenine, disappeared with time. They speculated on whether or not other alkaloids might once have been present in the Spruce material, concluding, "Our observation stresses the importance of storage-time in addition to knowledge of plant part, soil, season and climatic conditions, when alkaloid analysis is carried out on seeds and on the snuffs prepared from them" (Schultes et al. 1977: 283).

Smet and Rivier (1985), in a review of South American snuff use, reported the results of analyses of two ethnographical snuff samples. The first sample, which consisted of dry snuff lumps, was obtained from a European art dealer who had purchased the snuff and some snuff-taking paraphernalia of the Piaroa tribe from the missionary museum in Puerto Ayacucho, Venezuela. The equipment is now in a private collection. (Smet and Rivier 1985: 97)

The second consisted of a dry granular powder deposited in the Royal Museum of Central Africa, Tervuren, Belgium (coll. no. 74.76.594) said originally to have been collected "by a German named Baumgarter" sometime in the 1950s or 1960s. Quantitative analyses were performed using capillary column gas chromatography/mass spectrometry. In addition, pH measurements were made of an aqueous suspension of each snuff. The snuffs were found to be quite alkaline, with pHs of 9.4 and 9.2, respectively. It was suggested that this alkalinity may facilitate the diffusion of alkaloids through the nasal mucous membrane. Both samples were found to contain bufotenine, the former 1.0 percent and the latter only traces (<0.1 percent). The presence of bufotenine suggested the source of the snuffs to be an *Anadenanthera* species. The second sample was also found to contain traces of harmine, an alkaloid already reported to occur in snuffs by other researchers (Bernauer 1964; Holmstedt and Lindgren 1967b; Marini-Bettòlo et al. 1965). Smet and Rivier (1985: 99) concluded:

> [T]here is at last additional evidence that the Piaroa must have prepared snuffs not only from plants rich in tryptamines, but also from a vegetal source yielding harmine. This conclusion indicates that the tracing of Indian drug materials in European museums and private collections for chemical analyses may lead to interesting results.

In 1987, Smet and Rivier analyzed seeds said to be of the *paricá* tree originally collected by zoologist Johann Natterer from the Maué Indians during his travels in Brazil between 1817 and 1835, and deposited in the Museum for Ethnology, Vienna. These authors stressed the importance of tracing the seed sample because

> it has often been implied that the Maué and Mura Indians of the Brazilian Madeira River prepared *paricá* snuffs and enemas from *Anadenanthera* seeds. Up to now, however, these asser-

tions have not been supported by an early collection of the seeds (*vide* Schultes 1967). (Smet and Rivier 1987: 14)

Using capillary gas chromatography/mass spectrometry with selective ion monitoring, which increases the sensitivity of detection 20- to 50-fold, a single alkaloid—bufotenine—was found in 1.5 percent yield.

The oldest known samples of archaeological snuffs to be analyzed successfully for the presence of centrally active tryptamines came from an excavation at the site of Solcor 3, San Pedro de Atacama, Chile (Torres et al. 1991). Two snuff samples were found in burial number 112, which also contained a very well-preserved mummy bundle (Plates 46-48). The samples weighed 2.4 and 10.1 g, respectively. An alkaloid enrichment procedure involving chloroform extraction, partitioning into aqueous acid, removing neutral components with ethyl acetate, careful basefication (to pH 8-9) with 1.0*N* sodium hydroxide solution, and reextraction into chloroform provided a small residue, which was analyzed by the very sensitive technique of short-column gas chromatography-tandem mass spectrometry, in which a second mass spectrometer is used as a detector for selected ions generated by the first mass spectrometer (for a discussion of the technique, see McFadden 1973; Johnson et al. 1984; Johnson and Yost 1985). Estimates of detection limits for this technique are 0.5 to 1.0 nanogram for single components. Bufotenine, DMT, and 5-methoxy-DMT were detected in both snuff samples. The presence of bufotenine prompted the authors to attribute the source of the snuff to a species of *Anadenanthera,* possibly *A. colubrina* var. *Cebil.* This conclusion was strengthened by the finding of seeds identified as *Anadenanthera* in nearby burials corresponding to the period of the snuff samples.

BIOSYNTHESIS OF THE ANADENANTHERA *ALKALOIDS*

Once the structure of an alkaloid such as bufotenine has been determined and verified by laboratory synthesis, attention is often turned to the question of how the alkaloid was formed in the plant. This biosynthesis is defined as "the elucidation of the normal and usually unique route, the metabolic pathway, whereby the complex product is generated *in vivo*" (Pelletier 1970: 670). The basis of biosynthetic and metabolic pathways can be found in biogenetic theory. (Discussions of biogenesis can be found in specialized texts such as Meister 1965.) This theory seeks to define both the common cellular constituents from which, and the enzymatic mechanisms by which are derived alkaloidal precursors, the so-called primary metabolites. Primary metabolites consist of amino acids such as tryptophan, phenylalanine, tyrosine, and nicotinic acid, which in turn are derived from even smaller units such as mevalonic acid, acetate, pyruvate, anthranilic acid, shikimic acid, and glucose. Much of this theory is based on chemical reasoning, that is, that structural similarities of alkaloid skeletons can be related to common features of these primary metabolites (so-called obligatory intermediates) and that the formation of complex products from these cellular constituents can be explained in terms of "rational chemical mechanisms."

Many such biogenetically modeled syntheses have been carried out in the laboratory under "physiological" conditions, that is, in dilute aqueous solutions at room temperature and mild pH ranges. The successful outcome of these reactions, however, cannot be taken as proof of their existence in actual plant cells. Biosynthesis of secondary metabolites such as alkaloids must be determined experimentally for each species. The objectives of such studies are threefold: first, all intermediates in the metabolic pathway must be determined; second, enzymes and cofactors that catalyze each step must be characterized; and third, the kinetics, stoichiometry, and chemical mechanism for each step must be understood. Most published biosynthetic studies, however, are based only on precursor-product relationships, that is, step one. Even though incomplete, much useful information can be gathered from such studies. These experiments fall into one of two broad methodological categories: balance studies and radiolabeled tracer studies.

Balance studies consist of infusing a large amount of a putative precursor of the naturally occurring alkaloid into the plant in question and measuring the amount of end product formed at a future time. In theory, a major quantitative difference between what is produced under natural conditions and what is produced under precursor feeding should be measurable, thus establishing the precursor as a genuine naturally occurring (obligatory) intermediate. This method suffers from several difficulties. It does not take into consideration the existence of "rate-limiting steps" in the metabolic pathway. In controlling biosynthetic reactions, these steps will not allow the enhanced accumulation of products from an enhanced supply of precursor. Also, because individual plant specimens growing in the wild are subject to a great variation of natural conditions, the matching of experimental with control plants is very difficult.

The availability of radiolabeling techniques in organic synthesis has made possible far more accurate biosynthetic studies. This procedure involves feeding a suspected precursor that has been labeled at a specific site with a radioactive atom such as carbon 14 (the most abundant isotope of carbon has atomic weight 12), allowing the plant to grow for a limited time, extracting the product alkaloid, and measuring the incorporated radioactivity. Measuring radioactivity can be done either by chemical degradation or by instrumental means such as mass spectrometry or (as in the case of carbon 13) NMR spectroscopy. Even so, this technique cannot absolutely ascertain if the added precursor is indeed the natural, obligatory one. More evidence is needed from enzyme and kinetic studies. Several seemingly conflicting views exist regarding enzyme-catalyzed reactions in plants. Spenser (in Pelletier 1970: 677) has argued:

> There is no justification for assuming *a priori* that primary metabolic processes follow the same pattern in different living forms. Each species presents a unique set of metabolic problems . . . biosynthetic pathways which are proposed on the basis of incorporation studies freely invoke enzymatic reactions that are assumed to be of wide generality. . . . Assumption of unrestricted generality of such processes in biochemical systems is unjustified. Intracellular enzymes are of high substrate specificity.

The enzymatic reactions in question include transamination, decarboxylation, and oxidative deamination of alpha amino acids, oxidative decarboxylation of alpha-keto acids, and transmethylation from S-methyl methionine. However, Turner (1971: 21), in a discussion of biosynthetic pathways in fungi, noted that "microorganisms possess non-specific enzyme systems which will accept a wide variety of substrates." This nonspecificity of enzymes in fungi (and perhaps in higher plants) led Bu'Lock (1965) to propose the idea of a metabolic grid in which the same enzymes will each catalyze the reaction of more than one substrate such that there are several different pathways from a supposed precursor to the final product. Such a biosynthetic grid is illustrated in Figure 4.6 for the compounds under consideration here. Admittedly, one must take into account the vastly differing natures of microorganisms and green, flowering plants. However, one cannot deny that both specific and nonspecific enzymes exist throughout the living world. In any event, the reaction grid shown in Figure 4.6 may be useful to a discussion of the published experimental data regarding the biosynthesis of the elaborated indoles found in species of *Anadenanthera*.

At the outset, it must be appreciated that not all of the alkaloids shown in Figure 4.6 have been detected in species of *Anadenanthera*, that is, compounds 1 (tryptamine) and 7 (5-methoxytryptamine). This does not, however, preclude them as potential natural biosynthetic intermediates. Protein-bound substrates undergoing enzymatic reaction may be very difficult to detect under normal plant extraction and analysis techniques. Some of these intermediates might also be very short-lived, undergoing reaction as soon as they are

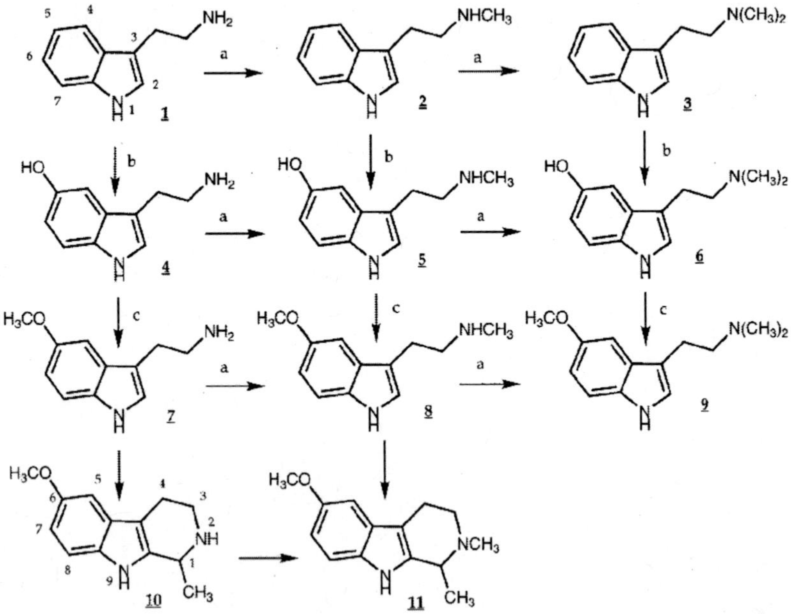

FIGURE 4.6. Biosynthetic grid of the *Anadenanthera* alkaloids.

formed. This phenomenon has been demonstrated in experiments in-volving genetic engineering. For example, in a study of the produc-tion of serotonin (compound 4, Figure 4.6) by root cultures of *Peganum harmala* (Syrian rue), Berlin and colleagues demonstrated a tenfold increase in serotonin yield upon introduction of a trypto-phan decarboxylase cDNA cloned from *Catharanthus roseus* (Berlin et al. 1993). The levels of tryptamine, the immediate product of tryptophan decarboxylase, were unchanged in these transgenic lines, indicating that it was used immediately after it was produced for enhanced serotonin biosynthesis.

Tryptophan, the presumed immediate precursor of tryptamine (1), is not shown in Figure 4.6. Neither is another possible key intermedi-ate, 5-hydroxytryptophan. With the inclusion of these compounds, one might envision not just a two-dimensional biosynthetic grid but a three-dimensional grid with a z axis as well as the shown x and y axes. Moreover, none of the cofactors that could mediate the enzymatic reactions are shown.

In the biosynthesis of 9 from 1, six reaction pathways involving three enzymatic reactions are shown. Hypothetically, all reaction pathways are possible, but not all are given equal importance. Some of the compounds may be better enzyme substrates than others. The enzymes involved in the sequence of *N*-methylation, aromatic hy-droxylation, and *O*-methylation are indicated by the letters a, b, and c, respectively, positioned over the reaction arrows. All of the enzymes that could effect such reactions are known to occur in the plant king-dom, although studies aimed at their isolation from species of *Ana-denanthera* are lacking. Certain broad assumptions can be made by analogy to other plant species. Preliminary discussions of certain as-pects of biosynthesis in this genus have already been mentioned (Fish, Johnson, and Horning 1955; Legler 1963).

Although these early works cannot properly be considered as biosynthesis studies, they provide useful information and insights into the type of reasoning that eventually results in an understanding of the metabolic pathways by which these alkaloids are formed. The observation that DMT *N*-oxide and bufotenine *N*-oxide are present in extracts of seeds of *P. macrocarpa* Benth. (*A. colubrina* var. *Cebil;* Fish, Johnson, and Horning 1955) prompted Fish and co-workers (1956) to investigate a mild ferric ion-induced rearrangement of these *N*-oxides as a model of biological *N*-dealkylation.

Although the conversion of tertiary alkylamines (such as DMT) into secondary amines by removal of a single methyl group had been known from the early twentieth century (Polonovski 1927) and actually studied for DMT itself (Ahond et al. 1970), reaction in the laboratory involved prolonged heating in boiling acetic anhydride, conditions far more severe than anything experienced in nature, although the natural occurrence of the agent acetyl phosphate had been invoked as a possible promoter of a "biological Polonovski" reaction (Bather et al. 1971). The reaction of DMT *N*-oxide with ferric nitrate in the presence of oxalic acid in aqueous solution first produced an unstable carbinolamine which rapidly underwent hydrolytic loss of formaldehyde to give *N*-monomethyltryptamine, a known *Piptadenia/Anadenanthera* alkaloid. These workers suggested that another possible product, *N*-methyltetrahydronorharman, might be formed from the intermediate carbinolamine under even milder conditions. Indeed, more than 20 years later (Schultes et al. 1977), this very compound was detected in seeds of *A. peregrina*. It was also claimed that work was proceeding on the rearrangement of bufotenine *N*-oxide "under circumstances where 6-hydroxy-*N*-methyltetrahydronorharman (2-methyl-6-hydroxy-1,2,3,4-tetrahydro-ß-carboline) can be detected" (Fish et al. 1956: 3669). No report of this investigation was published.

The work on oxidative *N*-dealkylation was presented in a biochemical format in an earlier publication (Fish, Johnson, Lawrence, and Horning 1955). In this paper, it was suggested that the reaction sequence DMT *N*-oxide → carbinolamine → *N*-monomethyltryptamine might also proceed in the reverse direction in nature, and if true, "the sequence is a model 'energy ladder' which may be useful in studying enzymatic methylation and demethylation reactions" (Fish, Johnson, Lawrence, and Horning 1955: 565). To test this hypothesis, the action on DMT of a mitochondria-free MAO system derived from mouse liver homogenates was investigated. Several transformation products were detected, among which were identified DMT *N*-oxide and indole-3-acetic acid. When a mitochondrial preparation of the same enzyme was studied, the only product seen was the latter acid. Added DMT *N*-oxide remained unchanged after incubation, from which it was concluded that the *N*-oxide was not an intermediate in the formation of indole-3-acetic acid, at least not in the mouse.

The work of Fish, Johnson, and Horning (1955), and the discovery of DMT *N*-oxide and 5-methoxy-DMT-*N*-oxide in another member of the Leguminosae, *Desmodium pulchellum* Benth. *ex* Baker, prompted study of the possible biosynthetic role of these compounds (Ghosal and Mukherjee 1966). When 5-methoxy-DMT-*N*-oxide was treated with an aqueous solution of ferrous sulfate and acetic acid, both 5-methoxy-*N*-monomethyltryptamine and 6-methoxy-2-methyl-1,2,3,4-tetrahydro-ß-carboline were isolated. This observation in conjunction with the known natural occurrence of DMT, bufotenine, gramine, 5-methoxy-*N*-monomethyltryptamine, and 5-methoxy-DMT as well as the above *N*-oxides in the same plant species led these authors to suggest, "The occurrence of several tertiary amine oxides in a single plant species is of considerable biogenetic interest because the amine oxides are probably the key intermediates in certain alkaloid biosynthesis" (Ghosal and Mukherjee 1966: 2285). Thus, a biosynthetic reaction sequence (starting from tryptophan) in which all of the observed indoles could be accounted for was envisioned, with the *N*-oxides playing a prominent role. These workers went so far as to postulate "a hypothetical biogenetic route common to all indole bases" (Ghosal and Mukherjee 1996: 2286) via the intermediacy of the *N*-oxides. Studies by both Ghosal and Agurell concluded that the tryptamine *N*-oxides were genuine, naturally occurring compounds and not artifacts produced under the conditions of extraction (Ghosal and Mukherjee 1966; Agurell et al. 1969).

The effects of bufotenine, DMT, harmine, harmaline, psilocybin, and the "laboratory alkaloid" lysergic acid diethylamide on the enzyme-catalyzed synthesis and catabolism of serotonin were investigated as part of a larger study of the alkaloids of Amazonian visionary plants (Hashimoto et al. 1970). The intermediates in this sequence were assumed to be tryptophan, 5-hydroxytryptophan, serotonin, 5-hydroxyindole-3-acetaldehyde, and 5-hydroxyindole-3-acetic acid. The enzymes invoked for these transformations were, respectively, tryptophan hydroxylase, 5-hydroxytryptophan decarboxylase, MAO, and aldehyde dehydrogenase. Harmine and harmaline were shown to be weak inhibitors of MAO and, along with bufotenine and DMT, also demonstrated an inhibition of tryptophan hydroxylase. None of the compounds studied inhibited 5-hydroxytryptophan decarboxylase.

In a study of psilocin biosynthesis (4-hydroxy-*N,N*-dimethyltryptamine, the positional isomer of bufotenine) in higher fungi, it was postulated that tryptophan- and tryptamine-epoxides are common intermediates in the formation of both psilocin and bufotenine (Chilton et al. 1979). These extremely labile "arene oxides" had been implicated (Kaubisch et al. 1972) in the monoxygenase-catalyzed hepatic metabolism of aromatic compounds. Such a hypothesis might be invoked for organisms such as certain fungi, in which both 4- and 5-hydroxytryptamines co-occur, although an equal abundance of each isomeric tryptamine might be expected from a nonregiochemical opening of a common arene oxide intermediate. However, although the co-occurrence of bufotenine and psilocybin in the single species *Panaeolus retirugis* was cited, they do not occur in equal abundance, and no other such co-occurrence has ever been reported for any other plant species. However, evidence for aromatic hydroxylation via the "arene oxide-NIH shift" mechanism has been experimentally verified for numerous plant and animal species (Jerina et al. 1971).

Rivier and Pilet (1971) also discussed the complexity of the biosynthetic relationships of the tryptamines and ß-carbolines as part of a review of the naturally occurring indole hallucinogens. They invoked certain common enzymatic pathways in the metabolism of these alkaloids starting from tryptophan, and their catabolism into indoleacetic acid and indolepyruvic acid derivatives. A reaction grid with tryptamine itself as a central feature was included.

The only relatively thorough investigation of alkaloid biosynthesis in *Piptadenia peregrina (Anadenanthera peregrina)* was carried out by Fellows and Bell (1971). Using both balance studies and radio-labeled precursor feeding, as well as "chemical reasoning" deduced from seed extraction results, these researchers discounted the suggestion of Fish, Johnson, and Horning (1955) that bufotenine was formed in the plant by peroxidic oxidation of DMT. Indoles in dormant seeds and in three-day-old germinated seedlings were analyzed by paper chromatography and high-voltage electrophoresis. Bufotenine, but not DMT or the *N*-oxides, was detected exclusively. After seven days' growth, however, the seedlings were found to contain serotonin (5-hydroxytryptamine), *N*-methylserotonin, and tryptophan in addition to bufotenine. A series of experiments were conducted in which both carbon 14 and tritium-labeled possible precursors D- and L-tryptophan, serotonin, 5-hydroxytryptophan, tryptamine, and DMT were incubated with etiolated stem tissue. After 15 hours, product makeup indicated that 80 percent of the label from the precursor serotonin was incorporated into bufotenine. In another experiment, only 20 percent of the labeled D- or L-tryptophan was incorporated. The unnatural D-isomer of tryptophan resulted in the formation, in good yield, of labeled indole-3-acetylaspartic acid, a compound apparently not found in wild *P. peregrina*. None of the label from precursor DMT was incorporated into bufotenine. Incubation with labeled tryptamine precursor led to incorporation of the label in serotonin, *N*-methyltryptamine, and bufotenine, but not in *N*-methylserotonin. Balance experiments in which high concentrations of serotonin were used led to higher accumulation of *N*-methylserotonin. The results of these experiments led the authors to conclude that bufotenine was formed by the sequence of steps: tryptophan → tryptamine → serotonin (5-hydroxytryptamine) → *N*-methylserotonin → bufotenine. They suggested that the key step, that is, the hydroxylation of tryptamine to produce serotonin, was due to a unique 5-hydroxylase enzyme present in *P. peregrina*. The partial incorporation of label from the precursor 5-hydroxytryptophan into bufotenine (via serotonin) was said to "merely reflect a lack of absolute specificity in the decarboxylase for which L-tryptophan is the normal substrate" (Fellows and Bell 1971: 2089). This precursor was not considered normal (obligatory) for formation of bufotenine.

Many of the limitations discussed at the beginning of this section apply to these studies. Although precursor-product relationships seem well established, enzyme studies for this genus are lacking. Further insights can be gained, however, from the pioneering studies into the biosynthesis of these tryptamines in species of *Phalaris,* a member of the Gramineae (grass family) from Australia, conducted by Slaytor and colleagues at the University of Sydney. In early work, Baxter and Slaytor (1972) invoked the metabolic grid concept to delineate the possible biosynthetic relationships among 12 alkaloids along the pathways from tryptophan to 5-methoxy-DMT, 7 of which had been detected in the plant. Elaborate feeding and trapping experiments eliminated only one of the six possible pathways, prompting the authors to quote Bu'Lock (1965): "[T]he more information which can be obtained from precursor-incorporation experiments then the fewer clear-cut conclusions there are to be drawn from them" (Baxter and Slaytor 1972: 2772).

However, with more than a decade of research and the emergence of new techniques such as affinity chromatography, enzymes that catalyzed decarboxylation, *O*-methylation, and *N*-methylation were isolated and characterized from species of *Phalaris*. More exacting techniques have demonstrated the presence of two very specific *N*-methyltransferases in *Phalaris,* one (primary indolethylamine methyltransferase) that produces *N*-monomethyltryptamine (and 5-methoxy-*N*-monomethyltryptamine) from tryptamine (and 5-methoxytryptamine), and a second (secondary indolethylamine *N*-methyltransferase) that subsequently produces DMT and 5-methoxy-DMT. Both enzymes utilize *S*-adenosylmethionine as a cofactor (Mulvena and Slaytor 1983; for a comprehensive discussion of methylation reactions in plant biochemistry, see Poulton 1981).

The biosynthetic origins of two reduced β-carboline alkaloids (compounds 10 and 11, Figure 4.6) in species of *Anadenanthera* are even more obscure than that of the tryptamines. They are included in Figure 4.6 to show their chemical relationship to the tryptamines. A direct biosynthetic formation of these compounds from the tryptamines 7 and 8 should not be implied. However, a number of possible biosynthetic routes to these compounds can be inferred from studies of other plant species and other closely related alkaloids. The structure of harmine (12, Figure 4.7), isolated from the seeds of *Peganum harmala* L. by Goebel (1841), was determined to be a cyclized tryptamine or β-carboline alkaloid (Perkin and Robinson 1919). Not long after, the latter workers (Kermack et al. 1921) proposed a biosynthetic origin for harmine (and harmaline, 15, Figure 4.7) involving the incorporation of a two-carbon fragment (acetaldehyde) into 6-methoxytryptamine, followed by a two-step oxidation sequence. Such reactions were known to proceed under "mild" conditions in the laboratory. However, experimental determination of the origin of this two-carbon fragment (carbons 1 and 10 in structure 12) was to prove elusive for the next 80 years. Slaytor and McFarlane (1968) conducted precursor feeding experiments with seedlings of *Passiflora edulis,* a species known to contain harman (14, Figure 4.7). The incorporation of radiolabeled *N*-acetyltryptamine into harman suggested that the two-carbon fragment arose by acetylation of tryptamine by acetyl Coenzyme A (CoA) followed by dehydrative cyclization to harmalan (17, Figure 4.7) and oxidation to harman. Later, however, the same researchers (McFarlane and Slaytor 1972; Nettle-

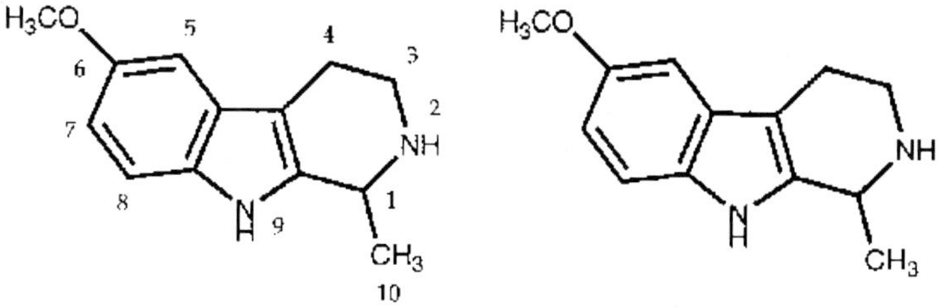

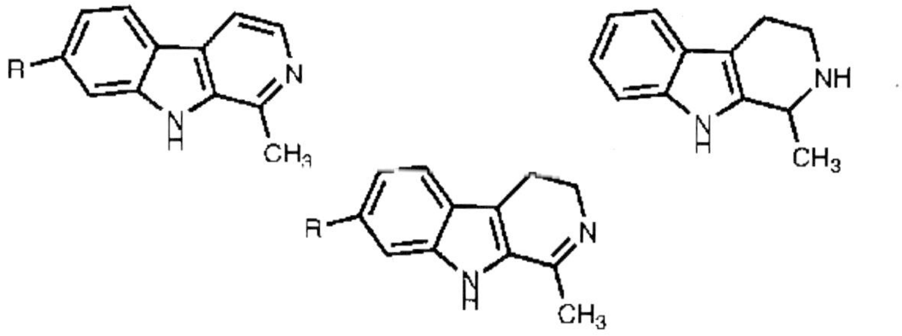

12 R=OCH₃, harmine
13 R=OH, harmol
14 R=H, harman
15 R=OCH₃, harmaline
16 R-OH, harmalol
17 R=H, harmalan
18 eleagnine or tetrahydroharman

FIGURE 4.7. Chemical relationship of *Anadenanthera* alkaloids 10 and 11 to other naturally occurring carbolines.

ship and Slaytor 1974) could not demonstrate the incorporation of *N*-acetyltryptamine into eleagnine (18, Figure 4.7) in seedlings of *Elaeagnus angustifolia* or into harmine in callus cultures of *Peganum harmala*. However, the co-occurrence of harman, eleagnine, and *N*-acetyltryptamine in *Prosopis nigra* (Gris.) Hieron. (Moro et al. 1975) suggested a possible biosynthetic role for such acetamides in some plant species. That the two-carbon fragment arose from pyruvate was suggested by labeled precursor feeding experiments with young plants of *P. harmala* (Stolle and Groger 1968).

Problems associated with the study of biosynthesis and enzymology of secondary plant metabolites through the use of radiolabeled precursor feeding experiments in whole intact plants can be partially alleviated through the use of cell suspension cultures or cultures of specific plant organs such as rootlets. In the laboratory such techniques can partially eliminate the variability of overall rates of biosynthesis and degradation associated with the stages of development of whole plants. Other influences on enzymatic activity and biosynthesis such as physical stimuli (light, temperature), injury, or infection can be controlled. Even so, such experiments with cultured cell lines also have certain limitations. Such limitations have been expressed by other researchers (Sasse et al. 1982: 318):

> Secondary metabolic pathways of higher plants are often not well expressed in cell culture systems. More biochemical knowledge especially on the interaction of primary and secondary pathways may be very helpful to overcome this behavior of cultured cells and may prove to be necessary for establishing more often high yielding cell culture strains. Such biochemical studies can be done by characterizing variant cell lines with different levels of secondary metabolites or by inducing secondary pathways in cultured cells.

A study of the biosynthesis of the ß-carboline alkaloids in hairy root cultures of *Peganum harmala* was only partially successful in identifying individual biosynthetic steps (Berlin et al. 1993). Although the levels of serotonin production were closely related to the level of tryptophan decarboxylase activity, there did not appear to be a direct correlation with ß-carboline formation. Only the last step in alkaloid formation, that is, the oxidation of harmaline to harmine, was identified with certainty.

Although close structural similarity of tryptamines and simple carboline and reduced carboline alkaloids combined with co-occurrence of both chemical classes in the same plant species suggests common biosynthetic pathways, more investigations of their mode of synthesis in nature and the enzymes involved are needed to clearly define the actual pathways.

BIOCHEMICAL SYSTEMATICS OF **ANADENANTHERA**

The study of comparative phytochemistry, biochemical systematics, or "chemotaxonomy" makes use of chemical constituents of plants as characters to be used along with morphological features such as flower, leaf, stem, and seed structures in taxonomy. Broadly defined, such study is concerned with evolutionary relationships among plants. Biochemical information, along with cytological and ultrastructural data, are relatively modern supplements to classical taxonomy. However, broad comparative phytochemistry has been used for centuries by herbalists and pharmacists in grouping medicinal plants according to their "virtues," qualities related to their active chemical constituents. Long before the isolation and structural elucidation of physiologically active principles from plants became routine, botanists, physicians, and herbalists recorded observations such as compatibility of grafts, bitterness, and resistance to insect attack as elements of chemotaxonomy. Today the main goal of chemotaxonomy is to determine how well the distribution of chemical constituents correlates with classical taxonomy. Ultimately, this discipline seeks to define the chemical structures of the plant genes themselves.

A chemist interested in plant chemical systematics concentrates on the secondary metabolites, constituents of intermediate occurrence in the plant kingdom. Primary metabolites, such as sugars, polysaccharides, and protein amino acids, which have a universal occurrence, are of little use in this endeavor. Similarly, seemingly unique chemical compounds that have rare occurrence in the plant kingdom are only of interest if they can be biogenetically related to similar compounds in other plants. The determination of biosynthetic pathways by which certain chemical constituents are formed is also of importance. This is particularly important when comparing obviously related plants that produce slightly different compounds having the same biogenetic origin. This phenomenon, known as homology (Hegnauer 1962), occurs, for example, when two complex structures differ from each other only by a single atom, for example, an oxygen atom replacing a nitrogen atom.

Many classes of naturally occurring compounds have been used in the study of chemotaxonomy. Some of these were discussed earlier in the context of general phytochemical investigations of *Anadenanthera*. Carbohydrates and certain unusual glycosides, complex phenols such as flavonoids, certain betacyanin and anthocyanin pigments, terpenoids, and of course alkaloids have all been studied as taxonomic markers within the plant kingdom. The alkaloids, of particular interest here, were one of the earliest groups of compounds to be so studied. This is partially true because of the physiological significance of many alkaloids and also because their basic nature simplifies isolation and purification.

The use of chemical constituents as potential taxonomic markers follows closely the classification scheme of the plant kingdom but is clearly not useful above the level of orders. *Anadenanthera* fits into botanical classification in the following way:

Division: Magnoliophyta
Subclass: Rosidae
Order: Fabales
Family: Fabaceae
Subfamily: Mimosoideae
Genus: *Anadenanthera*

Most chemotaxonomic studies concentrate on the level of family and below. For example, Hegnauer and Grayer-Barkmeijer (1993: 11) reviewed general trends in the occurrence of polysaccharides and flavanoids in the Leguminosae, noting that

> all three subfamilies [of the Leguminosae] are united by the possession of 5-deoxyflavanoids and C-glycosylflavanoids, and that there is more or less clear distinction between the Caesalpinioideae and Mimosoideae on the one hand, and the Papilionoideae on the other in a number of flavanoid characters.

Most chemotaxonomic studies, however, involve even lower levels of classification. In the current context, the occurrence of tryptamine alkaloids (with the exception of serotonin and 5-hydroxytryptamine) in the Leguminosae appears to be limited to nine genera of the subfamily Mimosoideae: *Acacia, Prosopis, Petalostylis, Piptadenia, Ana-*

denanthera, Mimosa, Desmodium, Mucuna, and *Lespedeza* (Mears and Mabry 1971; Smith 1977). Considering that there are approximately 13,000 species in the Leguminosae, such occurrence is definitely of taxonomic value.

A number of problems and limitations exist regarding the use of alkaloids as elements in taxonomy. Along with homology, subtle genetic variations within a population of plants can lead to differences in chemical constituents. Such phenomena as hybridization, in which members of two genetically distinct species of plants crossbreed, and introgression, in which a hybrid individual crosses back with one of the "parent" plants, lead to populations that contain various mixtures of genetic material. Since natural hybridization is not uncommon, and since such events are known, in some cases, to significantly alter the genetics of alkaloid formation, the use of alkaloids as chemical markers in two closely related species such as *A. peregrina* and *A. colubrina* or indeed, even between the genera *Anadenanthera* and *Piptadenia,* must be approached with caution. For a chemist studying chemical taxonomy, centuries-long human involvement with such genera, including deliberate cultivation and trade in seeds, makes awareness of these possible occurrences of acute importance.

Careful botanical documentation of plants being chemically studied is of utmost importance to the chemotaxonomist. Some have considered much of the chemical data gathered prior to the mid-twentieth century to be of little value in taxonomy. Mears and Mabry (1971: 74) have stated that "the major problem in using alkaloid reports for systematic studies is not that of the reliability of the chemical data; rather it is that the identity of plants studied before about 1965 can rarely be verified." Ettlinger and Kjaer (1968: 62) were even more acerbic:

The necessity of the mechanical features of systematic work, the collection and preservation of herbarium specimens and the assignment of correct names, tends to be disregarded by most chemists. They instinctively rebel, in the first place, against what is dimly imagined to be the arbitrary and prescriptive character of systematics. . . . Chemists rely on structures as primary symbols, seldom pondering names; they object to botanical nomenclature . . . because the Latin language and rules of priority make it seem antiquarian. Few chemists are at peace with a sense of history.

Assuming hat all botanical criteria for chemotaxonomic studies have been met, other chemical factors may also play a role. Up until now, we have only considered the qualitative nature of the chemical constituents of plants in the study of chemical systematics. The ability of a species to accumulate secondary metabolites may also be of importance to such studies. For example, although the alkaloid nicotine occurs as a trace component in many plants, only certain genera, such as *Nicotiana,* have the ability not only to synthesize but to store large quantities of this alkaloid. We have seen previously that such is also the case with the genus under review here. Reis Altschul (1964) suggested that the occurrence of large amounts of bufotenine and related alkaloids in the two species of *Anadenanthera* serves, along with morphological characters, as another indication of distinctness relative to earlier treatments of the genus and related members of *Piptadenia.* This quantitative factor may be far more important to the systematics of these members of the Mimosoideae than trace occurrences of these alkaloids in other leguminous genera. When a secondary metabolite, such as bufotenine, is an end product of a biosynthetic sequence instead of merely an intermediate of metabolism in a given species, certain limiting factors in its analysis are of less importance. Variations in alkaloid content due to stage of development of the plant or plant organs under investigation is of less concern. However, we have seen (Torres and Repke 1996) considerable variation in bufotenine concentration (from 3.5 percent to over 12 percent) in seeds from individuals of the same population of the same species collected from the same geographical region at approximately the same time of year. Although the seeds of three members of the genus *Anadenanthera* have been found to contain relatively (>1 percent) large amounts of bufotenine (*A. peregrina* var. *peregrina, A. colubrina* var. *Cebil,* and *A. colubrina* var. *colubrina*), the fourth member, *A. peregrina* var. *falcata,* contains a much smaller concentration of this alkaloid. Does this mean that the latter species should not be included in the genus *Anadenanthera*? Hardly; generic relationships cannot be established on the basis of one character alone, whether chemical or morphological. Yet on the basis of alkaloid content, the fourth species has more in common with the seven species of *Piptadenia* proper (see Appendix), which have been shown to contain low concentrations of bufotenine and other indole alkaloids. Should *A. peregrina* var. *falcata* be reclassified as a species of *Piptadenia*? Certainly not on the basis of the concentration of a single chemical character. Revisions of both genera will have to await further study. Perhaps more detailed investigations conducted by botanists and chemists working in close collaboration can solve some of the riddles of this most interesting topic.

APPENDIX: SPECIES OF PIPTADENIA FROM SOUTH AMERICA STUDIED FOR THE PRESENCE OF ALKALOIDS

Species	Alkaloids	Reference
Piptadenia paniculata	Unidentified tryptamines	Fish, Johnson, and Horning 1955
Piptadenia contorta	Bufotenine, DMT, unknown indole	Yamasoto et al. 1972
Piptadenia contorta Benth.	Alkalold positive	Reis Altschul 1964; Fish, Johnson, and Horning 1955
Piptadenia "leprostachya"	Theobromine, unknown indole	Yamasoto et al. 1972
Piptadenia leptostachya Benth.	Alkaloid positive	Reis Altschul 1964; Fish, Johnson, and Horning 1955
Piptadenia moniliformis	Bufotenine, unknown indole	Yamasato et al. 1972
Piptadenia excelsa	Bufotenine, bufotenine N-oxide, DMT	Iacobucci and Ruveda 1964
Piptadenia excelsa	"Quaternary alkaloid"	Stucker and Paya 1938
Piptadenia paraguayensis	Alkaloid positive	Iacobucci and Ruveda 1964
Piptadenia rigida	Alkaloid positive	Iacobucci and Ruveda 1964
Piptadenia viridiflora	Alkaloid positive	Iacobucci and Ruveda 1964
Piptadenia communis Benth.	Alkaloid positive	Reis Altschul 1964

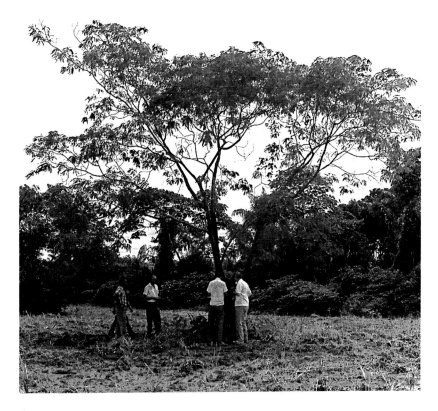

PLATE 1. *Anadenanthera peregrina*. Near Bôa Vista, Rio Branco, Brazil.
Source: Photo courtesy of Richard Evans Schultes.

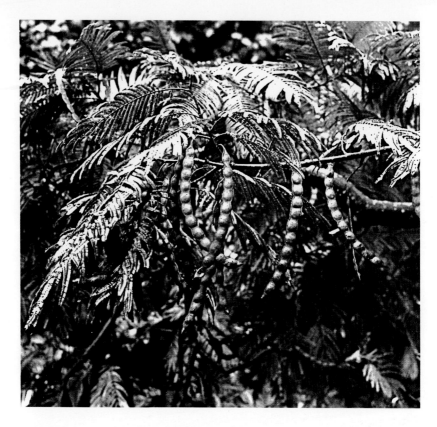

PLATE 2. *Anadenanthera peregrina* in fruit. San Juan, Puerto Rico. *Source:* Photo courtesy of Richard Evans Schultes.

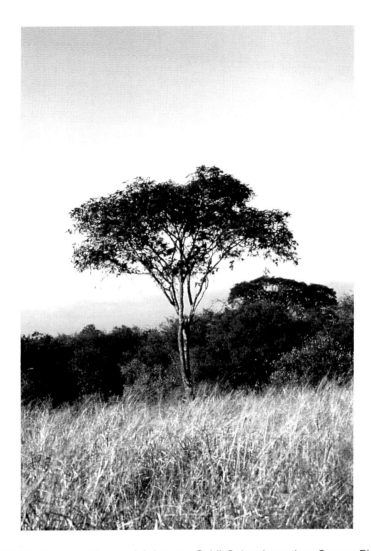

PLATE 3. *Anadenanthera colubrina* var. *Cebil,* Salta, Argentina. *Source:* Photo courtesy of Christian Rätsch.

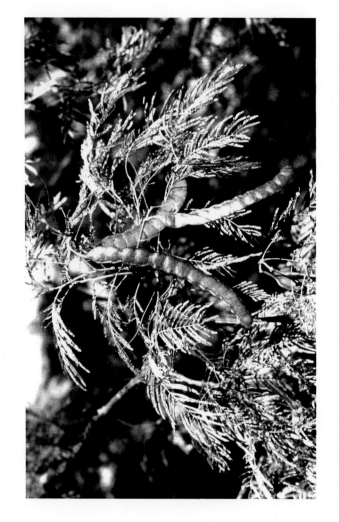

PLATE 4. *Anadenanthera colubrina* var. *Cebil*, in fruit. Cerro San Bernardo, Salta, Argentina. *Source:* Photo by Constantino M. Torres.

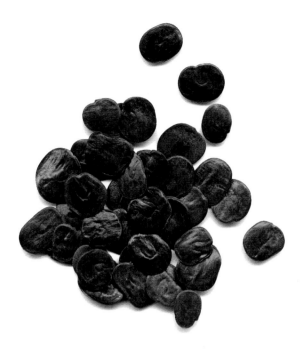

PLATE 5. *Anadenanthera colubrina* var. *Cebil,* pods and seeds. Misión Wichi, General Mosconi, Salta, Argentina. *Source:* Photo by Constantino M. Torres.

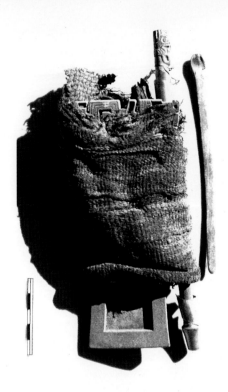

PLATE 6. Snuffing kit, Tomb 107, Solcor 3, ca. A.D. 570, San Pedro de Atacama, Chile. *Source:* Instituto de Investigaciones Arqueológicas y Museo, coll. #3811, Universidad Católica del Norte, San Pedro de Atacama, Chile. Reprinted with permission.

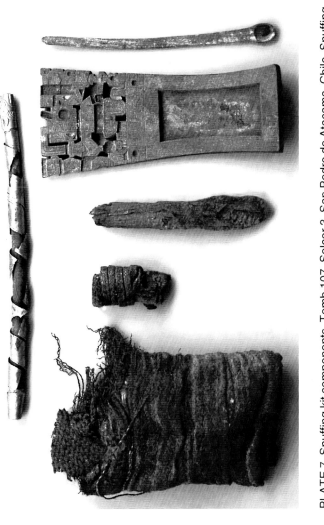

PLATE 7. Snuffing kit components, Tomb 107, Solcor 3, San Pedro de Atacama, Chile. Snuffing tube, wood with gold wrapping, 21.5 cm, coll. # 8431; wooden snuff tray with stone inlays, 16.1 × 7.3 cm, coll. #8432. *Source:* Instituto de Investigaciones Arqueológicas y Museo, Universidad Católica del Norte, San Pedro de Atacama, Chile. Reprinted with permission.

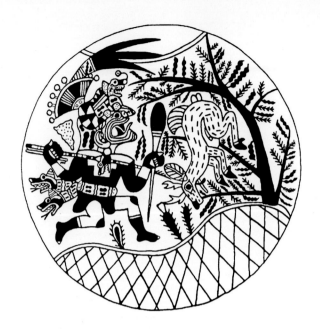

PLATE 8. Deer-hunting scene, pottery dipper, Moche, north coast, Peru. *Source:* Line drawing by Donna McClelland. Moche Archive, Fowler Museum, University of California, Los Angeles.

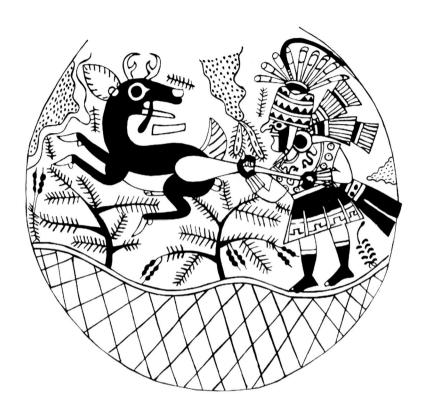

PLATE 9. Deer-hunting scene, pottery dipper, Moche, north coast, Peru. *Source:* Line drawing by Donna McClelland. Moche Archive, Fowler Museum, University of California, Los Angeles.

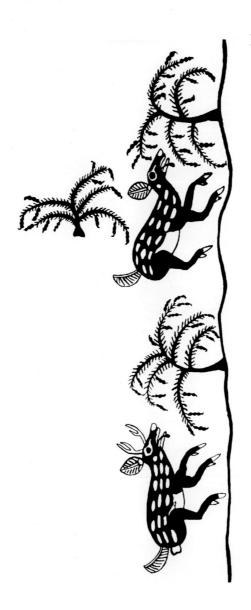

PLATE 10. Male and female spotted deer among probable *Anadenanthera* trees. Stirrup-spout vessel, Moche, north coast, Peru. *Source:* Line drawing by Donna McClelland. Moche Archive, Fowler Museum, University of California, Los Angeles.

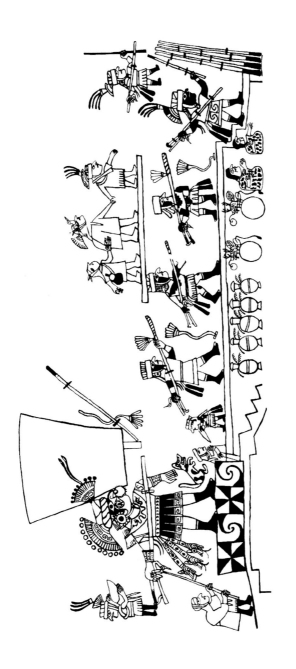

PLATE 11. Ritual scene from Moche stirrup-spout vessel. *Source*: Line drawing by Donna McClelland. Moche Archive, Fowler Museum, University of California, Los Angeles.

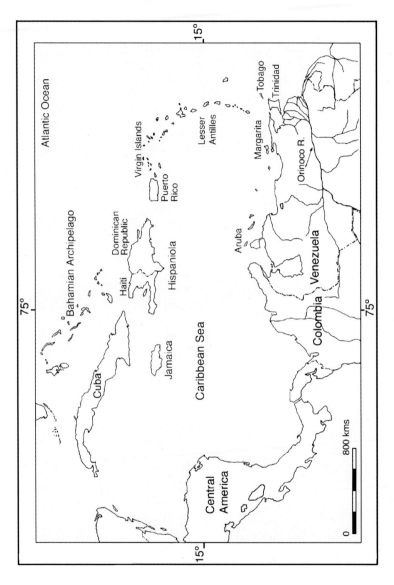

PLATE 12. Map of the Caribbean showing the area of Taíno occupation. *Source:* Map by Constantino M. Torres.

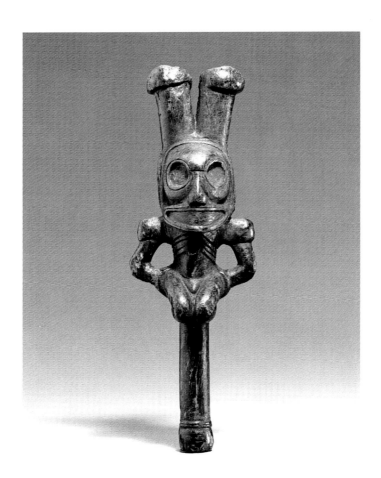

PLATE 13. Carved Y-shaped *cohoba* inhaler, wood, 15.3 cm, Taíno. Fundación García Arévalo, Santo Domingo, Dominican Republic. *Source:* Anthropomorphic Double Inhaler, Wood 15.3 cm, Taíno. Photograph © 1993 Dirk Bakker.

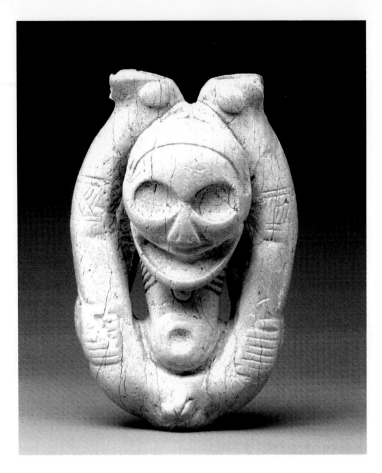

PLATE 14. "Acrobat" *cohoba* inhaler, manatee bone, 8.6 cm, Taíno. Fundación García Arévalo, Santo Domingo, Dominican Republic. *Source:* Anthropomorphic White Inhaler, Bone 8.6 cm, Taíno. Photograph © 1993 Dirk Bakker.

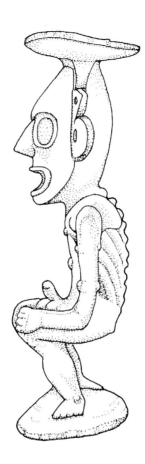

PLATE 15. *Zemí* with depiction of skeletonized human being, wood, 85 cm, Taíno. Private collection, Paris. *Source:* Line drawing by Donna Torres.

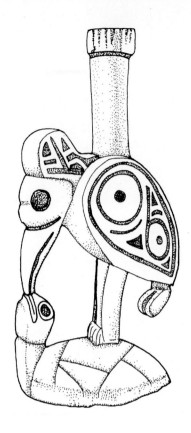

PLATE 16. *Zemí* with bird and turtle representation, wood, 66.5 cm, Taíno. British Museum, London. *Source:* Line drawing by Donna Torres.

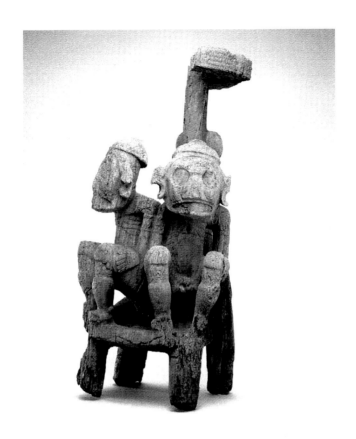

PLATE 17. *Zemí* with twin figures, wood, 77 cm, Taíno. National Museum of Natural History, Smithsonian Institution, Washington, DC. Reprinted with permission. *Source:* Double *Zemí* from Smithsonian Institution, Wood. Taíno. Photograph © 1993 Dirk Bakker.

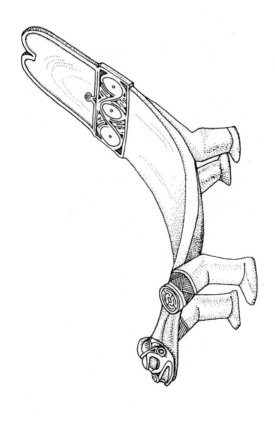

PLATE 18. *Duho*, wood, 78 cm, Taíno, Haiti. Musée de l'Homme, Paris. *Source:* Line drawing by Donna Torres.

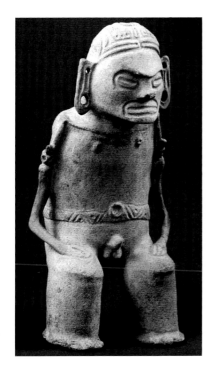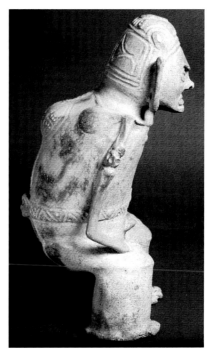

PLATE 19. Effigy vessel, ceramic, 41 cm, Taíno, Dominican Republic. *Source: Courtesy, National Museum of the American Indian, Smithsonian Institution (coll. # 05/3753) Washington, DC. Photo by David Heald. Reprinted with permission.*

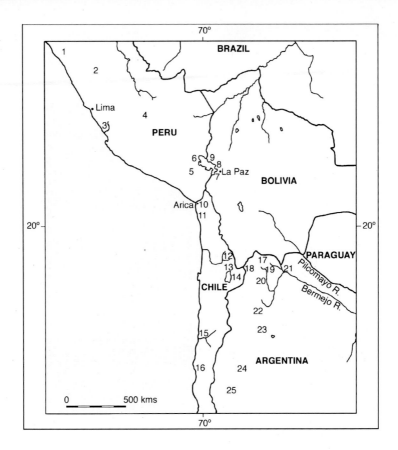

PLATE 20. Map of the central Andes showing location of the most important sites mentioned in the text. 1. Huaca Prieta, Chicama Valley, Peru. 2. Chavín de Huantar, Mosna River valley (Marañon tributary), Peru. 3. Asia, Omás River basin, Peru. 4. Huari (Wari), Ayacucho, Peru. 5. La Real, Aplao, Valle de Majes, Peru. 6. Pucara, north Lake Titicaca, Peru. 7. Tiwanaku, Bolivia. 8. Amaguaya, Depto. De La Paz, Bolivia. 9. Niño Korin, NE Lake Titicaca, Bolivia. 10. Arica, Chile. 11. Pisagua, Chile. 12. Caspana, middle Loa River basin, Chile. 13. San Pedro de Atacama, Salar de Atacama basin, Chile. 14. Toconao, Chile. 15. Coquimbo, Chile. 16. Copiapó, Chile. 17. Inca Cueva, Puna de Jujuy, Argentina. 18. Cusi Cusi, Puna de Jujuy, Argentina. 19. Pucará de Tilcara, Quebrada de Humahuaca, Argentina. 20. Ciénaga Grande, Quebrada de Humahuaca, Argentina. 21. Saladillo Redondo, El Piquete, Jujuy, Argentina. 22. La Paya, Calchaquí Valley, Salta, Argentina. 23. Tolombón, Yocavil Valley, Salta, Argentina. 24. Guandacol, La Rioja, Argentina. 25. Iglesia Valley, San Juan Prov., Argentina. *Source:* Map by Constantino M. Torres.

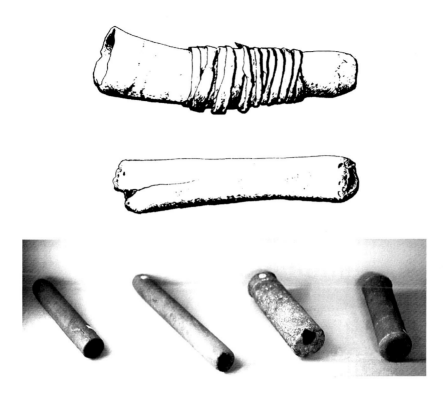

PLATE 21. (top) Tubular pipes, puma bone,13 cm and 11.2 cm, Inca Cueva (IC c7), Puna de Jujuy, Argentina. *Source:* After Fernández Distel 1980: Fig. 5. (bottom) Tubular pipes, Huachichocana (CH III), Puna de Jujuy, Argentina. Left to right: coll. # 2040, red sandstone, 27.8 cm; coll. # 2039, red sandstone, 34.7 cm; coll. # 2037, andesite, 23.8 cm; coll. # 2038, red sandstone, 22.7 cm; Museo Arqueológico, Tilcara, Jujuy, Argentina.

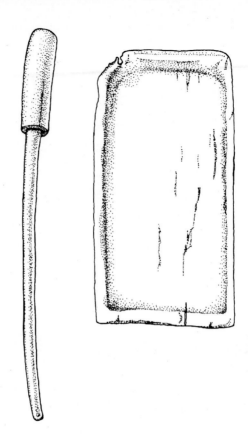

PLATE 22. Whalebone snuff tray, 11.7 × 6 cm, coll. # 41.2.4721; bird and fox bone snuff tube, 17.5 cm, coll. # 41.2.4722; Huaca Prieta, Chicama Valley, Peru. *Source:* American Museum of Natural History, New York. Line drawings by Donna Torres.

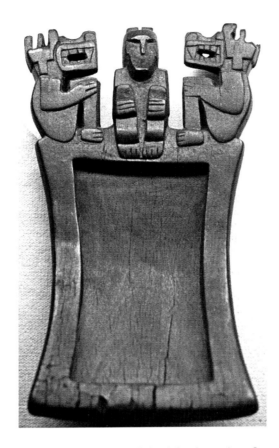

PLATE 23. Wooden snuff tray, 19 cm, Tolombón, Argentina. *Source:* Courtesy, National Museum of the American Indian, Smithsonian Institution (Heye Foundation, coll. # 15/1489) New York. Photo by Constantino M. Torres.

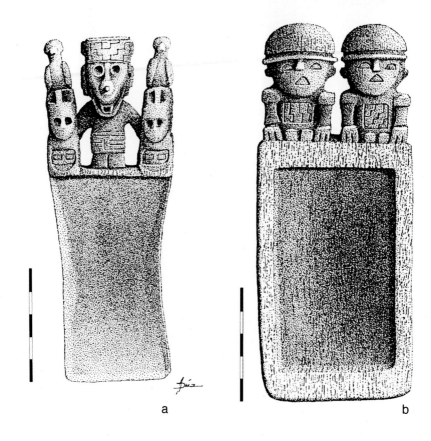

a   b

PLATE 24. Wooden snuff trays: (a) Tudcum, 15 cm, Instituto de Investigaciones y Museo, Tudcum, Departamento de Iglesia, San Juan Prov., Argentina; (b) Angualasto, 16.5 cm (private collection), Departamento de Iglesia, San Juan Prov., Argentina. *Source:* Gambier 2001: Figs. 2, 3. Reprinted with permission from Gambier, M. 2001. "The southernmost archeological evidence for snuffing in the Central Andes." *Eleusis* 5:153-157. Copyright 2001 by *Eleusis.*

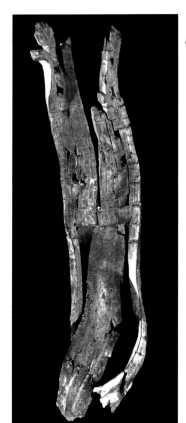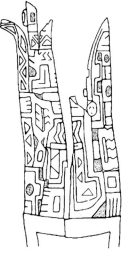

PLATE 25. Snuff tray, wood, decorated area approximately 9.5 cm, Toconao Oriente, t. 4229-30. *Source:* Instituto de Investigaciones Arqueológicas y Museo, Universidad Católica del Norte, San Pedro de Atacama, Chile. Photo by Constantino Torres. Line drawing by Donna Torres. Reprinted with permission.

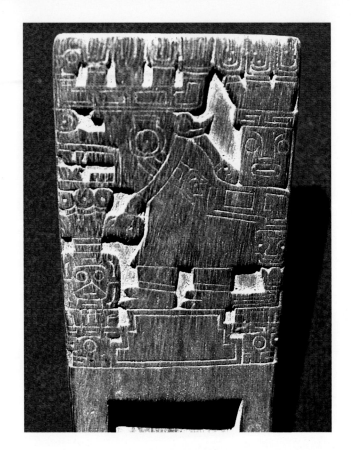

PLATE 26. Snuff tray with camelid representation, wood, 15.7 cm, Solcor 3, tomb 5. *Source:* Instituto de Investigaciones Arqueológicas y Museo, Universidad Católica del Norte, San Pedro de Atacama, Chile. Reprinted with permission.

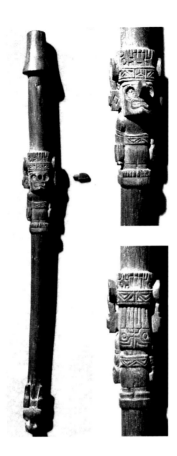

PLATE 27. Snuffing tube, figure with removable nose, wood, 19.6 cm, tomb 79, Solcor 3, San Pedro de Atacama, Chile. *Source:* Instituto de Investigaciones Arqueológicas y Museo, coll. # 2768, Universidad Católica del Norte, San Pedro de Atacama, Chile. Reprinted with permission.

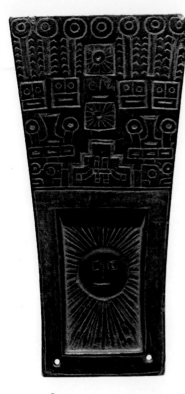
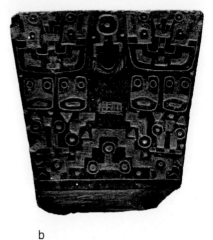

b

a

PLATE 28. (a) Stone snuff tray, 12.06 cm, Quiripuju, southern Lake Titicaca basin. University of Pennsylvania Museum, coll. # 35636. (b) Stone snuff tray, fragment, 7.3 cm, Cumana island, Lake Titicaca. University of Pennsylvania Museum, coll. # 35515. Collected by Max Uhle, University Museum Expedition, 1895.

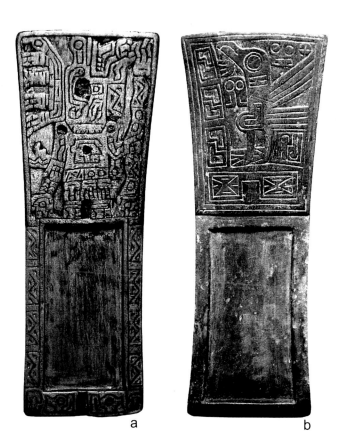

a   b

PLATE 29. (a) Wooden snuff tray, 18.5 cm, Niño Korin, Bolivia. Världskulturmuseet (Museum of World Culture), coll. # 70.19.1, Gothenburg, Sweden. (b) Wooden snuff tray with avian representation, 17 cm, Niño Korin, Bolivia. Världskulturmuseet (Museum of World Culture), coll. # 70.19.23, Gothenburg, Sweden. *Source:* Photos by Constantino M. Torres.

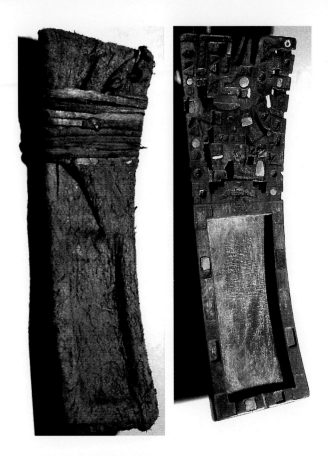

PLATE 30. Wooden snuff tray with gold and spondylus inlays, and its leather sheath, 24.6 cm. Amaguaya, Depto. La Paz, Bolivia. Museo Tiwanaku, La Paz, Bolivia. *Source:* Photos by Constantino M. Torres.

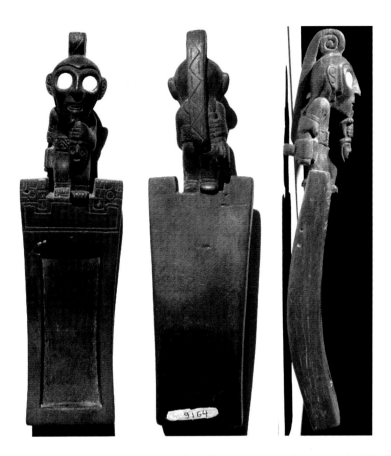

PLATE 31. Wooden snuff tray with Sacrificer representation, eyes inlaid with malachite, 18.1 cm, tomb 2196-98, Quitor 5, San Pedro de Atacama. *Source:* Instituto de Investigaciones Arqueológicas y Museo, Universidad Católica del Norte, San Pedro de Atacama, Chile. Reprinted with permission.

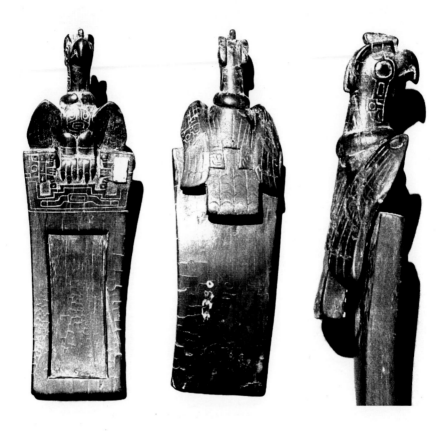

PLATE 32. Wooden snuff tray with condor representation, 17.8 cm, tomb 5334-41, Coyo Oriente, San Pedro de Atacama, Chile. *Source:* Instituto de Investigaciones Arqueológicas y Museo, Universidad Católica del Norte, San Pedro de Atacama, Chile. Reprinted with permission.

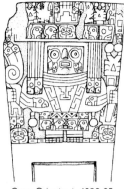

Coyo Oriente, t. 4093-95
San Pedro de Atacama, Chile

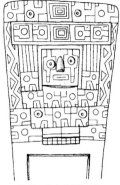

Quitor 5, t. 2183-84
San Pedro de Atacama, Chile

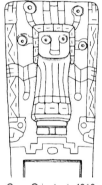

Coyo Oriente, t. 4010
San Pedro de Atacama, Chile

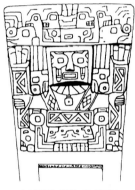

La Real, Valle de Majes,
Peru

PLATE 33a. Tiwanaku iconography in snuff trays from the south central Andes: frontal anthropomorphic representations. *Source:* Line drawings by Donna Torres; tray from La Real, after Garcia and Bustamante 1990: Fig. 3.

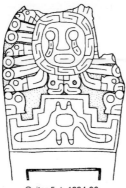

Quitor 5, t. 1994-96
San Pedro de Atacama, Chile

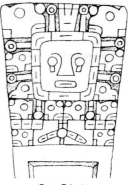

Coyo Oriente
San Pedro de Atacama, Chile

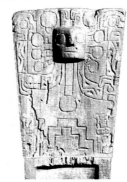

Sequitor Alambrado Oriental, t. 1618
San Pedro de Atacama, Chile

PLATE 33b. Tiwanaku iconography in snuff trays from the south central Andes: disembodied rayed head. *Source:* Line drawings by Donna Torres.

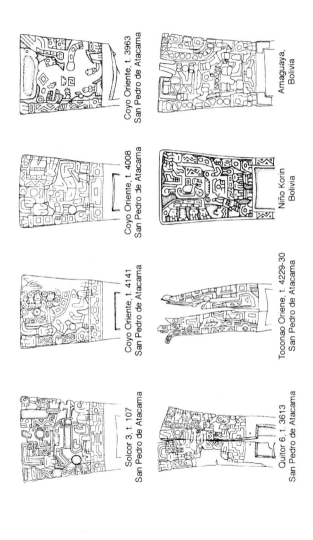

Coyo Oriente, t. 3963
San Pedro de Atacama

Amaguaya,
Bolivia

Coyo Oriente, t. 4008
San Pedro de Atacama

Niño Korin
Bolivia

Coyo Oriente, t. 4141
San Pedro de Atacama

Toconao Oriene, t. 4229-30
San Pedro de Atacama

Solcor 3, t. 107
San Pedro de Atacama

Quitor 6, t. 3613
San Pedro de Atacama

PLATE 33c. Tiwanaku iconography in snuff trays from the south central Andes: profile staff-bearing figure. *Source*: Line drawings by Donna Torres; tray from Amaguaya courtesy of Pablo Rendón.

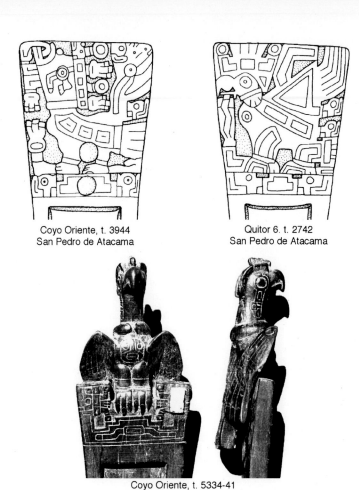

Coyo Oriente, t. 3944
San Pedro de Atacama

Quitor 6. t. 2742
San Pedro de Atacama

Coyo Oriente, t. 5334-41
San Pedro de Atacama

PLATE 33d. Tiwanaku iconography in snuff trays from the south central Andes: condor. *Source:* Line drawings by Donna Torres.

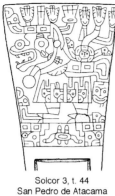

Solcor 3, t. 44
San Pedro de Atacama

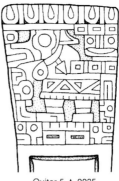

Quitor 5, t. 2235
San Pedro de Atacama

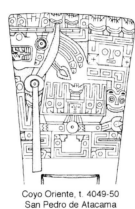

Coyo Oriente, t. 4049-50
San Pedro de Atacama

PLATE 33e. Tiwanaku iconography in snuff trays from the south central Andes: camelid. *Source:* Line drawings by Donna Torres.

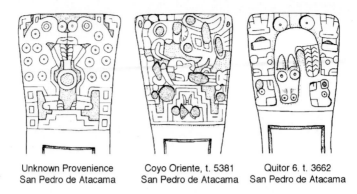

| Unknown Provenience
San Pedro de Atacama | Coyo Oriente, t. 5381
San Pedro de Atacama | Quitor 6. t. 3662
San Pedro de Atacama |

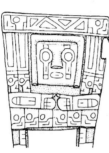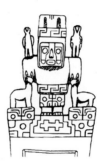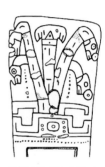

| Unknown Provenience
San Pedro de Atacama | Quitor 2, t. 3706
San Pedro de Atacama | Unknown Provenience
San Pedro de Atacama |

PLATE 33f. Tiwanaku iconography in snuff trays from the south central Andes: unique or infrequent thematic units. *Source:* Line drawings by Donna Torres.

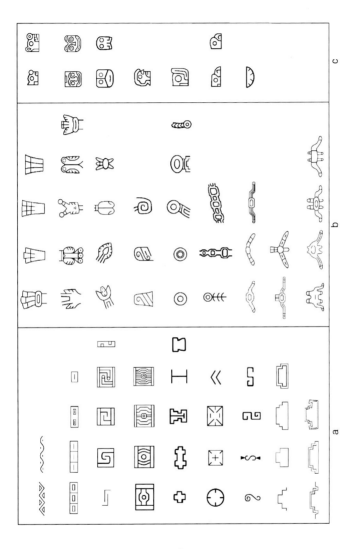

PLATE 34. Individual Tiwanaku motifs: (a) geometric; (b-c) biomorphic. *Source:* Line drawings by Donna Torres.

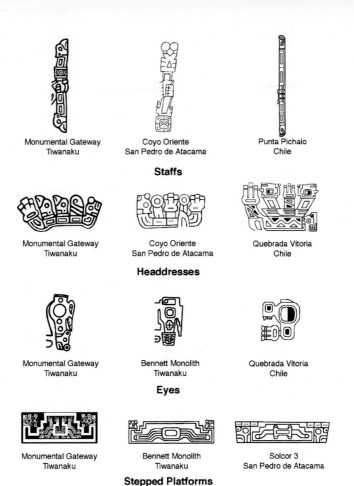

Monumental Gateway
Tiwanaku

Coyo Oriente
San Pedro de Atacama

Punta Pichalo
Chile

Staffs

Monumental Gateway
Tiwanaku

Coyo Oriente
San Pedro de Atacama

Quebrada Vitoria
Chile

Headdresses

Monumental Gateway
Tiwanaku

Bennett Monolith
Tiwanaku

Quebrada Vitoria
Chile

Eyes

Monumental Gateway
Tiwanaku

Bennett Monolith
Tiwanaku

Solcor 3
San Pedro de Atacama

Stepped Platforms

PLATE 35. Tiwanaku motif cluster samples. *Source:* Line drawings by Donna Torres.

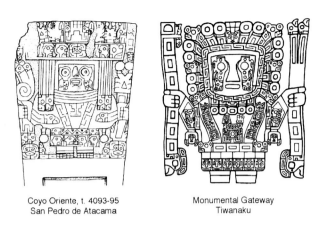

Coyo Oriente, t. 4093-95   Monumental Gateway
San Pedro de Atacama   Tiwanaku

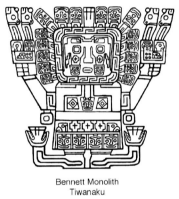

Bennett Monolith
Tiwanaku

PLATE 36. Comparison of frontal personages of diverse provenience. *Source:*
Line drawings by Donna Torres.

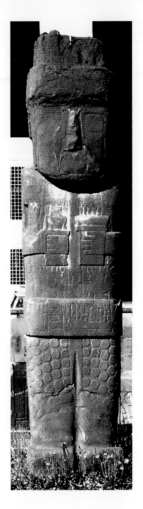

PLATE 37a. Bennett monolith, 5.5 m, Semisubterranean Temple, Tiwanaku, Bolivia. *Source:* Photo by Constantino M. Torres.

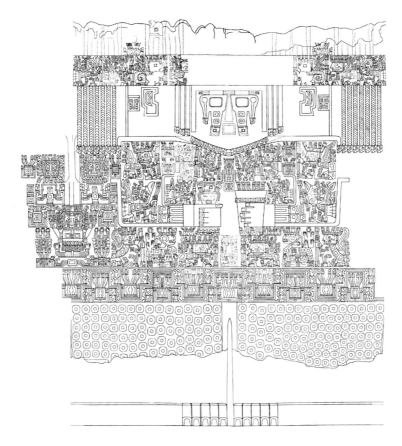

PLATE 37b. Rollout drawing of the Bennett monolith. *Source:* Adapted and revised after Posnansky 1945: Fig. 113a.

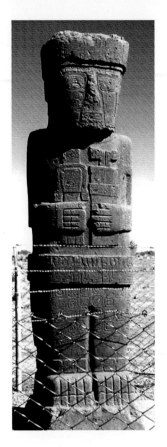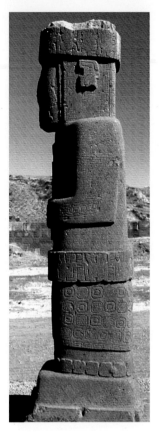

PLATE 38. Ponce monolith, 3.05 m, and details, central courtyard of the Kalasasaya, Tiwanaku, Bolivia. *Source:* Photo by Constantino M. Torres.

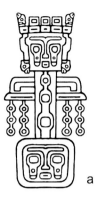

a

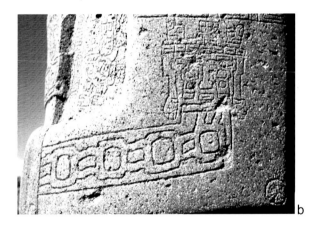

b

PLATE 39. (a) Chest pendant, detail, Bennett monolith. *Source:* Line drawing by Donna Torres. (b) Left arm, detail, Ponce monolith. *Source:* Photo by Constantino M. Torres.

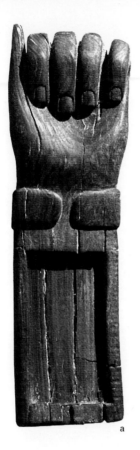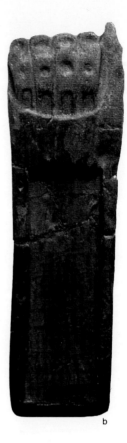

a   b

PLATE 40. Half-fist snuff trays: (a) Coyo Oriente, tomb 3974, wood, 15.7 cm, San Pedro de Atacama. *Source:* Instituto de Investigaciones Arqueológicas y Museo, Universidad Católica del Norte, San Pedro de Atacama, Chile. Reprinted with permission. (b) Niño Korin, Bolivia, 10.5 cm, Varldskulturmuseet (The Museum of World Culture), coll. # 70.19.33, Gothenburg, Sweden. *Source:* Photo by Constantino M. Torres.

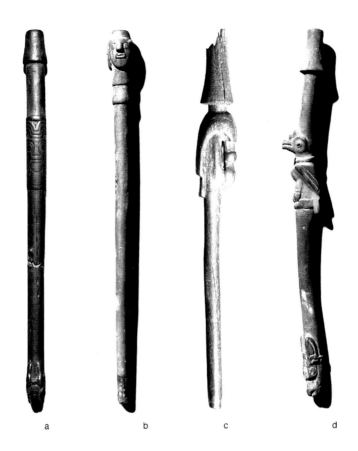

a   b   c   d

PLATE 41. Four wooden snuffing tubes: (a) Quitor 5, t. 1973, 21.9 cm; (b) Sequitor Alambrado Oriente, t. 1647, 21 cm; (c) Catarpe, 17.8 cm; (d) Solcor 3, tomb 50, 18.8 cm. *Source:* Instituto de Investigaciones Arqueológicas y Museo, Universidad Católica del Norte, San Pedro de Atacama, Chile. Reprinted with permission.

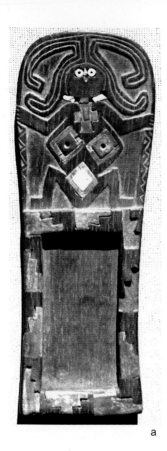 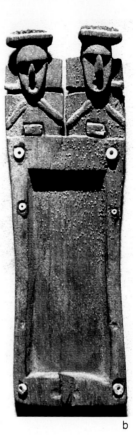

a b

PLATE 42. (a) Snuff tray with Heraldic Woman representation, wood with stone and wood inlays, 15.8 cm, San Pedro de Atacama, Chile (present location unknown). (b) Snuff tray with two anthropomorphic figures, San Pedro de Atacama. *Source:* Instituto de Investigaciones Arqueológicas y Museo, Universidad Católica del Norte, San Pedro de Atacama, Chile. Reprinted with permission.

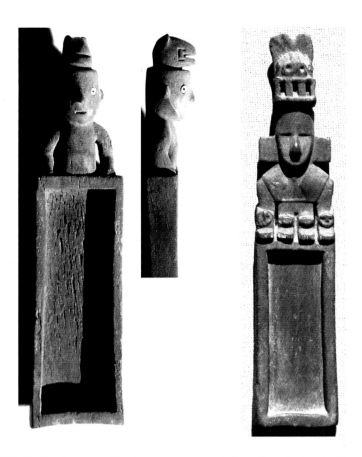

PLATE 43. Snuff trays with alter ego representation, San Pedro de Atacama.
Source: Instituto de Investigaciones Arqueológicas y Museo, Universidad Católica del Norte, San Pedro de Atacama, Chile. Reprinted with permission.

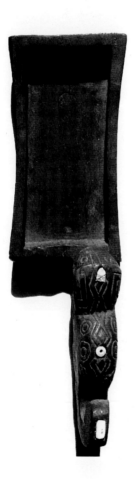
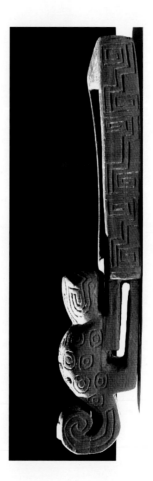

PLATE 44. Snuff tray with feline representation, wood, 18.7 cm, t. 2560, Quitor 5. *Source:* Instituto de Investigaciones Arqueológicas y Museo, Universidad Católica del Norte, San Pedro de Atacama, Chile. Reprinted with permission.

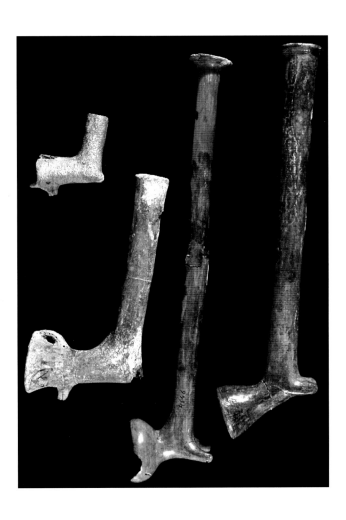

PLATE 45. Angular ceramic pipes, San Pedro de Atacama, Chile. Top to bottom: tomb 3817, Tchaputchayna, 6.9 × 7.5 cm h., coll. # 17105; tomb 4635, Toconao Oriente, 20.3 × 11.3 cm, coll. # 7308; tomb 4646, Toconao Oriente, 38.4 × 8.5 cm, coll. # 17107; tomb 4317, Toconao Oriente, 36.8 × 9.9 cm. *Source:* Photo courtesy of William Maguire. Instituto de Investigaciones Arqueológicas y Museo, Universidad Católica del Norte, San Pedro de Atacama, Chile. Reprinted with permission.

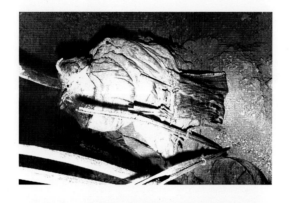

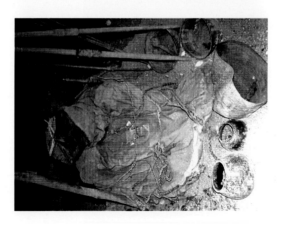

PLATE 46. Burial context, in situ, tomb 112, Solcor 3, San Pedro de Atacama, showing one of two snuffing kits found in this grave. *Source:* Instituto de Investigaciones Arqueológicas y Museo, Universidad Católica del Norte, San Pedro de Atacama, Chile. Reprinted with permission.

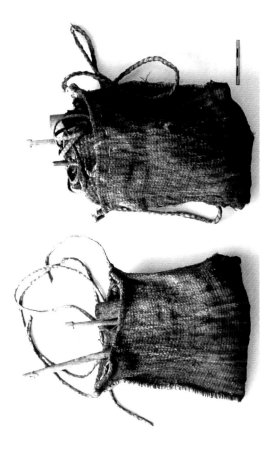

PLATE 47. Polychrome woolen bags containing snuffing kits, tomb 112, Solcor 3, San Pedro de Atacama. (left) 15.8 cm max. width, 15.9 cm max. height, coll. # 3901. (right) 15.4 cm max. width, 18.6 cm max. height, coll. # 3902. *Source:* Instituto de Investigaciones Arqueológicas y Museo, Universidad Católica del Norte, San Pedro de Atacama, Chile. Reprinted with permission.

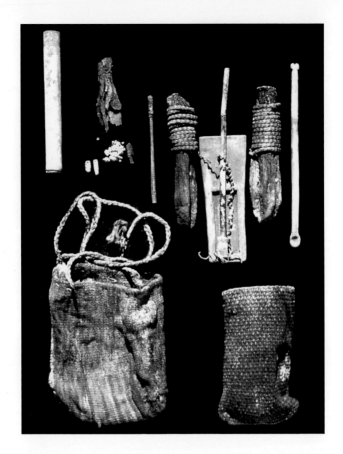

PLATE 48. Contents of bag # 3902, tomb 112, Solcor 3, San Pedro de Atacama. Leather pouches flanking the snuff tray contained the analyzed powders discussed in the text. *Source:* Instituto de Investigaciones Arqueológicas y Museo, Universidad Católica del Norte, San Pedro de Atacama, Chile. Reprinted with permission. Photo by Constantino M. Torres.

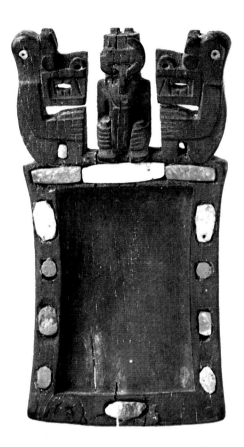

PLATE 49. Wooden snuff tray with stone inlays, 18 cm, Caspana, Chile. *Source:* Instituto de Investigaciones Arqueológicas y Museo, Universidad Católica del Norte, San Pedro de Atacama, Chile. Reprinted with permission.

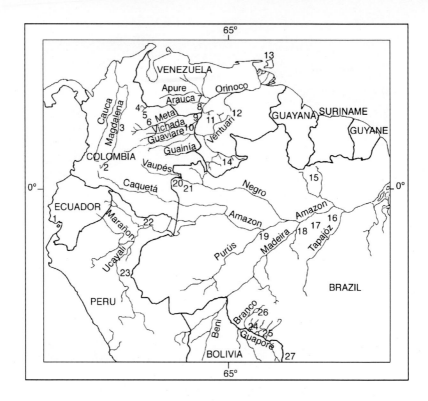

PLATE 50. Map of the northern Andes, Orinoquia and Amazonia, showing location of cultures discussed in the text. 1. San Marcos, Lower Colonche Valley, Ecuador. 2. San Agustín, upper Magadalena River, Colombia. 3. Muisca, middle Magdalena River, Colombia. 4. Tunebo, Arauca River, E. Colombia. 5. Airico, Meta Prov., Colombia. 6. Jirara, Meta Prov., Colombia. 7. Otomac, Venezuelan Llanos (between Orinoco, Apure, and Meta rivers). 8. Pumé, Arauca, Capanaparo, and Riecito rivers, Venezuela. 9. Cuiva-Guahibo, Meta, Apure, and Inirida rivers, Colombia. 10. Guahibo, Llanos Orientales, Colombia. 11. Piaroa, Ventuari, and Parguaza rivers, S. Venezuela. 12. Yecuaná, Upper Ventuari River, Venezuela. 13. Igneri, Trinidad. 14. Yanomamö (Waiká), Upper Orinoco, S. Venezuela, N. Brazil. 15. Kaxúyana (Cashuena), Cashorro River, tributary of Middle Trombetas, Brazil. 16. Maué, Tapajóz River, Brazil. 17. Mundurucú, lower Madeira and Tapajóz rivers, Brazil. 18. Mura, lower Madeira River, Brazil. 19. Catauixís (Katawishi), Purús River, Brazil. 20. Tuyuka, Tiquié River, Brazil. 21. Bará, Tiquié River, Brazil. 22. Omagua, mouth of the Napo River, Peru. 23. Piro, upper Ucayali River, Peru. 24. Arua, Rio Branco basin, Brazil. 25. Macurap, Rio Branco basin, Brazil. 26. Tupari, Rio Branco and Guaporé rivers, Brazil. 27. Bororo, upper Paraguay River, Matto Grosso, Brazil. *Source:* Map by Constantino M. Torres.

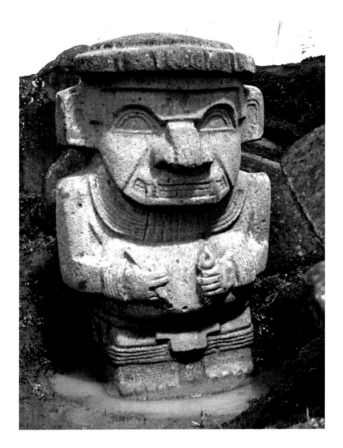

PLATE 51. Figure holding snail shell, 1.79 m, Mound 5, Alto de los Idolos, San Agustín, Colombia. *Source:* Photo by Constantino M. Torres.

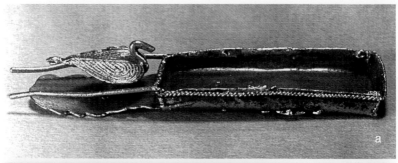

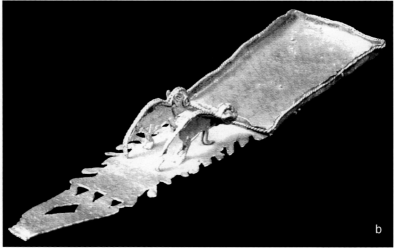

PLATE 52. Muisca gold snuff trays: (a) Vereda de Radamontal, Cogua, Cundinamarca, 6.1 cm, Museo del Oro, coll. # 8479, Banco de la República, Bogotá, Colombia. *Source:* Plazas and Falchetti 1979: Fig. 31. (b) Vereda El Roble, Gachancipá, Cundinamarca, 12.4 cm, Museo del Oro, coll. # 6784, Banco de la República, Bogotá, Colombia. *Source:* Torres 1994: 34. Reprinted with permission.

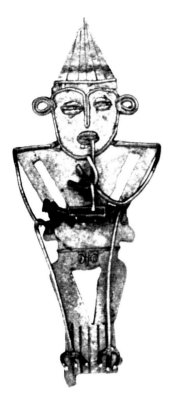
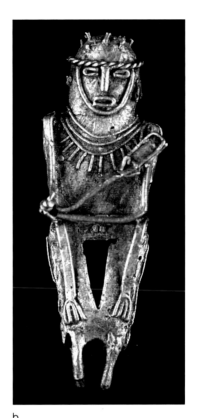

a   b

PLATE 53. *Tunjo* figurines holding snuff trays, gold and copper alloy *(tumbaga)*, Muisca, Colombia: (a) 7.8 cm. *Source:* Courtesy, National Museum of the American Indian, Smithsonian Institution (coll. # 13/1579), Washington, DC. Reprinted with permission. (b) Museo del Oro, Banco de la República, Bogotá, Colombia, coll. # 1867. *Source:* After Pérez de Barradas 1958, 2: Pl. 250. Reprinted with permission.

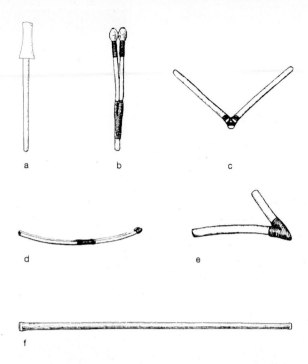

PLATE 54. Snuffing tube types: (a) Single-cylinder snuff tube for self-administration; (b) Y-shaped snuffing tubes for self-administration; (c) V-shaped snuffing tube, collaborative administration; (d) V-shaped snuffing tube for self-administration; (e) Double-parallel snuffing tube for self-administration; (f) Single-cylinder snuffing tube, collaborative administration. *Source:* Line drawings by Donna Torres.

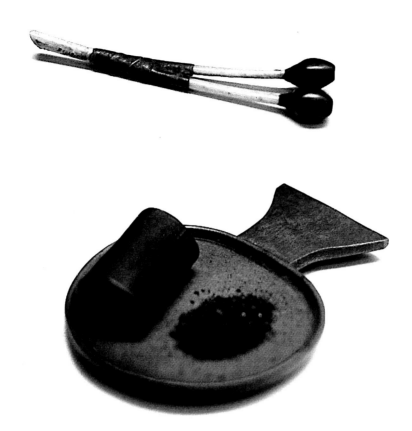

PLATE 55. Guahibo snuffing equipment, Meta and Vichada rivers, Colombia. Museo del Oro, Banco de la República, Bogotá. *Source:* Photo by Constantino M. Torres.

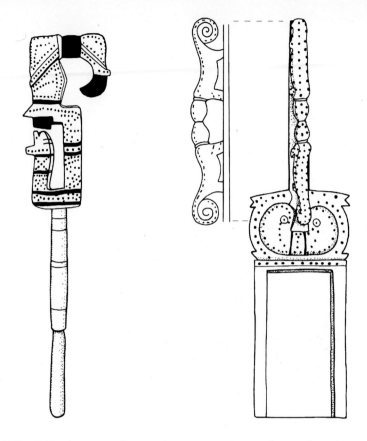

PLATE 56. Kaxúyana snuffing equipment: wooden snuff tray with avian and feline representations and staff with ophidian and avian representations. Franciscan Museum, Ipauarana, Paraíba State, Brazil. *Source:* After Wassén 1967a: Fig. 28.

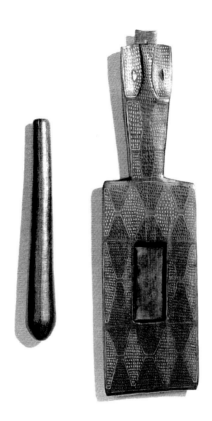

PLATE 57. Wooden snuff tray with reptilian representation, 37 cm, Maué, Brazil. Museum für Völkerkunde, Spix and Martius Collection, no. 534, Munich, Germany.

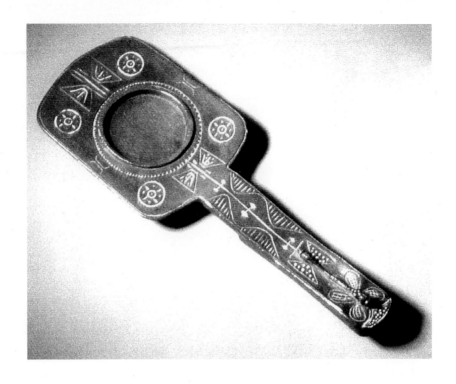

PLATE 58. Snuff tray with insect motifs, wood, 26 cm, Maué, Brazil. Kunsthistorisches Museum, Natterer Collection no. 1376, Vienna, Austria.

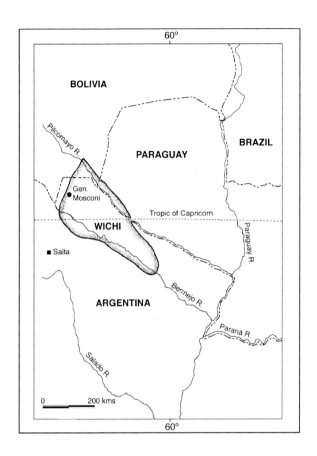

PLATE 59. Map of the Gran Chaco, showing location of Wichi territory. *Source:* Map by Constantino M. Torres.

Chapter 5

The Pharmacology of Bufotenine

Twelve indole alkaloids have been detected in the genus *Anadenanthera*. The distribution of these compounds in the various organs and vegetative parts of the plants is not uniform. Some are confined to the roots, bark, or leaves, others to the seed pods, still others to the seeds; many are found only in trace amounts (see Appendix). All 12 alkaloids have not been found in any single individual of any species of the genus. Although many of these compounds have exhibited biological activities in animals, this chapter reviews only the pharmacology of bufotenine, consistently detected as the major alkaloidal component of the seeds of every species in the genus, with a concentration ranging from 1 percent to over 12 percent of fresh weight. In most instances, *Anadenanthera* preparations used in traditional healing practices consist only of finely ground seeds. Occasionally, admixtures of other plants have been described and verified by chemical analysis. Other parts of *Anadenanthera* such as leaves or pods are rarely added to such preparations. Although DMT and 5-hydroxy-*N*-monomethyl-tryptamine also occur in these seeds, their concentrations are so low relative to bufotenine that it is unlikely they are of pharmacological significance in these preparations. One cannot overlook the possibility of synergism, however.

Pharmacological study of tryptamines occupies a large portion of the scientific literature, the study of bufotenine being third in rank, surpassed only by its parent compound, 5-hydroxytryptamine (serotonin) and its close analogue, DMT (*N,N*-dimethyltryptamine). This literature includes studies of the effects of bufotenine on organisms in both the plant and animal kingdoms, on isolated tissue systems, on natural and cloned neurotransmitter receptor systems, and on intact animals and primates, including human beings. Along with the last category, some of the more esoteric studies have included the effect of bufotenine on adenylate cyclase from liver flukes, sea urchin embryotoxicity, fish acetylcholinesterase activity, nerve cell action of the leech, tonic adductor activity in the clam, teratotoxicity of a planarian worm, egg-laying behavior in butterflies, brain activity in ants, fluid secretion of the Malpighian tubules of certain insects, and excitatory action on snail neurons. The controversy over the effect of bufotenine on human beings—cardiovascular toxin or psychoto-mimetic?—has occupied investigators for nearly 50 years. The advent of the phenomenon known as "toad smoking" or "toad licking" in the contemporary world has significantly broadened this debate. Another area of contention has been the possible role of bufotenine as an endogenous psychotoxin in certain disease states such as schizophrenia, childhood and adult autism, delusional paranoia, and sociopathic violence.

This chapter addresses the pharmacology of bufotenine under three broad (and often overlapping) categories: (1) whole animal research; (2) basic pharmacology, including receptor interactions and actions with other tissue preparations; and (3) human studies, including behavioral pharmacology. Within this framework, many of the previously mentioned studies are discussed.

WHOLE ANIMAL RESEARCH

Bufotenine was first isolated in pure form by Handovsky (1920) from extracts of the toad *Bufo vulgaris* L., hence its trivial name. The structure of bufotenine was determined by Wieland and co-workers (1934), who obtained 5.5 g of pure 3-[2-(dimethylamino)ethyl]-1H-indol-5-ol free base from extracts of the combined glandular secretions of 27,000 toads. Shortly thereafter, the structure of bufotenine was confirmed by synthesis (Hoshino and Shimodaira 1936). The identity of bufotenine with the alkaloid mappine first isolated from the *gelben Knollenblätterpilz, Amanita mappa* (Batsch. ex Lasch.) Quél. (*A. Citrina* Schaeff. ex S. F. Gray), was established by Wieland and Motzel (1953). This ubiquitous occurrence of bufotenine, especially the association with the highly toxic genera *Amanita* and *Bufo,* was to have an impact on its "perceived pharmacology" throughout the second half of the twentieth century.

Pharmacological studies of crude extracts of *Bufo* skin exudates began in the nineteenth century. Phisalix and Bertrand (1893) demonstrated that the host animal was not immune to the toxic effects of an injected dose of its own secretion. Within minutes of the injection of 1.0 milliliter of toad parotid-gland secretion, effects on the movement of the toads were observed. Within 15 minutes, the hind legs were completely paralyzed, breathing was shallow, heart activity was decreased, and pupils were dilated. It was concluded that the toads were not normally affected by the toxin because of compartmentalization within the glands. Since then, numerous investigations have demonstrated the presence of bufotenine (Erspamer et al. 1967) and related indolealklyamines (De Lima et al. 1991) as well as imidazole alkaloids (Roseghini, Erspamer, and Endean 1976; Roseghini, Endean, and Temperelli 1976; Roseghini et al. 1986), phenethylamines (Roseghini et al. 1986), cardioactive steroids (Wittliff 1968; Meyer 1966), and peptides, including a number of bradykinins (Roseghini et al. 1989) in nearly 300 amphibian species worldwide. Bufotenine has also been found as a constituent of viperid, crotalid, and elapid snake venoms (Welsh 1966). The antimicrobial activity of certain of these secretions has been partially related to the presence of bufotenine (Habermehl and Preusser 1970). Occurrence of bufotenine in amphibians is not confined to skin secretions. It is also present in the brain and retina of *Bufo bufo,* but neither in liver nor pancreas (Axelsson et al. 1971). Protection from predation due to toxicity may not be the only role played by these amphibian glandular secretions. The effects of bufotenine and related indoles on the skin pigmentation and blanching process and on the melanin granule aggregation of the frog *Rana tigrina* have also been studied (Bhattacharya et al. 1971).

Observations of gross pharmacological effects of crude snuff preparations and extracts of *Piptadenia peregrina* seeds on animal physiology began in the mid-twentieth century. Henker and Huston (1950) studied the effects of a hot water extract of the snuff *yopo.* Rats given an intraperitoneal injection of this extract displayed signs of central nervous system depression. Within 15 minutes of administration, rats were lethargic and unable to walk. An analgesic effect was measured by the rat "tail pinch" method. The same lethargy was noted upon administration to frogs, which was accompanied by a much reduced heart rate. Raymond-Hamet (1956) demonstrated the hypertensive and respiratory stimulant effects of a 10 percent aqueous extract of the seeds of *P. peregrina* (obtained from Fish, Johnson, and Horning 1955) on the chloralose-anesthetized dog. These effects were aug-

mented by pretreatment with adrenaline and antagonized by yohimbine. A crystalline picric acid salt (presumably bufotenine picrate)
isolated from the aqueous extract duplicated the pharmacological actions of the crude extract.

Granier-Doyeux (1965) reported on studies carried out in 1947 in
which *yopo* snuff was administered intranasally to rats and mice.
Along with gross behavioral effects, marked dyspnea (irregular breathing) and intense nasal irritation were noted: "As well as the signs of
drunkenness . . . the rats scratched themselves all over; they seemed to
be suffering from acute generalized itching, with slight multilocular
paresthesi" (Granier-Doyeux 1965: 32). Mice showed difficulty in
walking, and "dragged their bellies along the floor of the cage." Overall, the effects of the snuff were likened to "a state of drunkenness"
with a torpid condition and semilethargy noted in the later stages,
much as had been reported by Henker and Huston (1950).

The same observation of hind limb paralysis and ataxia was later
noted by Evarts et al. (1956) in monkeys. This study also commented
on the initial anesthesia following injection. Evarts suggested that
these effects were centrally mediated and related to a disorder of
proprioceptive sensation. In mice, intraperitoneal injection of an
aqueous extract of *Amanita citrina,* shown to contain bufotenine, serotonin, and 5-hydroxytryptophan, also decreased motility (Andary
et al. 1978). In the same study, the LD_{50} for intraperitoneal bufotenine was found to be 200 mg/kg.

A fairly detailed study of the effects of pure bufotenine and its quaternary derivative, bufotenidine, was reported by Alvares-Pereira et
al. (1963). Both compounds caused a marked rise in blood pressure
when administered to anesthetized dogs, bufotenidine being about
seven times more active than bufotenine. This hypertensive effect
was accompanied by an initial bradycardia followed by a dose-
dependent tachycardia. Lethal doses caused respiratory arrest. The
effects of these drugs appeared to be antagonized by both cholinergic
(atropine) and adrenergic (dibenzyline) blockade. Bufotenidine was
much more active in all experiments than bufotenine, exhibiting a cu-
rare-like action on an isolated rat diaphragm-phrenic nerve preparation (Alvares-Pereira et al. 1963).

Other researchers studying bufotenine noted the pressor effect in
anesthetized rats (Gessner et al. 1960), an antidiuretic effect in rats
and dogs (Franzen 1961), oxytocic effect in cats (Gessner et al.

1961), hyperthermia in rabbits (Jacob and Robert 1966), and a depressed patellar reflex (knee jerk) in cats (Weidmann and Cerletti 1959, 1960). These last two effects of substituted tryptamines were suggested to be related to psychotropic activity in humans (Cerletti et al. 1968; Brimblecombe 1967). In rats, bufotenine was found to produce a hypothermic effect that could be blocked by xylamidine (Winter 1972). A similar drop in body temperature was produced by intracerebral injection of bufotenine in mice and was not potentiated by noradrenaline (Ratcliffe 1971), suggesting that the drug acted by a centrally mediated adrenergic antagonism. Bufotenine was also shown to inhibit bronchospasms induced by serotonin-aerosol administration to guinea pigs (Courvoisier and Leau 1958), possibly indicating that the drug also had serotonin antagonist properties. Bufotenine and serotonin were shown to produce an increase in pulmonary perfusion as a result of pulmonary vasoconstriction in the dog (Hageman et al. 1973). The mechanism of this effect was said to be different from that of the known vasoconstrictors noradrenaline and histamine.

Electrophysiological experiments showed the similarity of bufotenine to the catecholamines in stimulating the reticular arousal system and depressing the mediothalamic system (Monnier et al. 1960). This effect was also shared by caffeine; similar experiments were performed using cats (Evarts et al. 1955). Electrophysiological recordings were made using electrodes implanted in three brain regions. Optic tract responses to light stimuli, lateral geniculate responses to electrical stimulation, and cortical responses to supramaximal electric shock to the geniculate radiation fibers were measured. Bufotenine and lysergic acid diethylamide (LSD) were found to decrease the postsynaptic spike in the geniculate but had no effect on the cortical response. LSD (but not bufotenine) reduced the response to retinal photic stimulation. Bufotenine, but not LSD, was also shown to produce a marked, but transitory, increase in blood pressure. At higher doses (10 mg/kg), bufotenine produced respiratory arrest. In similar experiments with rabbits, Himwich (1967) demonstrated that intravenous bufotenine in conjunction with intracarotid injection of the serotonin precursor 5-hydroxytryptophan produced a sustained alert pattern in seven brain regions after transection of the spinal cord at the first cervical segment.

In an extensive electrophysiological analysis of a number of psychoactive drugs measuring the transcephalic direct current potential in anesthetized rats, LSD, DMT, bufotenine, adrenochrome, and d-amphetamine were shown to increase frontal negativity in a dose-dependent manner (Cowen et al. 1973). Vasoactive substances such as serotonin and norepinephrine produced different effects. The conclusion was that these drugs produced this direct current effect by altering nucleic acid metabolism in the frontal cortex. The results compared favorably with voltage phenomena obtained from human beings after administration of hallucinogens, suggesting that such use produced either long-lasting or permanent changes in brain function. Other electrophysiological experiments (Bradley and Briggs 1974) suggested that bufotenine (and allied compounds) were 5-hydroxy-tryptamine (5-HT) antagonists rather than receptor agonists. Central 5-HT mechanisms were also invoked to explain the bufotenine-mediated decreases in ponto-geniculo-occipital waves in cats induced by the tryptophan hydroxylase inhibitor 4-chlorophenylalanine (Ruch-Monachon et al. 1976; Haefely et al. 1976).

A prolonged stimulation of prolactin secretion was observed following intracerebroventricular injection of bufotenine into the lateral ventricle of rats (Seeman and Brown 1985). The close structural congener 5-methoxy-DMT was found to be more active and DMT less active than bufotenine. That this was a central nervous system–mediated effect was demonstrated by the slower onset of prolactin release when the drugs were given by peripheral routes.

Many of these experiments and reports utilized the direct application of bufotenine to central nervous system regions. Other experiments had shown that peripherally administered bufotenine does not readily pass the blood-brain barrier (Sanders and Bush 1967; Takahashi et al. 1985) and that it is rapidly metabolized. Among the metabolites are 5-hydroxy-indoleacetic acid (rat, Ahlborg et al. 1968; human, Sanders-Bush et al. 1976) and bufotenine-O-glucuronide (rabbit, Vigdorchik et al. 1984). Urinary metabolites of DMT and bufotenine-O-methyl ether (5-methoxy-DMT) in the rat included significant quantities of their respective N-oxides (Sitaram, Lockett, Blackman, et al. 1987) as well as bufotenine and bufotenine glucuronide (Agurell et al. 1969). Incubation of 5-methoxy-DMT with rat liver, kidney, and brain tissue preparations has also been shown to produce bufotenine as one of the metabolites (Sitaram, Talomsin, et al. 1987; Sitaram, Lockett, McLeish, et al. 1987). Intraperitoneally injected bufotenine was found to pass the blood-brain barrier in rats pretreated with the MAO inhibitors pargyline or tranylcypromine (Narasimhachari et al. 1979). One study (Fuller et al. 1995) examined tissue distribution and metabolism of subcutaneously injected bufotenine in rats. After one hour the concentrations of bufotenine were highest in lungs and hearts while those in brains and livers were lower. The concentration and rate of metabolism of bufotenine in blood was similar to those in the heart. The half-life of bufotenine was about the same in all tissues studied, that is, two hours, with clearance from all tissues complete by about eight hours. Distribution differences of bufotenine across four different brain regions one hour postdose were found to be relatively small. The order of decreasing concentrations was found to be hypothalamus > brain stem > striatum > cortex. The major metabolite in all tissues was found to be 5-hydroxyindole-3-acetic acid arising by oxidative deamination. *N*-methylserotonin, which could arise by enzymatic mono *N*-demethylation of bufotenine, was not detected in any tissue after any dose. Pargyline pretreatment significantly reduced 5-hydroxyindole-3-acetic acid concentrations in all tissues suggesting a major role for MAO-A in the metabolism of bufotenine.

The low concentration of bufotenine in brains relative to hearts and lungs suggested that the drug did not easily cross the blood-brain barrier. Nevertheless, these authors noted some significant behavior changes in the studied rat population following bufotenine injection. The animals were slightly stimulated for 5 to 10 minutes and showed some "head searching":

> At 15-20 minutes, rats remained in the center of the cage in a flat posture and exhibited some ptosis, leg weakness, vasodilation, occasional head searching and sniffing. . . . At 60 minutes, rats were slightly depressed and showed some vasodilation and piloerection with little ptosis remaining. (Fuller et al. 1995: 801)

Such gross behavioral changes induced in animals by drugs like bufotenine have been studied extensively. Disruption of trained behavior induced by bufotenine has been taken as a measure of its central activity. Mahler and Humoller (1959) showed that bufotenine and LSD were effective in prolonging the climbing time of rats trained to climb a pole. This effect was said to be inhibited when brain levels of serotonin were altered by pretreatment with 5-hydroxytryptophan and potentiated by pretreatment with reserpine and iproniazid. Using rats in a conditioned-avoidance response (CAR) experiment, Gessner and Page (1962) demonstrated that bufotenine and DMT were less active than 5-methoxy-DMT and LSD. This observation, along with the assumption that abnormal *O*- and *N*-methylating enzymes might be present in mammals, prompted these investigators to suggest that abnormal tryptophan metabolism could result in mental disturbance. This study was further refined and expanded with a statistically significant CAR study of a number of variously substituted tryptamines, including a supposed "prodrug" of bufotenine, 5-acetoxy-*N,N*-dimethyltryptamine (Gessner et al. 1968). A dose-response curve for this compound was established and showed an effect significantly different from saline even at 5 micromoles/kg.

Glennon and colleagues (1979) studied the effects of a series of bufotenine esters including the acetate on the 5-HT receptors in rat stomach fundus strip preparation (Vane 1959). The ability of these esters to inhibit the 5-HT-induced contraction of the strip was taken as a measurement of receptor affinity. The order of potency (pA_2 values) was acetate > pivalate = bufotenine = isobutyrate > *n*-butyrate > propionate > 5-methoxy-DMT > DMT. The pivalate ester was said to be about one-fifth as active as 5-methoxy-DMT in a rat discriminative stimulus assay, although the former had about a half-log order more potency at the fundus strip. All of the esters had a higher chloroform-pH 7.4 buffer partition coefficient exhibiting from 40 to 300 times more lipid solubility than bufotenine, suggesting easy central nervous system (CNS) penetration from peripheral administration.

Using a type of CAR known as the swim maze, it was demonstrated that bufotenine was much less active than 5-methoxy-DMT in prolonging the swim time of trained rats. However, both drugs equally antagonized the reserpine-induced decrease in motor activity. Bufotenine was significantly less toxic than the other drugs studied, showing an LD_{50} of 290 mg/kg in mice (Ho et al. 1970).

The effects of bufotenine (and LSD) on nonhuman primates has been previously documented (Evarts et al. 1956). Studying maximally effective doses of both drugs on nine observable behavioral parameters, Evarts concluded that they share a syndrome characterized by "gross sensory disorder in the absence of a clear defect in muscle power, and by a marked degree of tameness" (Evarts et al. 1956: 51). The only observable difference between the two drugs was that bufotenine produced a hyperactivity in deep tendon reflexes of 15 minutes duration, commencing about one minute after injection.

Geyer and co-workers (1975) compared the effects of intraventricularly infused (thus avoiding the complications of the blood-brain barrier) serotonin and bufotenine on the air-puff-induced startle response in rats. This type of experiment was said to be useful in assessing such phenomena as reactivity, sensitization, and habituation. Serotonin was found to reduce and bufotenine to increase the magnitude of the response in a statistically significant manner. The effects of bufotenine were similar to those elicited by LSD and DMT, suggesting that all three activated a septal-hippocampal serotonergic system involving a decrease in the firing rate of serotonergic raphe cells. This further suggested a functional antagonism between bufotenine and serotonin in these systems.

Dose-dependent myoclonic jerking in guinea pigs induced by bufotenine and other tryptamines was shown to be of central origin (Luscombe et al. 1982, 1984). This effect was suggested to result from stimulation of an indole-selective brainstem 5-HT receptor (called the 5-HT_1 receptor), since the nonindolic 5-HT agonist quipazine failed to elicit the response. Bradley and Briggs (1974) had previously shown that bufotenine antagonized the excitatory action of 5-HT upon the lower brainstem by a non-receptor-mediated event. Bufotenine has also been shown to produce an increase in motor response in young chickens (Rauzzino and Seifter 1967; Mandell and Spooner 1969), a species said to be exquisitely sensitive to CNS stimulants (Dewhurst and Marley 1965).

Other behavioral effects of bufotenine elicited in animals, such as an influence on feeding in rats (Uluitu et al. 1976), gait and postural effects in rats (Nir et al. 1974), and anxiogenesis (Bhattacharya et al. 1996; Spencer and Traber 1987) have been correlated with binding potencies at specific serotonin (5-HT) receptor subtypes, such as 5-HT_{1A} and 5-HT_2 (Spencer et al. 1987). Reduced aggression was an interesting effect of bufotenine on mice (Kostowski et al. 1972). Among the indoles studied, only ibogaine increased muricidal (rat murder) activity. Similar results were reported in a study of stress-induced behavior in rats (Winocur et al. 1971). We address this topic further in the discussion of tryptamines and mental illness. An indirect sympathomimetic effect of bufotenine on rabbit heart (Fozard et al. 1978) was said to be mediated by a 5-HT receptor. Although both bufotenine and serotonin (5-HT) were found to be powerful stimulants of rate and force of cardiac contraction, the former was found to be more potent in causing atrial and ventricular tension. Bufotenine was also found to activate cholinergic nerves in guinea pig ileum (Fozard and Mobarok 1976a, 1976b).

Most of these studies encompass classic pharmacology. In a broad sense, the goals of such work are threefold: (1) to understand the mechanisms by which drugs exert their effects, (2) to determine how natural processes in animals (including humans) are effected and controlled, and (3) to use this knowledge to develop medicinal agents to treat said processes when they become abnormal. Although much can be learned from whole animal studies from the observation of cause and effect of drug action, the finer tuning of experimental design might lead to a corresponding increase in the understanding of drug action on the molecular level. The evolution of receptor theory attempts to address this finer understanding.

BASIC PHARMACOLOGY

The receptor theory of drug action arose just before and during the turn of the twentieth century from the notion that the actions of any given drug upon a biological system were a function of its chemical constitution (Crum Brown and Fraser 1889). In its simplest form, receptor theory can be expressed as the "key and lock" hypothesis. For any given drug (the key) to exert an action, it must fit into a specific area (the lock) on, in, or near a cellular structure such as an enzyme. This defines a receptor as a macromolecular "pocket," the stimulation of which with an extracellular chemical messenger will elicit a specific cellular response.

During the first half of the twentieth century, the study of pharmacology underwent a series of evolutionary changes. Progress toward an understanding of drug action in molecular terms led Langley (1905) to propose a "specific receptive substance" in biological systems with which drug molecules were supposed to react. Erlich further refined this idea with the concept of structural complementarity between receptor and drug molecules in which the former were considered to be "small, structurally discrete areas from which a biological response emanated following interaction with a complementary foreign molecule" (Bloom 1970: 108).

Clark (1937) was the first to use a mathematical description of the quantitative nature of drug-receptor interaction. This interaction was seen as a consequence of mass action between drug and receptor, that is, that one drug molecule occupies one receptor and that "the drug is present in sufficient excess so that its concentration remains effectively unchanged during complex formation" (Bloom 1970: 109). This treatment, known as *occupancy theory* (Ariens 1954), defined *agonists* as drugs with high intrinsic activity, that is, with the ability to readily produce the observed biological responses. *Antagonists* were seen to be drugs that bind strongly to receptors but are devoid of activity. This apparent difference between drugs that supposedly could occupy the same receptor can be explained by *rate theory* (Paton 1967), in which agonists are defined as drugs in which the rates of association and dissociation with the receptor complex are fast and in which drug action takes place as a series of impulses within a discrete period of time. Antagonists differ in that their rate of associations with the receptors are fast, dissociations being slow (Korolkovas 1970).

Further refinements of receptor theory have included the idea that receptors are not rigid entities but rather flexible protein biopolymers that can undergo conformational changes as a result of drug interactions (Belleau 1964). Agonists are seen as molecules that can, for example, transform a receptor on an enzyme from a resting state to one in which the enzyme becomes active. Antagonists are said to bind to this site in such a way that a conformationally inactive state results, inhibiting the role of the enzyme. Such a concept presumes that these receptor sites can (and do) interact not only with exogenously applied drugs but also with bioactive molecules produced by the organism itself. Indeed, modern receptor nomenclature is often based upon the names of known natural transmitter substances such as the alpha- and beta-adrenoceptors (adrenaline), cholinergic receptors (acetylcholine), and the 5-HT receptors (5-hydroxytryptamine, serotonin).

The nature of the physicochemical interactions between receptors and either natural transmitter substances or exogenous drugs is beyond the scope of this work. The reader is referred to works such as that of Korolkovas (1970). However, the measurement of this interaction is the major goal of radioligand binding experiments (Williams and Lefkowitz 1979). In the laboratory, these experiments are carried out by incubating a receptor-containing tissue preparation with a solution of radiolabeled drug and subsequent separation and quantitation of bound versus unbound radioactive material. Radioligands of high receptor specificity can also be used in competitive binding experiments in the following way. A constant concentration of radioligand is incubated along with varying concentrations of unlabeled drugs under equilibrium binding conditions. Measurement of the resulting bound radioactivity results in the quantitative determination of binding affinity for the series of test drugs. A direct correlation for antagonists can be obtained in this way, and agonists can be determined via so-called functional assays, in which changes in receptor-mediated cell function are measured.

Serotonin (5-HT) has been called an ancient neurotransmitter (Hartig 1997). It is released from fiber tracts originating in primitive brainstem regions. It has been found in ancient species such as *Drosophila* (fruit fly) and *Aplysia,* and phylogenetic comparisons suggest the earliest 5-HT receptors may have appeared 700 million years ago (Peroutka 1994). Serotonergic involvement in a wide range of CNS functions such as thermo- and motorregulation, pain, appetite, sleep, sexual function, aggression, mood, anxiety, and neuronal development (Keane and Soubrie 1997) has been reported. The role of serotonin and 5-HT receptors in the mechanism of action of hallucinogenic drugs has been the subject of intense and wide-ranging study since the discovery that LSD antagonized the effects of serotonin on smooth muscle (Wooley and Shaw 1954).

Gaddum (1953; Gaddum and Picarelli 1957) was the first to demonstrate the existence of two separate types of 5-HT receptors in guinea pig ileum preparations. The first was called the D receptor because contraction of the strip induced by application of 5-HT was blocked by dibenzyline. The so-called M receptor was blocked by morphine. Other drugs that antagonized the effects of 5-HT on the D receptors included LSD, dihydroergotamine, and 5-benzyloxygramine. These substances also were found to antagonize the effects of 5-HT on rat uterus and rabbit ear preparations, suggesting that the D receptors were on smooth muscle. Drugs that blocked M receptors such as cocaine, atropine, and methadone indicated that it was associated with nerve ganglia or other nerve fibers.

Currently, seven families and at least 14 subtypes of 5-HT receptors have been classified (Hoyer et al. 1994; Hartig 1997). These receptor families are defined by binding and effector-coupling properties. The 5-HT group includes both ligand-gated receptors (5-HT$_3$) and G protein-coupled receptors. The latter category consists of three classes, depending on the second messenger system to which the receptor is coupled. The 5-HT$_2$ subfamily is coupled to the activation of phospholipase C, whereas the 5-HT$_1$ family interacts negatively with adenylate cyclase, and the 5-HT$_4$, 5-HT$_6$, and 5-HT$_7$ families interact positively with adenylate cylase (Choi et al. 1994). Some of the 5-HT receptors are specific to certain animal species; others are ubiquitous. Many 5-HT receptors are found in both the peripheral and the central nervous system, some in specific brain regions. The distribution of 5-HT receptors in rat brain has been reviewed (Mengod et al. 1997). Other receptors, such as 5-HT$_{2B}$, occur in both humans and rodents, although their absolute identity has not been established. They are said to exhibit about 90 percent homology. Receptor nomenclature is just as fluid and subject to revision as is botanical nomenclature. Synonymy is also an important consideration in both disciplines. For example, 5-HT$_{1C}$ appears identical with 5-HT$_{2C}$.

It is known that many serotonergic neuronal cell bodies are clustered in the raphe nuclei and that the processes of these neurons are highly branched, that is, the 5-HT neurons of the raphe innervate all brain structures. This distribution means that neuromodulation can be exerted over widespread cerebral areas. The differential CNS regional distribution of 5-HT$_1$ subtypes was measured using autoradiography (Boulenguez et al. 1991). In this study, bufotenine was found to have a higher affinity for the 5-HT$_{1A}$ sites in the dentate gyrus than for the 5-HT$_{1B}$ sites in the substantia nigra, both anatomical regions in the mesencephalon. The authors suggested that specific ligands "could be of great interest for the study of both localization of the subtypes at the electron microscope level and of the behavioral implications of 5-HT" (Boulenguez et al. 1991: 97). Rats have been shown to exhibit stereotypic behavior upon administration of agents known to affect 5-HT receptors, specifically mescaline and certain methoxylated amphetamines (Kulkarni 1973).

A number of symptoms in this "5-HT syndrome" can be ascribed to selective activation of certain 5-HT subtypes. For example, in rats, activation of 5-HT$_{1A}$ results in the appearance of lower lip retraction; activation of 5-HT$_{1C}$ results in penile erection; and activation of 5-HT$_2$ produces "head shakes" (Berendsen et al. 1989). Subcutaneous injections of bufotenine (and 5-methoxytryptamine) were shown to induce hind limb scratching in rats (Berendsen and Broekkamp 1991). This effect was attributed to specific activation of a peripheral 5-HT$_{1D}$ (or a 5-HT$_{1D}$-like) receptor. A series of experiments with other centrally active 5-HT agents ruled out the involvement of 5-HT$_{1A}$ B-Hydroxy-*N*, *N-dipropyl-2-aminotetralin (DPAT) and 5-HT$_{1C}$/5-HT$_2$* (2,5-Dimethoxy-4-iodoamphetamine [DOI] and quipazine). The conclusion was that bufotenine and other tryptamines were acting as peripheral 5-HT$_{1D}$ agonists.

In a study of the pharmacological differentiation of 5-HT receptor subtypes, Eglen and collegues (1992) demonstrated the utility of 15 tryptamine agonists in delineating the presence of specific 5-HT receptor subtypes in five different tissue preparations. Bufotenine (but not 5-methoxy-DMT) was found to have agonist properties at the 5-HT$_4$ receptor in both guinea pig ileum and rat esophagus. However, bufotenine was shown to have little selectivity between 5-HT$_1$-like (canine saphenous vein), 5-HT$_2$ (rabbit aorta), or 5-HT$_4$ receptor subtypes. Bufotenine did exhibit somewhat selective agonist activity at 5-HT$_3$ (guinea pig ileum) sites.

McKenna and colleagues (1990) conducted radioligand competition binding studies with 21 variously substituted tryptamines. Three 5-HT receptor subtypes were investigated: 5-HT$_{1A}$ from rat cortex (labeled with tritiated DPAT), 5-HT$_{2A}$ from rat cortex (labeled with ^{125}iodine-DOI), and 5-HT$_{2B}$ from bovine cortex (labeled with tritiated ketanserin). Bufotenine and psilocin were found to be equipotent at 5-HT$_{2A}$ sites (bufotenine, IC$_{50}$ = 3.5 nM), but the former displayed about a hundred times more potency than the latter at the 5-HT$_{1A}$ receptor (bufotenine, IC$_{50}$ = 4.9 nM; psilocin, IC$_{50}$ = 190 nM). All of the compounds studied exhibited much less activity at the 5-HT$_{2B}$ receptor (bufotenine, IC$_{50}$ = 370 nM).

A study of possible heterogeneity of rat and human cortical 5-HT$_2$ receptors suggested that differential binding of bufotenine and psilocin (4-hydroxy-DMT) could be explained by the difference in amino acid residue number 242 in transmembrane domain 5, serine being present in human 5-HT$_2$ and alanine in rat 5-HT$_2$ receptors (Gallaher et al. 1993). Psilocin was found to have a much higher specific affinity for human (Ki 340 nM) versus rat (Ki 5100 nM) 5-HT$_2$, while bufotenine had Ki 300 nM (human) versus 520 nM (rat; tritiated ketanserin as ligand).

The $5\text{-}HT_2$ receptor family has been shown to be of importance in a wide variety of central and peripheral functions of serotonin. Central nervous system effects include mediation of visionary effects of LSD and related amphetamines and neuronal sensitization to tactile stimuli. Cardiovascular effects include change in platelet shape and contraction of blood vessels. The pharmacological characterization of a human liver $5\text{-}HT_{2B}$ receptor transfected in COS-1 cells was investigated by Choi et al. (1994). This particular receptor was also found to be expressed in human lungs and hearts and was thought to be useful for investigating cardiovascular pharmacology in therapeutic drug development. Pharmacologically, there was a strong correlation between this receptor and rat $5\text{-}HT_{2B}$, although agonist affinities correlated almost as well with mouse $5\text{-}HT_{2B}$ and human $5\text{-}HT_{1D}$. Comparison of rat, human, and mouse $5\text{-}HT_{2B}$ receptor protein sequences showed little homology. In this preparation, bufotenine was found to be an antagonist in competitive binding experiments against radiolabeled DOI (4-iodo-2,5,-dimethoxy amphetamine). The authors concluded by stating:

> The implications of this work for drug design are profound: the same receptor protein in various mammalian species differ so greatly in expression sites and in pharmacological properties that a particular non-human receptor may be of very little value in the design of human therapeutic agents. (Choi et al. 1994: 398)

A study of the ability of $5\text{-}HT_3$ agonists to modulate the release of serotonin from superfused rat spinal cord synaptosomes found that bufotenine was capable of increasing basal neurotransmitter (5-HT) efflux (Monroe et al. 1994). This release was found to be calcium ion independent, indicating that this action of bufotenine was not receptor mediated. Bufotenine was also found to compete for sites labeled with tritiated citalopram, a known 5-HT uptake inhibitor. The evidence suggested that bufotenine was acting directly on the 5-HT neuronal membrane transport carrier. Thus, bufotenine gains access to the nerve terminal by mimicking 5-HT at the active transporter. The authors commented, "The ability of bufotenine to inhibit the carrier mediated uptake of 5-HT into the neuron, while in the same concentration range promote carrier mediated release of 5-HT out of the neuron, may appear paradoxical" (Monroe et al. 1994: 281). The paradox was explained by invoking the fact that the transport carrier is partially driven by the concentration gradient across the membrane. Since bufotenine disrupts 5-HT storage, a cytosolic concentration is produced that is sufficient to promote 5-HT efflux.

The implication that the 5-HT_4 receptor subtype mediates tachycardia was explored in the piglet isolated right atrium (Medhurst and Kaumann 1993). A number of tryptamines, including bufotenine, were found to act as partial agonists at the piglet sinoatrial 5-HT_4 receptor. The log of the concentration necessary to produce 50 percent of the maximum increase in heart rate for bufotenine was found to be 5.95, slightly higher than that for 5-methoxy-DMT (4.69) and slightly lower than for 5-HT itself (7.13). The authors concluded that the pharmacological profile for the piglet heart 5-HT_4 receptor compared favorably with results from other 5-HT_4 preparations from rat esophagus, guinea pig ileum and colon, mouse embryonic colliculi neurones, and human atrium.

Treatment of migraine with selective 5-HT_{1D} agonists derived from *N,N*-dialkyltryptamines (such as sumatriptan, 5-methylaminosulfonylmethyl-DMT) has added another dimension to the medicinal and pharmacological study of tryptamines (Humphrey 1991). Although the precise mechanisms are unclear, both neuronal and vascular hypotheses have been advanced to account for the pathophysiology of migraine (Ferrari and Saxena 1995). Studies have shown that 5-HT_{1D} receptor agonists constrict the large cerebral arteries during attacks, thus decreasing blood flow in these vessels. Nonselective 5-HT agonists such as ergotamine have been used to treat migraine, but agonist potency at 5-HT_{2A} receptors leading to coronary vasoconstriction and a host of undesirable side effects, including a rise in blood pressure, have limited their utility. A study (Glen et al. 1995) of potential new antimigraine drugs ("hemicranolytics," Muehldorf and Repke, personal communication, 1997) included bufotenine in a 5-HT agonist assay. The selectivity of bufotenine for the 5-HT_{1D} over the 5-HT_{2A} receptor was marginal, with $p[A_{50}]$s (a measure of agonist potency; large numbers are better) of 7.3 and 6.8, respectively.

The trifluoromethylsulfonyl ester of bufotenine (bufotenine triflate) and a homologous series of *N,N*-dialkyl analogs were studied as possible antimigraine drugs (Barf et al. 1996). Although all of the triflate esters examined displayed agonist affinities for 5-HT_{1D} receptors, the dimethyl analog exhibited a 10- to 12-fold preference for cloned 5-

$HT_{1D\alpha}$ versus $5\text{-}HT_{1D\beta}$ subtypes. These compounds also showed a substantial affinity for the $5\text{-}HT_{1A}$ receptor in an in vitro assay, although an in vivo study of the dimethyl analog in the rat failed to demonstrate a change in the turnover rate for 5-HT, an effect said to be mediated by central $5\text{-}HT_{1A}$ receptors. However, in the guinea pig, bufotenine triflate did show a pronounced decrease in central 5-HT accumulation after systemic doses, indicating good CNS penetration. Unlike sumatriptan, bufotenine triflate also caused a significant hypothermia in the guinea pig, a response attributed to central $5\text{-}HT_{1D}$ receptors. It was also shown to produce small decreases in heart rate (bradycardia) and arterial blood pressure in the pig. These effects were said to be mediated by central $5\text{-}HT_{1A}$ and $5\text{-}HT_{1D}$ mechanisms. Its possible utility in the treatment of migraine was demonstrated by its ability to constrict porcine carotid arteriovenous anastomoses (Saxena et al. 1996).

The receptor binding profile of alnitidan, a nonindolic antimigraine drug, at 14 native and cloned 5-HT receptors has been documented. In this thorough study, binding affinities for 12 indolic 5-HT agonists including bufotenine at a native $5\text{-}HT_{1D}$ (calf substantia nigra) and two cloned human ($5\text{-}HT_{1D\alpha}$ and $5\text{-}HT_{1D\beta}$) receptors (against tritiated 5-HT) were also reported. Bufotenine did not show selectivity between the native and cloned subtypes. However, the equilibrium inhibition binding constant in the substantia nigra preparation showed an eight-fold higher activity for bufotenine over DMT. Interestingly, D-lysergic acid had about the same binding affinity as alnitidan in all three binding assays (Leysen et al. 1996).

The human $5\text{-}HT_{1D}$ receptor is complex partly because it is encoded by a subfamily of two distinct genes located on different chromosomes, which also show a selective tissue distribution (Jin et al. 1992; Peroutka and Howell 1994). A certain amount of confusion with regard to the nomenclature of the $5\text{-}HT_{1D}$ complex also exists. The $5\text{-}HT_{1D}$ receptor is synonymous with $5\text{-}HT_{1D\alpha}$, and $5\text{-}HT_{1D\beta}$ is also designated as $5\text{-}HT_{1B}$. However, human $5\text{-}HT_{1D}$ and $5\text{-}HT_{1B}$ receptor subtypes are distinct molecular entities that mediate serotonergic neurotransmission, although the precise function of each remains to be defined. Pharmacological study is further complicated since rodents have a $5\text{-}HT_{1B}$ receptor distinct from the human receptor. Human $5\text{-}HT_{1D}$ receptors are highly expressed in brain raphe nuclei and $5\text{-}HT_{1B}$ in striatum, suggesting distinct functional roles for each. Some investigators believe it is the 5-HT_{1B} receptor that is responsible for the contractile response of human cerebral arteries, although the target for antimigraine drugs has been the 5-HT_{1D} subtype. Others think the two subtypes can be distinguished pharmacologically only if both the receptor-binding affinities and functional activities of a series of compounds are taken into account (Pauwels et al. 1996). Comparison of intrinsic agonist activities and corresponding binding affinities at cloned human 5-HT_{1D} and 5-HT_{1B} receptors along with the measurement of inhibition of forskolin-stimulated cyclic adenosine monophosphate (cAMP) formation provided evidence that supported a distinct pharmacology for the two subtypes. Bufotenine was shown to be a nonselective efficacious agonist, that is, one with agonist potency close to its binding affinity. At both receptor subtypes, bufotenine showed a binding affinity (as measured by the equilibrium concentrations for inhibition of tritiated 5-carboxamidotryptamine) three times higher than tryptamine and equipotent with the antimigraine drug sumatriptan.

Jakab and Goldman-Rakic (1998) studied the cellular and subcellular distribution of 5-HT_{2A} receptors in the cerebral cortex of the macaque monkey. Using both light and electron microscopy and immunocytochemical techniques, these receptors were detected in all five layers of the cortex. The majority of intensely stained (i.e., regions of high receptor density) areas were associated with pyramidal neurons. This suggested that the "apical dendritic field proximal to the pyramidal cell soma" is the "hot spot" for 5-HT_{2A} receptor-mediated actions relevant to normal and psychotic functional states (Jakab and Goldman-Rakic 1998: 739). The 5-HT_{2A} receptor density was found to predominate over 5-HT_{2B} and 5-HT_{2C} receptors in the cortex. The authors suggested that "the gating mechanisms of apical dendritic ion channels may be dysfunctional in psychotic behavior states occurring in the acute 'positive' phase of schizophrenia or induced by 5-HT_{2A} agonist drugs" (Jakab and Goldman-Rakic 1998: 739).

Krebs-Thomson, Paulus, and Geyer (1998) studied the influence of 5-HT_{2A} and 5-HT_{2C} receptors on locomotor and investigatory activity in rats. Pretreatment of the test animals with 5-HT antagonists specific for each receptor subtype demonstrated that for certain hallucinogens such as DOI, only contributions from 5-HT_{2A} receptors were important, while for LSD, both 5-HT_{2A} and 5-HT_{2C} receptor interactions accounted for behavioral effects. In addition, a significant contribution from 5-HT_{1A} receptors was found to be involved in the locomotor activity induced by LSD.

Competition-binding experiments were conducted using either tritiated LSD or tritiated serotonin as radioligand as part of a study of binding affinity, agonistic potency, and efficacy of a series of ligands at the cloned 5-HT_6 receptor derived from rat striatum (Boess et al. 1997). Agonist efficacy was determined by measurement of cAMP accumulation in a cell preparation using the HEK293 cell line. Several important experimental variables were examined. Binding affinities for the tryptamines studied were significantly higher (tenfold) than for other drugs when $[^3\text{H}]$-5-HT was used as ligand. Bufotenine exhibited one of the highest affinities, with a pK_i (negative log of the inhibitory concentration) of 8.35. By contrast, against $[^3\text{H}]$-LSD, the pK_i for bufotenine was 6.95. Several explanations of these results were offered. High-affinity ligands such as LSD and 5-HT may exhibit differences in their mode of interaction with some receptors; for example, at the 5-HT_6 receptor, LSD acts as partial agonist. Temperature differences between these two binding assays may also have played a role. The $[^3\text{H}]$-5-HT studies were conducted at $4°$ instead of the usual $37°$ to improve the signal-to-noise ratio. It was suggested that a lower temperature-stabilized receptor conformation might lead either to higher affinity for certain classes of compounds or lower affinity for the radioligand used. The rank order of agonist potency in the stimulation of cAMP formation for the tryptamines studied was N-monomethyl-5-hydroxytryptamine > bufotenine = 5-methoxytryptamine > 5-HT > tryptamine. Overall results suggested that a 5-hydroxyl group was necessary for full agonist activity at this 5-HT_6 receptor preparation. The 5-HT_6 receptor has also been found in humans, and other evidence suggests its presence in a mouse neuroblastoma cell line, mouse embryonic striatal neurons, and pig caudate membranes. More recent research suggests that the 5-HT_6 receptor may be of importance in memory and cognition function, an area of interest in Alzheimer's disease (Russell and Dias 2002).

Site-directed mutagenesis of cloned and expressed human 5-HT_{2A} and 5-HT_{2C} receptors were used in an attempt to differentiate receptor selectivities for a series of psychoactive and nonpsychoactive serotonergic agents, including bufotenine (Almaula et al. 1996). If it is assumed that the initial actions of such drugs occur at the level of receptor interaction, then their receptor selectivities in humans may play an important role. However, the demonstration that human potency of known psychoactive drugs correlates with binding affinities for rat brain 5-HT$_{2A}$ (Glennon et al. 1984) should not be taken to indicate a definitive role for the same receptor in humans. We have already seen that significant differences in ligand affinities exist between rat and human 5-HT$_{2A}$ receptors. A single amino acid difference between the two receptors has been shown to account for significant pharmacological differences (Johnson et al. 1994). Similarly, human 5-HT$_{2A}$ and 5-HT$_{2C}$ receptors also differ by a single amino acid residue, serine in the former and alanine in the latter in transmembrane domain 5. In theory, exchange mutations at this point in each receptor could allow the measurement of differential effects of the mutations on affinity and selectivity of a series of ligands. The nonpsychoactive compound mesulergine showed a higher affinity for wild-type (nonmutated) 5-HT$_{2C}$ than for wild-type 5-HT$_{2A}$ or mutant 5-HT$_{2C}$. The opposite was seen for LSD, with higher affinity for wild-type 5-HT$_{2A}$ and the mutant 5-HT$_{2C}$. By contrast, neither bufotenine nor psilocin showed any significant selectivity or affinity differences between the wild strains of either receptor. Bufotenine and psilocin did show significant decreases in affinities for mutant 5-HT$_{2A}$ receptors. DOI showed higher affinity for both wild-type receptors and a decrease in affinity for both mutant strains. The goal of this study to determine the role of the point mutation locus in the selectivity of 5-HT hallucinogens was only partially met. Of the known psychoactive drugs studied, bufotenine, psilocin, DOI, and LSD, only LSD exhibited any selectivity consistent with an important binding site at the serine-alanine mutation. The authors concluded:

> This *locus* may play an important role in determining the neurobehavioral effects of hallucinogens of the ergoline class. . . . The current results illustrate the potential difficulties of extrapolating those [rat] results to humans. . . . This is especially intriguing because the pharmacological actions of hallucinogens of this [ergoline] chemical class have been characterized with rat models. (Almaula, Ebersole, Ballesteros, et al. 1996: 41)

Bufotenine was also used as a high-affinity ligand for 5-HT$_{2A}$ receptors in another point-mutation study of the 5-HT binding pocket in this receptor (Almaula, Ebersole, Zhang, et al. 1996). A previous site-directed mutagenesis study had shown that an interaction between the basic nitrogen of the ligand and the carboxyl side chain of the third transmembrane helix domain (TMH 3) stabilized ligand binding. Furthermore, a three-dimensional computer model of the ligand-receptor interaction had suggested a complex array of interactions between TMH 3 side chains and specific ligands such as 5-HT. The amino group of serotonin was found to bind both with a TMH 3 aspartate residue and to form a hydrogen bond with a nearby serine. It was predicted, and borne out by experiment, that the tertiary amine function of bufotenine could not form this second hydrogen bond with serine, that is, bufotenine bound with equal affinities at both wild and mutant 5-HT$_{2A}$ receptors.

A similar study (Roth et al. 1997) of site-directed mutagenesis involving native and cloned 5-HT$_{2A}$ receptors tested the concept that high-affinity agonist binding (intrinsic activity) was essential for second messenger production (efficacious agonism). The introduction to this study stated, "The molecular mechanisms by which agonists bind to and activate G protein-coupled serotonin (5-HT) receptors remain major enigmas for modern pharmacologists" (Roth et al. 1997: 576). In agreement with previous reports, a point mutation (in this case of a highly conserved phenylalanine residue in transmembrane domain 6) resulted in a range of intrinsic activities and efficacies for several tryptamines, including bufotenine. The data also suggested that 5-HT$_{2A}$ receptors exist in both high and low affinity states (conformations). No correlation was found between the percentage of high-affinity sites and the ability of selected agonists to activate second messenger production (phosphoinositide hydrolysis). Bufotenine and 2,5-Dimethoxy-4-methylamphetamine (DOM) were shown to be full agonists at the cloned receptor, while DMT and 5-methoxy-DMT behaved as partial agonists. Bufotenine also exhibited a 90 percent decrease in efficacy at the cloned receptor. By contrast, amphetamines such as DOI showed diminished affinities (and numbers of high-affinity sites) without corresponding losses of agonist efficacies between the native and cloned 5-HT$_{2A}$ receptors. The authors concluded, "[W]e demonstrate that the relationship between high-affinity agonist binding states and second messenger production is more complicated than previously suggested for 5-HT$_{2A}$ receptors" (Roth et al. 1997: 582). These types of experiments and the refinement of techniques and technology in several related disciplines such as microbiology, computer modeling, and receptor pharmacology add to our understanding of the second goal of pharmacology, that is, to determine how natural processes are effected and controlled. Site-directed mutagenesis of receptors expands our knowledge of the nature of drug-receptor interactions, dynamics of changes in receptor conformations brought about by drug and transmitter stimuli, and the receptor transition states by which agonists induce the production of second messengers.

Are the psychoactive effects of tryptamines such as bufotenine, DMT, 5-methoxy-DMT, and psilocin/psilocybin mediated by a single receptor? Does this putative "psychotropic receptor" also account for the effects of other visionary drugs of the phenethylamine and ergoline types? Nichols (1997) reviewed the evidence from animal receptor studies (particularly rat) and showed that the 5-HT_{2A} receptor is intimately involved in visionary phenomena generated by certain tryptamines, by the potent DOM and related amphetamines, and to a certain extent by LSD. Other investigations have also determined that many tryptamines and other psychoactive drugs possess relatively high affinities for the 5-HT_{2C} receptor. Earlier thought to be primarily associated with the choroid plexus, it has been shown to be the principal 5-HT receptor in rat brain, occurring along with 5-HT_{2A} receptors in distinct but overlapping brain regions (Pompeiano et al. 1994). Tryptamine and ergoline (but not phenethylamine) psychoactive drugs also share significant affinities for the 5-HT_{1A} receptor. The 5-HT_{1A} receptor is located almost exclusively on the cell membranes of serotonin neurons in the raphe nuclei. Although these powerful 5-HT_{1A} agonists inhibit raphe cell firing, this cannot account for the complete mechanism of action of these drugs, since a number of nonpsychoactive 5-HT_{1A} agonists also share this property (Sprouse and Aghajanian 1988). Although many serotonin receptor interactions might account for qualitative differences between the various classic hallucinogens, quantitative differences are harder to rationalize. Significant differences in behavioral potency exist between LSD and the tryptamines DMT and psilocin, yet all three drugs exhibit comparable affinities for 5-HT_1 and $5\text{-HT}_{2A/2C}$ receptors. The prototypic psychedelic LSD shares a similar clinical profile with the amphetamine derivative DOM. Although DOM has high affinity for only two monoamine receptors, $5\text{-HT}_{2A/2C}$, LSD is a very "dirty" ligand, having affinity for seven 5-HT receptors, two dopamine receptors, and modest affinity for the two alpha-adrenergic receptors. It is quite possible that the interaction of LSD with these other receptors modulates or potentiates its effects. These findings indicate that while affinity for certain 5-HT receptors such as 5-HT$_{2A}$ may be a necessary component for visionary activity of certain drugs, it may not be a sufficient component for all known agents.

Sophisticated anecdotal accounts (Hofmann 1980; Shulgin and Shulgin 1991, 1997; Strassman 1994; Repke et al. 1985; Gómez-Jeria et al. 1987) of human experiences with psychoactive compounds such as LSD, mescaline, DOM, and psilocin, which exhibit the full spectrum of psychedelic effects, suggest that administration of even minute amounts of these materials can evoke a complex array of CNS events. The onset, time course, duration, and nature of these effects have been described as unique in the world of known psychopharmaceuticals (Nichols 1997). It is clear that a single receptor-mediated event alone cannot account for the actions of materials such as mescaline as described by Lewin (1924) in his work *Phantastica,* or of LSD as discussed by Freedman (1968: 331):

> [O]ne basic dimension of behavior, compellingly revealed in LSD states is "portentiousness," the capacity of the mind to see more than it can tell, to experience more than it can explicate, to believe in and be impressed with more than it can rationally justify, to experience boundlessness and "boundaryless" events, from the banal to the profound.

Nichols (1997: 564) has also commented on the fact that the hallucinogens "do not obey regular dose-response relationships": "[H]igh doses do not simply produce effects similar to low doses, but of greater intensity. Furthermore, identical doses given to the same individual on different occasions may provoke dramatically different responses." Grof (1975: 32) stated, "I consider LSD to be a powerful unspecific amplifier or catalyst of biochemical and physiological processes in the brain." Although receptor-mediated events may be part of the spectrum of the action of these drugs, it is more likely that they precipitate a series of neurochemical events that might be called a neuronal cascade, in which a specialized and sophisticated sequence of receptor activation/deactivation, neurotransmitter release, pre- and postsynaptic chemical and electrical events, axoplasmic and other cellular transport mechanisms, enzyme activation, and perhaps ion efflux/influx as well as other membrane phenomena occur on a specific and well-established (but poorly understood) time scale. Even more amazing is that little or no disruption of life-sustaining autonomic processes occur even as the cascade unfolds in the higher regions of the CNS.

Hints that such a concept might be so come from electrophysiological measurements. Data from such experiments can be obtained from single neuron recordings using implanted microelectrodes (in animals), from neuronal populations following artificial stimulation (evoked potentials), or from electroencephalographic (EEG) studies, that is, the recording of spontaneous electrical activity in the entire cortex and related subcortical structures, using either implanted macroelectrodes or, in the case of human subjects, sensors applied directly to the cranium. Some information about the effect of LSD (and bufotenine) has been gathered from single neuron studies of the lateral geniculate, cerebral cortex, pyriform cortex, and dorsal raphe nuclei. A reduction of firing frequency of neurons in these areas upon microapplication of LSD was the most common occurrence. In the lateral geniculate, bufotenine was found to be more potent than LSD or psilocybin in exhibiting this decrease in firing rate (Goldstein 1975). However, such effects are also seen to occur with the nonpsychoactive ergoline BOL (2-bromo-LSD). Studies using evoked potentials at the level of the optic nerve have shown that both LSD and mescaline (Chweitzer et al. 1937; Koella and Wells 1959) cause marked decrease in amplitude of these potentials in both the lateral geniculate and the visual cortex. When the site of stimulation is the eye itself, an enhancement of the recorded potentials is noted along with a striking "decrease in the variability of the latency of the change as well as for the amplitudes of the successive evoked waves" (Goldstein 1975: 410). This reduction of variability in evoked potentials is a consistent finding with all hallucinogens studied. The use of LSD in EEG experiments both in animals and human beings has demonstrated a marked induction of arousal through stimulation of the ascending mesencephalic reticular formation. This increase of incoming signals to the cortex

> might result in a number of distortions of the function of the reticular formation and, by extension, of the whole brain. . . . As in any other biological system, both the reticular formation and the cortex have upper limits in their capacities to handle incom-

ing signals. In the case of overload, profound modifications of the functional systems occur. (Goldstein 1975: 412-413)

Modern recording instruments coupled to computer analysis have made possible the collecting of EEG data from hundreds of cranial sites, thus producing topographical brain maps representing a complex array of brain electrical fields. A statistically significant EEG study (Don et al. 1998) of the effects of ayahuasca (see Ott 1994) on humans demonstrated enhancement of the 40 hertz power band from recordings from eight scalp sites over the cortex. Although the measured activation of the visual cortex and associated sites could not be easily correlated with verbal descriptions of phenomenological experiences during the intoxication, the findings suggested that future studies could examine a possible systematic relationship between EEG effects and drug-induced phenomena. Indeed, it has been proposed that the 40 hertz EEG band may serve as a means for embodiment of internal sensory and cognitive mental activities (Basar et al. 1984). Other evidence supporting the neuronal cascade theory comes from positron emission tomography studies of the psilocybin-induced changes in brain function in humans (Vollenweider 1998). Data from such research suggests that sensory gating deficits characterized by a cortico-striato-thalamo-cortical loop model result in cognitive fragmentation and sensory overload of the cortex.

A number of conclusions about the biological activities of bufotenine can be ascertained from the foregoing discussion. Data from receptor studies indicate that bufotenine is not a "clean" 5-HT ligand, that is, that it has very little selectivity for any single 5-HT receptor. It acts on both peripheral and central subtypes in human beings and other animals. Its activity at these receptors has been described as agonist, partial agonist, and in some cases as antagonist. In some cases, the affinity of bufotenine for these receptors is higher than for other tryptamine serotonergic agents, including 5-HT itself, and in other cases lower. The activity of bufotenine is not limited to the 5-HT family of receptors. Antagonism to central adrenergic receptors has been suggested.

In many cases, the receptor affinities of bufotenine are not tissue selective. Physiological actions of bufotenine include dose-dependent effects on both the force and rate of heart contractile responses. Constriction (and in some cases vasodilation) of blood vessels in both the CNS and periphery have been noted along with effects on blood platelet morphology. The lethal dose (LD_{50}) of bufotenine in rodents has been determined to be between 200 and 300 mg/kg, death occurring by respiratory arrest. By contrast, the LD_{50} for methamphetamine in mice is 70 mg/kg, for morphine 200-300 mg/kg IV, for strychnine about 1.0 mg/kg in rats. Hyperthermic and hypothermic effects have been attributed to bufotenine, perhaps involving peripheral and/or central vasculature. Mild MAO inhibitory action has been reported for bufotenine. The release and inhibition of serotonin reuptake in spinal cord synaptosomes via effects upon the 5-HT active transport carrier have been demonstrated. Although it is generally assumed (and verified by experiment) that bufotenine has poor blood-brain barrier penetration following peripherally administered doses, a number of clearly centrally mediated effects of the drug so administered have been reported. Some of these are species dependent, such as general depression and lethargy in monkeys, stimulation and hypermotor activity in chickens, reduced aggression in mice, and anxiogenesis in rats. Direct applications of bufotenine to CNS regions in animals show marked stimulant-like effects as well as stereotypic behavior, especially in rodents. Electrophysiological experiments have demonstrated that bufotenine causes a marked state of arousal in many regions and levels of the CNS in a number of animal species. Moreover, several esoteric biological actions of bufotenine have been reported that do not fall into convenient categories.

Using 5-HT–stimulated liver fluke adenylate cyclase as a model for predicting hallucinogenic activity in humans, Northrup and Mansour (1978) studied the effects of a number of ergolines and tryptamines on this activation. Affinity for an apparent 5-HT receptor paralleled intrinsic activity. Affinity of LSD for this receptor was about 200-fold higher than that of bufotenine. A rank order of affinity among tested tryptamines was 5-methoxy-DMT = bufotenine > DMT > *N*-methyltryptamine > 5-methoxy-tryptamine.

The development of fungal pathogens on the surface of host plants is influenced by many factors, including the role played by chemicals that are leached by rain from the plants themselves (Brown 1922). These substances can affect several phases in the development of these organisms, including spore germination, germ-tube growth, and the formation of infectious structures known as appressoria. The species *Colletotrichum musae* (Berk. & Curt) Arx. produces particularly distinctive appressoria that cause a latent infection in green bananas, eventually producing anthracnose lesions in ripe bananas. In an experiment to determine if chemicals leached from banana skins stimulated this fungus, Swinburne (1976) studied the growth of *C. musae* on the Valery clone of Cavendish bananas imported into Northern Ireland from Ecuador. Leachate from the fruits was obtained in the laboratory by spraying a fine water mist on the hanging bunches ("hands") of bananas and collecting the runoff. This leachate was shown to greatly enhance both germination and appressoria formation on conidia of *C. musae.* Two compounds were isolated and identified from the ether-soluble extract of this leachate. The first was anthranilic acid, which was positively identified by comparison with a known standard. The other was tentatively identified as bufotenine. Although the ether-soluble fraction could not account for the total activity of the leachate in promoting appressoria growth, the isolated material presumed to be bufotenine did have a positive effect on such growth.

Mammals and plants are not the only organisms on which the effects of bufotenine have been studied. A number of reports on insect physiology have included such research. The identification of serotonin in the nervous systems of insects, including arthropods, prompted Kostowski et al. (1972) to investigate the effects of several tryptamine derivatives, including bufotenine, on the concentration of 5-HT and bioelectric activity in the ant, *Formica rufa.* Injection of bufotenine into the abdominal cavity was found to increase the level of 5-HT in ant brain significantly over control values. The effect of bufotenine on ant brain EEG patterns, however, was not clear. In some cases, the amplitude measured in the lobi optici was increased, with no change in the frequency. In other cases, the amplitude was decreased, with a corresponding increase in the frequency. Interestingly, a close analog of bufotenine, 5-hydroxy-6-methoxy-tryptamine, was found to reduce the brain content of 5-HT. The work concluded with the observation that ant brain contained higher baseline concentrations of 5-HT than vertebrates (or other arthropods) and that higher concentrations of 5-HT correlated well with increases in the amplitude of brain EEG patterns.

Bufotenine has also been found to have a diuretic effect in the insects *Rhodnius prolixus* (known as the "kissing bug") and *Carausius morosus* (Maddrell et al. 1969), nerve stimulatory activity in the subesophageal ganglia of the African giant snail, *Achatina fulica* (Ku and Takeuchi 1984), heart stimulatory activity in the tobacco horn-worm, *Manduca sexta* (Platt and Reynolds 1986), and the decapod crustaceans *Astacus leptodactylus* and *Eriphia spinifrons* (Florey and Rathmayer 1978), and teratotoxicity in the planarian worm *Dugesia tigrina* (Lenicque 1973). This teratogenic effect was particularly striking, with the formation of abnormal regeneration blastema including genuine "janus heads," that is, regenerated animals without tails or pharynx. The parasitic protozoan *Entamoeba histolytica* is a common cause of diarrhea in humans. The *E. histolytica* lysate-induced alteration of active electrolyte transport in rabbit ileum and rat colon was found to be inhibited by bufotenine and stimulated by serotonin (McGowan et al. 1983). In these preparations, bufotenine was shown to decrease both sodium ion and chloride absorption.

Among other components isolated from the leaves of the mandarin orange, *Citrus unshiu,* 5-hydroxy-*N*-methyltryptamine, bufotenine, and its *O*-glucoside were found to contribute to the stimulation of egg-laying behavior in the swallowtail butterfly, *Papilio xuthus* L., a species that feeds upon its leaves. Bufotenine was found to be a potent synergist, with a mixture of four flavanoids that stimulated this oviposition (Nishida et al. 1990). The concentration of bufotenine in the leaves was reported to be 10 µg/g of leaf. Subsequent work (Ohsugi et al. 1991) demonstrated that these host-plant stimulants are species specific, and that female butterflies can detect the essential ingredients through chemoreceptors on their forelegs. This contact chemical stimulus was found to be more important than visual and olfactory clues.

The involvement of serotonin and related tryptamines in the regulation of photoperiodic events in such distant taxa as arthropods, angiosperms, and vertebrates has been well established. The mammalian pineal substance melatonin (*N*-acetyl-5-methoxytryptamine) acts as a mediator of information concerning temporal position and duration of darkness (Reiter 1985). This pineal-mediated circadian rhythmicity not only participates in the determination of day length but has also been implicated in reproductive cycles (Reiter 1980). The unicellular dinoflagellate *Gonyaulax polyedra* has been shown to undergo a well-defined photoperiodic-induced resting cyst formation (Balzer and Hardeland 1992) mediated by the presence of melatonin. Deviation in the accuracy of time measurement in *Gonyaulax* has been shown to be less than two minutes per day, making this organism ideal for the study of photoperiodism. An interruption of the encystment produced by an abnormal photoperiod (short days, light/dark cycle 11 hours/13 hours) can be overcome by the administration of certain tryptamines. At a concentration of 10^{-4} molar, bufotenine was shown to provoke cyst formation even when given one hour prior to darkness. Similar experiments using the isolated eyes of *Aplysia* species (Corrent and Eskin 1982) demonstrated that serotonin and to a lesser extent bufotenine induce a rhythmic phase shift of light-induced responses, suggesting a role for 5-HT as a neurotransmitter in the circadian time-keeping mechanism in *Aplysia*.

HUMAN STUDIES

Perhaps no more confusing area about the effects of bufotenine exists than that of the human use of extracts of members of the toad genus *Bufo,* the original source of the drug. A fair body of literature exists detailing the supposed ancient Mesoamerican, Asian, and contemporary Western use of such materials. The reader is referred to review articles (Davis and Weil 1992; Lyttle et al. 1996) for a thorough discussion of this subject. One thing is clear from research on this topic: *Bufo* species are veritable chemical factories whose cutaneous exudates contain a host of bioactive substances, of which bufotenine is a minor component. Physiological effects of total extracts can mostly be attributed to the presence of many toxic cardioactive steroids such as bufogenin and bufotoxin.

A report detailing the analysis of material considered to be an alleged West Indian aphrodisiac thought to be responsible for a number of deaths in New York City found it to be linked to toad exudates (Barry et al. 1996). Originally thought to be of plant origin (Chamakura 1994), the gas chromatographic elution profile of this "Love Stone" was found to be identical to that of "Chan Su," an ancient Chinese medicinal preparation also derived from toads. Levels of bufotenine found in the samples ranged from 0.3 to 1.2 percent. Significant quantities of at least five cardiotoxic bufadienolides were also detected in "Love Stone." An intriguing, but unsubstantiated statement appeared in this paper: "Bufotenine is currently being used as both an hallucinogen and an aphrodisiac, and is the latest recreational drug of abuse appearing in the New York City area" (Barry et al. 1996: 1072).

The idea that certain endogenous *N*- and/or *O*-methylated tryptamines could be causative factors in mental illness has been persistent (Gaddum 1953; Wooley and Shaw 1954; Benington et al. 1965; Mandell and Segal 1973; Gillin, Kaplan, et al. 1976). Three lines of evidence seemed to suggest that this might be so. First was the discovery of "psychotomimetic" *N*- and *O*-methylated tryptamines such as DMT, bufotenine, and 5-methoxy-DMT, which were structurally closely related to the mammalian transmitter serotonin (5-HT; Erspamer and Asero 1952; Rapport et al. 1948) and the natural amino acid tryptophan. Second, enzymes (*N*-methyltransferase, hydroxy *O*-methyltransferase, and catechol *O*-methyltransferase) were discovered (Axelrod 1961; Osmond and Smythies 1952) in both rabbit lung and human brain that were capable of biologically producing these "abnormal" compounds from serotonin and tryptamine. Third, a bufotenine-like substance was detected in the urine of schizophrenics but not controls (Fischer et al. 1961). This aspect of the theory was studied by several groups. Investigating the quantitative variations in urinary indoles, Brune and Himwich (1962) found that schizophrenic patients periodically eliminate larger amounts of indoles, not primarily in relation to the underlying mental illness but in relation to "momentary changes of intensity of certain psychotic symptoms" (325).

One problem that would have to be accounted for if the overall theory was to have credence is the short-acting nature and rapid metabolism of substances such as bufotenine. Since it had been shown that the enzyme responsible for the metabolism of bufotenine and DMT in humans was MAO-A, then an abnormality in the activity of this enzyme in mentally ill patients relative to "normals" would have to be demonstrated (Sanders and Bush 1967; Szára 1956). Subsequently, the activity level and substrate specificity of MAO in the brains of schizophrenics was found to be similar to those of "normals" (Domino et al. 1973). However, platelet MAO activity was shown to be higher in a group of depressed patients (Nies et al. 1971) and lower in a bipolar group (Murphy and Weiss 1972). The confirmation that chronic overproduction of bufotenine and related compounds in the human brain could lead to schizophrenia or other mental illness faced many obstacles.

The conclusion drawn in a review of two decades of research on this question was that the relationship between schizophrenia and *N*-methylated tryptamines was tenuous (Luchins et al. 1978). Some increase in transmethylation in mental illness could scarcely be substantiated. Exacerbation of symptoms in schizophrenia by loading (with "methyl" donors) experiments could not be attributed to an increase in the production of methylated tryptamines, and elevated concentrations of these substances in schizophrenics could not be conclusively demonstrated.

A study of urinary excretion of bufotenine in a population of violent male criminals who had committed or attempted murder or "other grave assaults" showed statistically higher rates of bufotenine excretion than did a reference group of laboratory personnel (Räisänen et al. 1984). Quantitative variation in bufotenine excretion was seen across this small population, with higher levels detected in patients with paranoid symptoms and especially high levels in those with a history of violence against family members. Clinical assessment was done without prior knowledge of the results of the bufotenine analysis.

This study was expanded (Karkkainen et al. 1995) to a larger population (112) of violent offenders who had been referred by courts to the Psychiatric Clinic of Helsinki University. Urinary bufotenine excretion levels were correlated with a number of personality variables as determined by the Karolinska Scales of Personality index. Suspiciousness was positively and socialization was negatively correlated with bufotenine excretion. Highest excretion levels were found in patients considered to be violent and to have paranoid personality traits. Other factors in this population, such as a history of drug use, were taken into consideration. Patients who were on prescription antidepressants were also found to excrete higher levels of bufotenine. In summation, the investigators noted:

> On the basis of the present investigation, it is unlikely that the tissue bufotenine levels in the suspicious violent offenders were the cause of paranoid or other abnormal behavior. . . . The role of the transmethylation pathway of indoleamine metabolism in the mechanism of drug action or in the etiology of psychiatric disease is completely unknown at present. (Karkkainen et al. 1995: 151)

The MAO inhibitor nialamide was found (Karkkainen and Raisanen 1992) to significantly increase the urinary excretion levels of bufotenine in a "normal" male. Blood plasma levels required for such high excretion in urine were said to be not far from those that produce psychic symptoms in humans.

An unusual serotonin metabolic degradation pathway in the Japanese toad, *Bufo bufo japonicus,* leading to high brain concentrations of bufotenine in toad brains (Takeda et al. 1995) was reported. It was suggested that this toad could be an animal model for the study of such aberrant (for human beings) metabolism, possibly leading to an understanding of some forms of mental illness. For example, it was possible to distinguish autistic patients from controls from an examination of chromatography patterns of substances excreted in the urine. Among these substances, bufotenine was consistently found at higher levels in autistic patients (Takeda et al. 1995). The severity of symptoms of the disease were found to positively correlate with these levels.

One report (Farber et al. 1998) explored the possible protective role of serotonergic agents in a special kind of schizophrenia, that induced by the N-Methyl-D-aspartic acid (NMDA) antagonists phencyclidine and ketamine. This drug-induced syndrome, thought to be mediated by NMDA receptor hypofunction, involves a complex mechanism of disruption of both the NMDA excitatory system and the gamma-aminobutyric acid A ($GABA_A$) inhibitory transmitter system. Since it is known that serotonergic innervation of GABAergic systems occurs via $5\text{-}HT_{2A}$ receptors, it was postulated that activation by $5\text{-}HT_{2A}$ agonists might restore inhibition to this network and prevent neuronal injury. This hypothesis was verified when it was demonstrated that the $5\text{-}HT_{2A/2C}$ agonists LSD, DOM, DOI, and 2,5-Dimethoxy-4-bromoamphetamine (DOB) afforded protection in a rat model of NMDA antagonist-induced neurotoxicity. The nonpsychoactive ergoline compund lisuride, a selective $5\text{-}HT_{2A}$ agonist, also afforded protection, suggesting that the visionary effects of LSD and the other agents were mediated solely by $5\text{-}HT_{2C}$ receptor agonism, thus resolving the apparent contradiction that known hallucinogens might alleviate the symptoms of NMDA antagonist-induced psychoses.

The study of the effects of bufotenine on human beings is a long and often twisted road spanning the last half of the twentieth century. Only now, at the beginning of a new century, with renewed interest in the study of current shamanic use of bufotenine-containing snuffs from South America, have we come full circle: not that the study of this interesting molecule, nor the controversy surrounding its human effects, will end with the beginning of the twenty-first century, but perhaps some of the pharmacological mythology and misunderstandings can be put to rest.

The first reported human "clinical" trial of pure bufotenine (Fabing and Hawkins 1956) took place on October 12, 1955, using four young, healthy prisoners at the Ohio State Penitentiary. The drug was supplied by chemists from Upjohn Laboratories who had recently developed a convenient synthesis of the molecule (Speeter and Anthony 1954). Much of the short paper by Fabing and Hawkins bears quoting here, because of its firsthand descriptions of the effects of bufotenine. Four of the subjects received single intravenous doses of 1, 2, 4, and 8 mg bufotenine as the creatinine sulfate derivative in sterile distilled water. The second subject, who had been given the 2 mg dose, was given an additional 16 mg 90 minutes later.

Within one minute of the beginning of the injection (1 mg, but before the injection was finished) the first subject complained of "a tight feeling in the chest" and a prickling sensation in his face "as if he had been jabbed by nettles." This was accompanied by a "fleeting sensation of pain in both thighs and a mild nausea." The effects passed within six minutes, and no significant change in blood pressure nor pulse was noted. (Reprinted with permission from Fabing, H.D., and J.R. Hawkins. 1956. "Intravenous bufotenine injection in the human being." *Science* 123: 886-887. Copyright 1956 AAAS.)

The second subject (2 mg) received the injection over the same three-minute period. Within the first minute he felt "a tightness in his throat" and the sensation of a racing pulse, although measurement of the pulse remained at the base rate of 84. Tightness in the stomach, tingling in both pretibial areas, and the development of a purplish hue about his face all passed in about seven minutes. Again, blood pressure and pulse rate remained near normal.

The third subject (4 mg) reported much the same initial effects. In addition, he complained of "chest oppression" and stated, "a load is pressing down from above and my body feels heavy." A "numbness of the entire body" and "a pleasant Martini feeling—my body is taking charge of my mind." Pupils were dilated and bilateral nystagmus was present. Within a minute after the injection he reported, "I see red and black spots—a vivid orange-red—moving around." The spots changed in size and shape and persisted for two minutes. His face perspired and became "purplish," a color that persisted for about 15 minutes. After the experience, the subject stated that it was difficult to concentrate, but that he "had a feeling of great placidity during the experiment" (Fabing and Hawkins 1956: 886). No significant blood pressure nor pulse rate changes were seen.

The fourth subject (8 mg) developed an immediate sense of light-headedness, a burning sensation in his face, which turned purple, nausea, and a transient hyperpnea (labored breathing). His pupils were "grossly dilated" and moderate nystagmus was present. As the needle was withdrawn, the subject "blurted":

> I see white straight lines with a black background. I can't trace a pattern. Now there are red, green, and yellow dots, very bright, like they were made out of fluorescent cloth, moving like blood cells through capillaries, weaving in and out of the white lines. (Fabing and Hawkins 1956: 886)

This visual experience was "present with eyes both open and closed, facial sweating and purpling was intense, nausea had abated, and the subject felt calm." The visual phenomena were fleeting and disappeared after two minutes. Eleven minutes later the subject appeared normal and stated, "Even at the height of this, my mind felt better and more pleasant than usual." There was no significant change in blood pressure nor pulse rate during this experiment.

Undaunted by the apparent transient episode of respiratory arrest in subject 4, the investigators pressed on. Subject 2 was given a second dose (16 mg) 90 minutes after receiving the 2 mg dose. A burning sensation in his mouth, generalized body tingling, a "livid purple" face, and nausea were apparent almost immediately. During the third minute, the subject vomited and stated "my chest feels crushed." As the needle was withdrawn, "he saw red spots passing before his eyes and red-purple spots on the floor, and the floor seemed to be very close to his face" (Fabing and Hawkins 1956: 887).

Within two minutes these visual components were gone, but they were replaced by a yellow haze, as if he were "looking through a yellow lens filter." His attempt to subtract serial 7s from 100 was abandoned because of many errors. His face "remained deeply purple and sweating was profuse." Nine minutes into the experiment, the subject stated, "Words can't come. I can't express the way I feel. My mind feels crowded." At 12 minutes there was a "fleeting return of red spots before the eyes." At 16 minutes he said, "When I start on a thought, another one comes along and clashes with it, and I can't express myself clearly" (Fabing and Hawkins 1956: 887). At the twenty-fifth minute, "I feel dopey but not sleepy. I feel physically tense and mentally clouded. I am here and not here." At 40 minutes, "I feel better, but I still feel like I want to walk it off—like a hangover." His face assumed a normal color after 60 minutes. Again, no significant changes in blood pressure or pulse rate were noted. The investigators correctly summed up the overall experiment:

> . . . that the drug is hallucinogenic, that there is a linear progression in symptoms as dose increases, and that its effects are reminiscent of LSD and mescaline but develop and disappear more quickly, indicating rapid central action and rapid degradation of the drug. (Fabing and Hawkins 1956: 887)

This experiment, especially the 16 mg dose, would today be deemed clinically improper. Some have used the word "shoddy" and have criticized this study at great length. However, apart from two troubling aspects, those of the potential for respiratory arrest and the purple faces, indicating serious peripheral vasoconstriction and anoxia, the descriptions of the effects of bufotenine are congruent with those of other classic hallucinogens, DMT, mescaline, LSD, psilocin, and DOM. The early body sensations, pupil dilation, the colored visions, distortion of surroundings, loss of words, alteration of time and space perception, a "rush" of thoughts, a general feeling of well-being, mild hyperthermia, and (at the higher dose) a "waxing and waning" of effects, even the desire "to walk it off," are all part of a classic hallucinogenic experience.

Turner and Merlis (1959) conducted a clinical study of the effects of *Anadenanthera* snuff preparations and pure bufotenine (and DMT), using schizophrenic patients at the Central Islip State Hospital in New York. In addition, one of the authors tested the effects of the snuff on himself. The possible connection between mental illness and these tryptamines, particularly bufotenine, served as the impetus for this study. The authors stated:

It might be reasoned . . . that the nonschizophrenic has enzyme systems . . . which are capable of rapid destruction of a trypto-phan-containing polypeptide . . . and that this destruction goes on via serotonin in these persons, whereas in schizophrenia this does not occur. Under these conditions it might not be possible to render a normal person the equivalent of a schizophrenic [by administering "psychotomimetics"]. . . . On the other hand, the introduction to the already burdened schizophrenic of a sub-stance which would specifically increase his metabolic load might aggravate . . . a psychosis. (Turner and Merlis 1959: 122-123. Reprinted with permission from Turner, W. J., and S. Merlis. 1959. "Effect of some indolealkylamines on man." A.M.A. Archives of Neurology and Psychiatry 81: 121-129. Copyrighted © 1959, American Medical Association. All Rights reserved.)

Two samples of indigenous snuffs thought to be from *Anadenanthera* seeds and an "artificial" snuff prepared by pulverizing seeds, ob-tained from the National Institutes of Health from the same batch studied chemically by Fish and known to be from that species, were utilized (Fish, Johnson, and Horning 1955). The largest dose of snuff employed by one of the investigators was half a gram, containing about 6 mg bufotenine. At this dose, no discernible intoxication could be induced. Since it was known at the time that native peoples rou-tinely ingested 10 g of snuff containing perhaps 100 mg of alkaloid (mostly bufotenine) in a single dose, the outcome of Turner's experi-ment is not surprising. The native use of this snuff must have been an "acquired taste" since the investigators reported, "It [the snuff bolus] could be retained [in the nostrils and sinus cavities] only for about three minutes before violent gagging, coughing, and sneezing led to rejection of most of the mass" (Turner and Merlis 1959: 123). The na-sal inhalation of 6 to 10 mg of pure bufotenine (as the creatinine sul-fate) likewise did not cause inebriation, although symptoms similar to the early phase of IV studies reported by Fabing were noted, that is, "a feeling of fear, associated with flushing of the face, lacrimation, tachycardia and tachypnea." A letter from Dr. Harris Isbell (from the U.S. Public Health Service Hospital in Lexington, Kentucky) sum-marizing his own experiments, was quoted: "No subjective effects were observed after spraying [intranasally] with as much as 40 mg of bufotenine (creatinine sulfate)" (Turner and Merlis 1959: 123. Re-printed with permission from Turner, W. J., and S. Merlis. 1959.

The IV injection of bufotenine into schizophrenic patients was another matter. The administration of 20 mg bufotenine to one subject over a 77 minute interval produced (as one would expect) no psychological changes. Minor physiological changes were limited to a "slight decrease of *alpha* voltage and the appearance of some 5- to 7-cycle activity in the EEG." When the same subject received a 10 mg dose over a 50 second period, "the effects were extreme":

> At 17 seconds there was flushing of the face. At 22 seconds there was maximal inhalation followed by maximal hyperventilation, as to both rate and volume. This persisted for about two minutes, during which time the patient was unresponsive to stimuli, her face was reddish blue ("plum-colored"), and she became slightly restless. . . . There was intense salivation . . . the present subject could have . . . drowned in her own saliva and had to be turned on her side. (Turner and Merlis 1959: 124)

The subject's pulse rate rose slightly without much change in blood pressure.

Several patients were given IV doses of bufotenine as they were coming out of insulin-induced coma or following electroconvulsive therapy on the assumption that "fear associated with the injection could be avoided." Several others were given bufotenine in conjunction with doses of reserpine and chlorpromazine. These experiments nearly proved fatal (by respiratory arrest) and the details need not be reiterated here. In summation of the bufotenine experiments, Turner noted:

> Psychologically, we have not noted any evidence that the patient's psychosis was aggravated, or relieved, either immediately following injection or later. It is true that at higher doses patients became frightened to an extreme degree, and one might expect thereafter accentuation of their defenses; but this did not occur. (Turner and Merlis 1959: 124)

However, it was known at the time that most chronic schizophrenic patients do not report visual hallucinations after intravenous administration of mescaline. A further quote from a letter from Dr. Isbell reported that "elementary visual hallucinations after intramuscular doses of 10 to 12.5 mg (bufotenine) . . . consisted of a play of colors, lights, and patterns" (Turner and Merlis 1959: 124).

Intramuscular doses of 5 to 50 mg *N,N*-dimethyltryptamine were also given in this study. Low doses (10-25 mg) produced many of the same peripheral and physical symptoms as bufotenine, including facial flushing and mydriasis, some anxiety, and restlessness. A near-fatal episode occurred following the intramuscular injection of 40 mg DMT into one patient. Symptoms included extreme tachycardia, a rapid fall in blood pressure, extreme cyanosis, and auricular fibrillation. A brief cardiac arrest necessitated vigorous cardiac massage in order to save the subject. At 50 mg, however, one patient noted:

> [T]he injections made her feel like an animal; she saw the nurses as rubber dolls and the walls as crumbling paper. This was like she had felt six years before, when she had come to the hospital; lately she had been better and did not like to have these things happen again. (Turner and Merlis 1959: 125)

Control injections with saline apparently did not produce such effects. The investigators could obviously draw no conclusions about theories of schizophrenigenesis from this study, and certainly none regarding the pharmacology of *Anadenanthera* snuffs. They did state, however:

> [T]he difficulties become so great that we must reject bufotenine and DMT as capable of producing the acute phase of *cohoba* intoxication. . . . In a field where experience may be so fallacious and judgment so difficult, we do not feel justified in making further statements. (Turner and Merlis 1959: 127-128)

The experiments that were made by these investigators were, however, enough to put the lid on human experimentation with bufotenine for the next 20 years.

The work of Turner, and to a lesser degree that of Fabing, could be considered unethical and experimentally flawed. Fabing clearly showed, through anecdotal reports, that bufotenine was hallucinogenic, although not without troubling side effects. It is not known to what degree the patients in the Turner study were compromised by other psychopharmaceuticals that might have been prescribed for them during their confinement in the institution. Turner's experiments also showed that bufotenine had some central effects, although in the end he ignored the letter from Isbell containing comments about "colored visions."

The experiments by Fabing and Hawkins and Turner and Merlis have convinced many authors (Brimblecombe and Pinder 1975; Chilton et al. 1979; Davis 1988; Holmstedt and Lindgren 1967b; Kety, in Osmond 1956; Lyttle et al. 1996; Mandell and Morgan 1971; Migliaccio et al. 1981; Repke et al. 1981; Shulgin 1981a) that bufotenine is simply a cardiovascular and respiratory toxin. Perhaps the appalling nature of these studies involving the use of prison inmates and the mentally ill have reinforced this negative view and prevented a more rational appraisal of the actual results. The Turner study also reported a number of experiments using DMT and LSD, one of which proved as nearly fatal as the bufotenine/chlorpromazine episode. One wonders why the negative stigma of this work firmly attached itself to bufotenine and not to DMT. Perhaps those who wished to embrace and promote "psychedelic culture" sought to distance bufotenine from the supposedly more sacramental and benign DMT. The association of bufotenine with toads (Lyttle et al. 1996) and European witchcraft (Harner 1973), its connection to the poisonous mushroom genus *Amanita,* dubious association with Viking berserkers (Fabing 1956), and the possible implication of bufotenine as an endogenous psychotoxin conspired with these clinical studies to taint this "black sheep" of the tryptamine family.

In a study of the metabolism of carbon-14–labeled bufotenine, low doses (0.2 mg and 1.0 mg) of the drug were administered to two human volunteers (Sanders-Bush et al. 1976). The major metabolite (in urine) was found to be 5-hydroxyindole acetic acid. The subject receiving the 1 mg dose described a brief "tingling sensation in arms and hands," symptoms that had also been reported with a similar dose by Fabing (Sanders-Bush et al. 1976: 1409).

Thirty years after Fabing's experiment, McLeod and Sitaram (1985) published a report on IV administration of bufotenine to a "medically trained volunteer subject." The work was conducted at St. Vincent's Hospital, University of Melbourne, and had been prompted by an earlier finding by the same group of a compound tentatively identified as bufotenine in the urine of schizophrenics. Intranasal application of 2 to 16 mg bufotenine (as the oxalate salt) produced no symptoms other than a degree of intense local irritation. Intravenous injection of 2 to 4 mg bufotenine produced moderate anxiety, while injection of 8 mg over a three-minute period produced

> profound emotional and perceptual changes, involving extreme anxiety, a sense that death was imminent, and a visual disturbance which was associated with color reversal and distortion, such as might be seen in a photographic negative. (McLeod and Sitaram 1985: 447. Reprinted with permission from McLeod, W. R., and R. R. Sitaram. 1985. "Bufotenine reconsidered." *Acta Psychiatrica Scandinavica* 72, 5: 447-450. Copyright 1985 by Blackwell Publishing.)

Intense facial flushing but no difficulty in breathing was noted. Following the report of the subject (a transcript of which was included as an addendum to this paper), it was decided the "further experimentation on this, or any other subject, would not continue" (McLeod and Sitaram 1985: 447). The administered dose of bufotenine was found to be rapidly eliminated from the bloodstream with a concomitant rapid appearance in urine. Some of the verbatim transcript follows:

> I had an experience of panic unlike anything I had ever experienced before. . . . As the injection proceeded I had yet again the sense of wanting to call a stop. . . . The faces around me remained the same, but were at the same time different. Each seemed to have a transparent mask, smaller than the face itself, superimposed over it, giving . . . even a sense of evil. . . . Artificial panelling on the cupboards seemed somehow more intense. . . . At the same time I was aware that my speech was slurred and that I seemed detached from my surroundings. Not only did my surroundings appear unreal, but I also had the sense of being unreal in some undefinable way. . . . I was aware that I was transfixed . . . and my hands were pulsing and even seemed to be increasing with size with each pulse beat. (McLeod and Sitaram 1985: 449-450. Reprinted with permission from McLeod, W. R., and R. R. Sitaram. 1985. "Bufotenine reconsidered." *Act Psychiatrica Scandinavica* 72, 5: 447-450. Copyright 1985 by Blackwell Publishing.)

This report, like that of Fabing, clearly identifies bufotenine as a short-acting visionary substance.

Field studies and laboratory analyses of snuffs and smoking preparations derived exclusively from seeds of *Anadenanthera colubrina* var. *Cebil,* currently used in traditional healing practices in the Argentine Chaco, have been reported (Torres and Repke 1996). The isolation of 12.4 percent pure bufotenine from a seed sample directly linked to unadulterated shamanic inebriants and the eyewitness accounts of both the preparation and use of these materials led the authors to conclude that bufotenine was solely responsible for the observed central activity of these preparations. It was calculated that a single cigar of crushed *Anadenanthera* seeds and tobacco might contain approximately 196 mg bufotenine. The weight of the powdered seeds necessary to obtain the given dose was only 1.5 g, considerably less than the 10 g said to be ingested by natives according to Turner and Merlis (1959).

One problem of bufotenine-induced psychoactivity in human beings remains to be resolved. Visionary effects for bufotenine have only been demonstrated clinically by either intravenous or intramuscular injections. Such modes of administration are obviously unknown in South American shamanic practice. In traditional healing, bufotenine-containing preparations are administered by three known routes: insufflation of finely ground seeds, smoking pulverized seeds often mixed with tobacco, and by enemas (Smet and Rivier 1985). Early clinical investigations have failed to elicit psychoactive effects in human beings, whether by inhalation of authentic snuffs or by direct nasal application of as much as 40 mg bufotenine (as the creatinine sulfate). The lack of effects seen in these studies can be explained by the fact that in the clinical setting, only a subthreshold dose of bufotenine (about 1.5 g of snuff containing 6 mg bufotenine; Turner and Merlis 1959) was applied. It is clear from observations of animal behavior that peripherally administered bufotenine does produce dose-dependent centrally mediated effects. Pharmacokinetic considerations, such as rapid metabolism, suggest that a larger nasal dose relative to the injection route would be required. By injection, an effective dose has been shown to be between 4 and 8 mg of bufotenine (molecular weight 204) free base, which on a molar basis equals 8 to 16 mg bufotenine creatinine sulfate (molecular weight 413). Analyses of native snuffs suggest that approximately 100 mg bufotenine (as the base) are ingested at one time (Torres and Repke 1996; Turner and Merlis 1959). The largest dose of bufotenine (as the creatinine sulfate) employed in a clinical setting was 40 mg (Isbell in Turner and Merlis 1959), equaling only 20 mg bufotenine free base. Clearly, this would be a subthreshold intranasal dose. We can estimate that the threshold intranasal dose of bufotenine free base is between 20 and 50 mg and that a fully effective dose is between 50 and 100 mg. Confirmation of this estimate will have to await further clinically controlled study. Such a study will have to take into account not only the psychoactive effects of bufotenine but also any possible toxic side effects of the drug, namely its pulmonary vasoconstrictive action. It might be assumed that this effect would be more pronounced when the drug is administered by intravenous injection than by nasal administration. Seasoned traditional healers do not seem concerned with this, nor are they overcome by symptoms of respiratory arrest.

A delightful anecdotal account of a self-administered dose of powdered seeds of Argentine *Anadenanthera colubrina* var. *Cebil* has been reported by a European investigator (Rätsch 1996). The detailed translation follows:

> In January 1996 I had the opportunity to take the snuff. I insufflated approximately one half gram in two portions (one per nostril) [Representing about 22 mg bufotenine]. The next morning I wrote down the following account: We drew the blinds in our rain forest bungalow. The powder was inhaled with relative ease and without untoward event. It does not have the same burning properties as other snuffs (e.g., *Anadenanthera peregrina*). A mild stinging sensation on the mucosa was deemed acceptable. Initially I noted that my body felt heavier. Particularly the arms and legs assumed a leaden weight, but the sensation in the body was characterized by a quite pleasant warmth. . . . I closed my eyes in a state of excited anticipation of the impending drug action. After about five minutes I grew aware of swirling, dancing phosphenes in my visual field. At this point they were bright pinpoints on a deep blue backdrop. The darting points of light associated into flowing, liquid forms and patterns. It was as though the flood gates of the Universe had been thrown open. A rushing tumult of patterns poured across my visual field. Every point was the source of streams and rivers of

braided ropes of light. These braided and unbraided themselves in a vast tangle. All this took place at breakneck speed. A panorama of flowing designs—the exact patterns depicted in the nimbus surrounding the head of the Chavín deity! I marveled for minutes at the interlocking tessellation of these geometric shapes. They possessed a multiple interlocking penetrated arrangement which matched the characteristic style of Tiahuanaco artwork. At that moment I was convinced that the Tiahuanaco artists used this snuff to inspire their work. The rapidly shifting array of patterns transformed itself into a chaotic current of spermatozoa. These teemed and writhed in all directions at once, giving the sensation that they were on an (almost aggressive) mission to fertilize the entire cosmos. This tableau was followed by geometric forms which projected from the depths of the room and assembled themselves into a visual tunnel. To this point I had seen no color. Presently subtle colorations became apparent. The speed of visual effects began to ease—and suddenly they were over. I opened my eyes in the darkened room and had the sensation of an abrupt change in ambient light level. I briefly felt faint nausea; I belched and then felt fine. It was a truly novel visionary experience. (Rätsch 1996: 60-61. Reprinted with permission from Rätsch, C. 1996. "Eine Erfahrung mit dem Mataco-Schnupfpulver *Hataj*." Y*earbook for Ethnomedicine and the Study of Consciousness* 5: 59-65, Verlag für Wissenschaft und Bildung, Berlin. Copyright 1996 by Verlag für Wissenschaft und Bildung.) [Duration of effects was approximately 25 minutes.]

Clearly, bufotenine is a many-faceted physiologically active substance possessing short-term visionary effects in human beings. The mechanisms of this action, like those of other psychoactive tryptamines, are not clearly understood. Studies of the involvement of serotonin, mediated by the complex central 5-HT receptor systems, offer some insight into this problem (Marek and Aghajanian 1998). However, a mechanism of psychotropic action common to all known agents, at least of the major chemical classes, remains elusive. Perhaps we should view drug-induced hallucinosis as the unfolding of a wide-ranging process requiring a well-developed, time-sequenced, multisite model (such as a neuronal cascade). Reductionist investigations of unimolecular events at the receptor level need to be integrated with an understanding of information processing in neural ensembles. In addressing this latter matter, Deadwyler and Hampson (1997: 218) stated, "A key missing concept in our appreciation of how the brain functions . . . is an understanding of the nature of the spatio-temporal impulse flow that constitutes the fabric upon which . . . critical events are tailored."

The operation of neural networks requires multiple nonlinear processes occurring at the synaptic, cellular, and network levels (Getting 1989). It will be challenging to devise and perfect experimental techniques that will allow measurement of such dynamic processes in large segments of vertebrate central nervous systems without damaging neural interconnections. No doubt the twenty-first century will witness such advances. An account from the first chemical examination of the brain stated:

> [T]he brain is certainly that part of the animate body in which the subtlest and most penetrating substance alone is received . . . the brain is truly the throne of the soul and the abode of wisdom. . . . Hence its nature and what emerges from its constituent parts concerning temperament, disposition, number and mixture deserves to be investigated a little more exactly. (Hensing 1719, in Tower 1983: 249)

After nearly 400 years of research and with the help of the study of psychoactive drugs, we are presently a bit closer to understanding "exactly" how our brains work.

APPENDIX:
CHEMICAL STRUCTURES
OF ANADENANTHERA-
BASED DRUGS

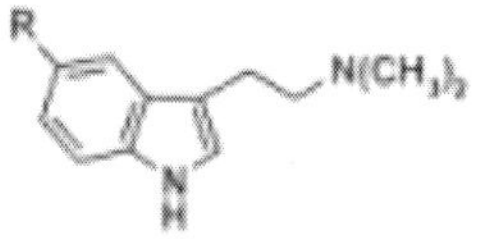

R=H; *N,N*-dimethyltryptamine (DMT)
R=OH; bufotenine
R=OCH$_3$; 5-methoxy-DMT
R=OCOCH$_3$, acetoxy-DMT

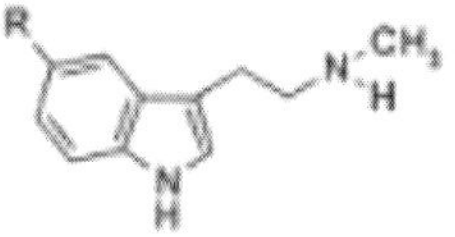

R=CH$_3$; 5-hydroxy-*N*-methyltryptamine
R=H; serotonin

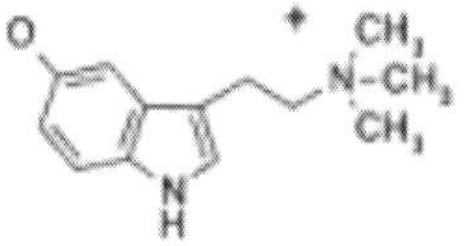

bufotenidine

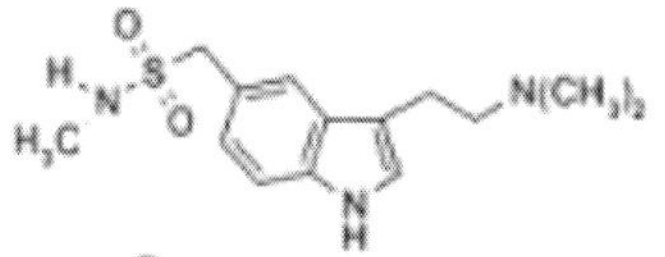

sumatriptan

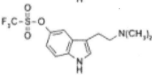

bufotenine triflate

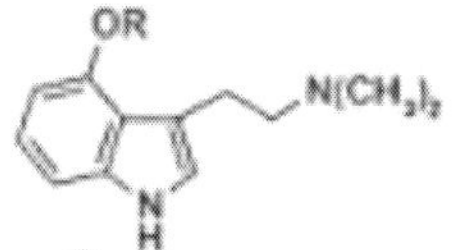

R=H; psilocin
R=P(O)$_2$OH; psilocybin

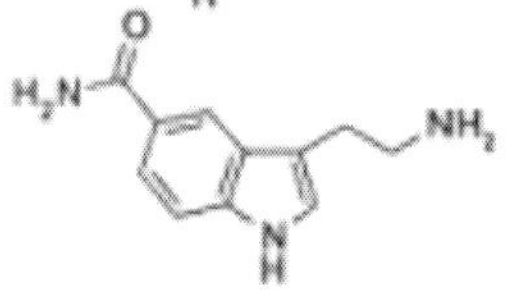

5-carboxamidotryptamine (5-CT)

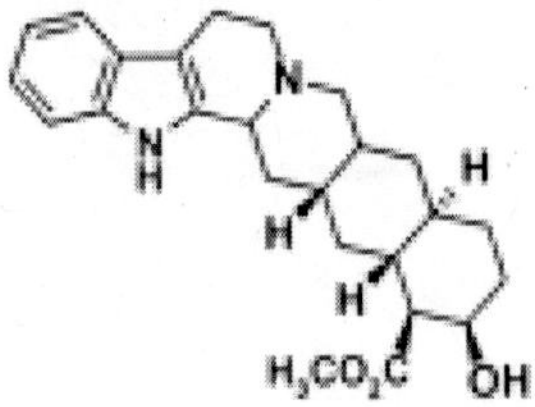

yohimbine

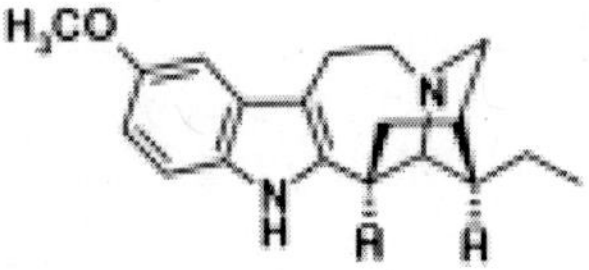

ibogaine

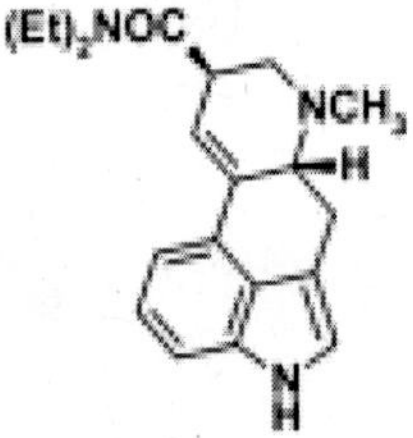

LSD

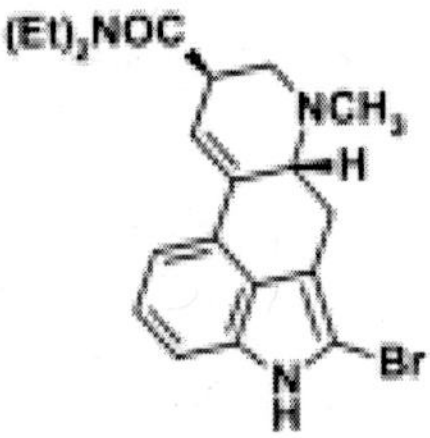

BOL

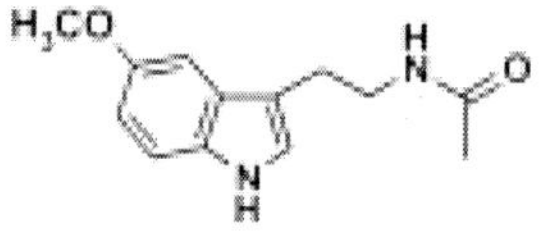

melatonin

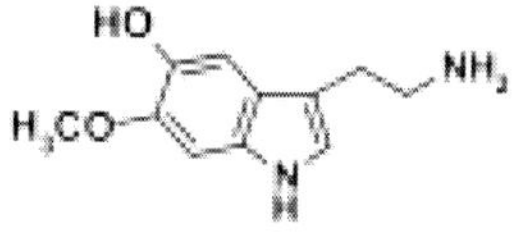

5-hydroxy-6-methoxytryptamine

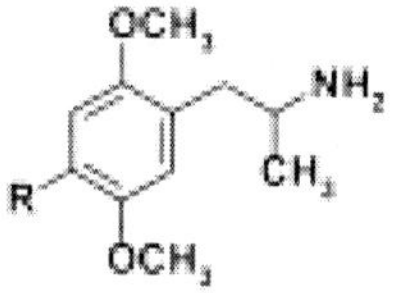

R=I; DOI
R=CH$_3$; DOM

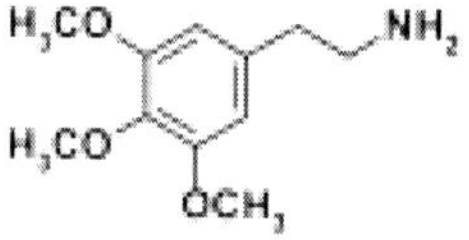

mescaline

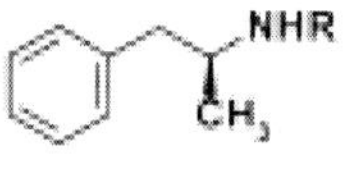

R=H; d-amphetamine
R=CH$_3$; d-methamphetamine

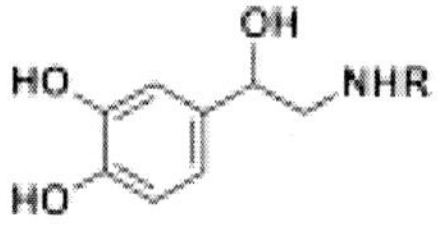

R=H; norepinephrine
R=CH$_3$; adrenaline

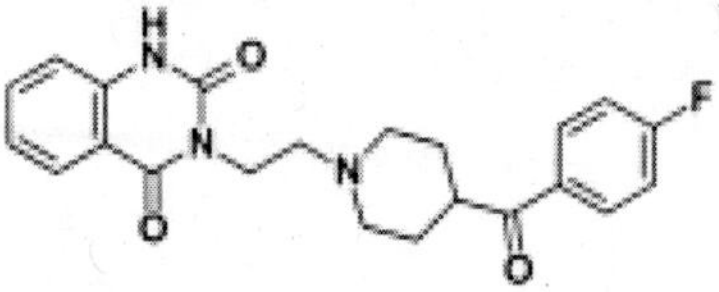

ketanserin

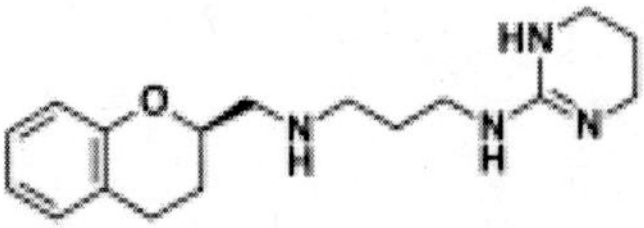

alnitidan

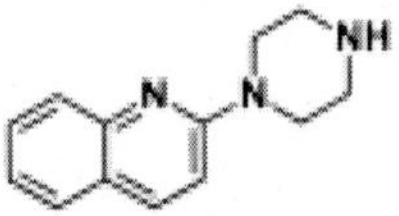

quipazine

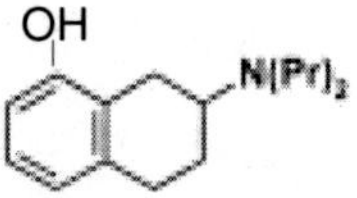

DPAT

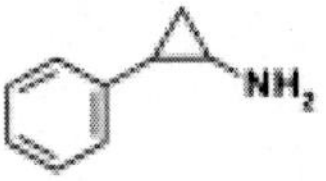

tranylcypramine

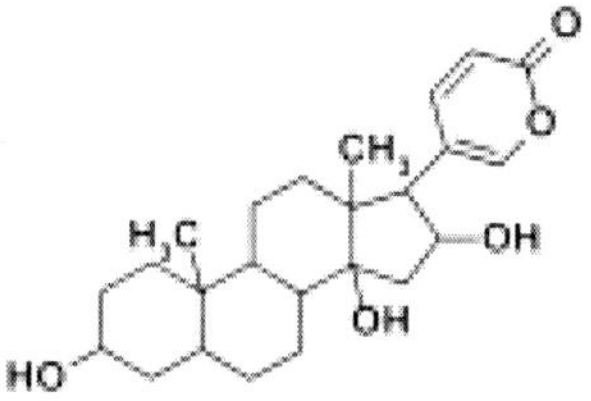

bufogenin

bufotoxin

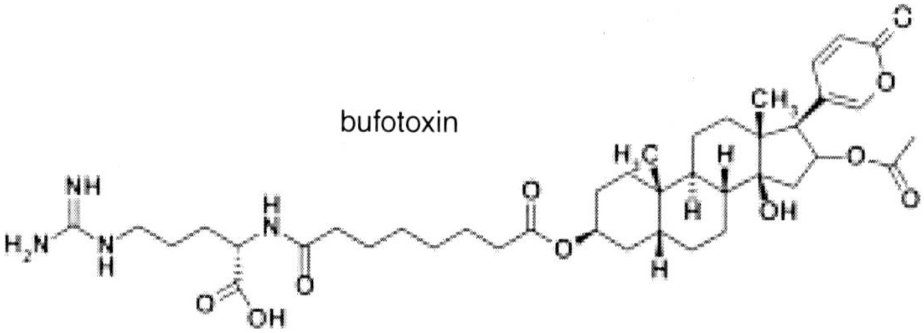

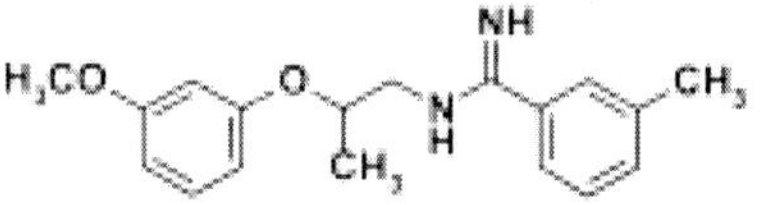

xylamidine

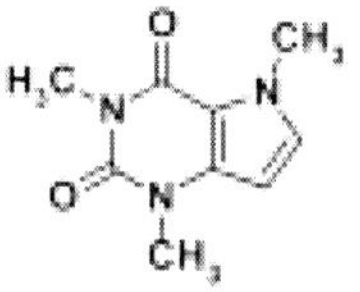

caffeine

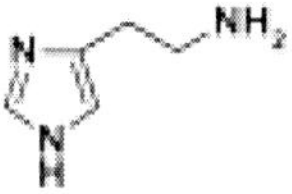

histamine

Chapter 6

Summary and Conclusion

Anadenanthera is a genus of arborescent legumes that currently consists of two species, *A. peregrina* (L.) Speg. and *A. colubrina* (Vell.) Brenan. Each of these has two varieties: *A. peregrina* (L.) Speg. var. *peregrina* von Reis Alt. and *A. peregrina* (L.) Speg. var. *falcata* (Benth.) von Reis Alt. *A. colubrina* (Vell.) Brenan var. *colubrina* von Reis Alt. and *A. colubrina* (Vell.) Brenan var. *Cebil* (Griseb.) von Reis Alt. Originally classified by Bentham (1840) as section *Niopo* of the much larger genus *Piptadenia,* the species of *Anadenanthera* differ sufficiently in a number of morphological characters to warrant separate classification. Among these are flower structures, such as presence or lack of anther glands and shape of anthers, and pod or seed characteristics such as dehiscence of pods along one suture, or suborbicular seeds, narrow or not winged, lacking endosperm. Elements of wood anatomy, including the presence of nonseptate fibers and wide, typically 4- to 5-seriate rays, also serve to separate *Anadenanthera* from *Piptadenia.* In addition, Reis Altschul (1964) distinguished the two species of *Anadenanthera* based on the presence or absence of anther glands, the position of the involucre surrounding the peduncle, pod texture, and geographical location.

Although botanists rarely accept chemical markers when classifying plants, especially on the level of species, there are cases where consistent trends in the chemical makeup of botanically closely related plant groups might help to delineate sections. Rarer still would be the acceptance of a single chemical as a unique character when classifying genera, let alone the establishment of a new genus. The presence of relatively large quantities of bufotenine in the seeds of both species and varieties of *Anadenanthera* was considered as an ancillary feature of distinctness when the last revision of the genus was made (Reis Altschul 1964). This was based strictly on a quantitative, not merely qualitative, analysis since bufotenine has also been found to occur in species formally belonging to *Piptadenia*. Bufo-tenine content in the two species of *Anadenanthera* has consistently been found to be between 1 percent and 12 percent of the weight of seeds, whereas occurrence of this alkaloid in *Piptadenia* proper is usually much less than 1 percent.

The genus *Anadenanthera* continues to have a significant role in society and culture in South America. Historically, these trees have been part of the economic, medicinal, and spiritual development of the region. Among their economic uses were lumber, paper pulp pro-duction, and the tanning and dyeing of leather. Logging of both natu-ral and cultivated *Anadenanthera* forests continues to this day, al-though on a much reduced scale relative to the early twentieth century. Medicinally, the tannin from species of *Anadenanthera* has been used to produce a less bitter-tasting antimalarial preparation of quinine. Along with its adhesive properties, *angico* gum derived from these trees has been used in the treatment of respiratory illness. The chemical composition of *angico* has been shown to consist of poly-saccharides derived from galactose, ribose, arabinose, xylose, and rhamnose.

Chemical analyses of species of *Anadenanthera* have been thor-ough. Every part of the plants has been examined. A number of ste-roids such as β-sitosterol and its palmitic ester, as well as several triterpenoids (lupeol and lupenone) and neoflavanoids (dalbergin and Kuhlmannin) have been detected in heartwood (Miyauchi et al. 1976). The leaves have been shown to contain the C-flavanosides orientin and vitexin (Figure 4.3), a number of cyclitols (inositol, pinitol, bornesitol, ononitol, and quebrachitol; Plouvier 1962), sev-eral rare amino acids, such as 5-hydroxypipecolinic acid, L-albizzin, and djenkolic acid (Krauss and Reinbothe 1973), and a host of indole alkaloids (Figure 4.4). The last are by far the most studied chemical substances in *Anadenanthera*. A dozen tryptamine and β-carboline alkaloids have been detected in leaves, seeds, pods, seedlings, roots, bark, and twigs (Schultes et al. 1977). The seeds contain the largest quantities of the three main alkaloids, bufotenine, *N,N*-dimethyl-tryptamine, and 5-hydroxy-*N*-monomethyltryptamine. No single in-dividual of any species has been shown to contain all twelve alkaloids.

Methods of preparation and additives are so variable that it would be senseless to endeavor to establish fixed or specific recipes. The seeds are usually roasted and powdered; they can be ingested as the sole ingredient, but most frequently an alkaline substance is added to the powdered seeds. The alkaline component is obtained from calcined and powdered snail shells or ashes from burned tree bark or stems. Tobacco leaves are also a frequent admixture. The most common method of administration is by snuffing, although *Anadenanthera* seeds are often mixed with tobacco and smoked as a cigar or in pipes, or even administered as enemas (Califano 1976; Métraux 1947; Nimuendajú 1948b; Reichel-Dolmatoff 1944; Spruce 1970). Snuffing is accomplished two ways: self-administered and collaborative. Self-administration is done via a variety of implements, usually made of bird bones. The shapes include single tubes, double parallel tubes, and Y- and V-shaped inhalers (Plate 54). The collaborative modality is usually achieved with a long bamboo or bird bone tube that is preloaded with the powder, one individual blowing the snuff into the nose of another. Some groups such as the Maué and Kaxúyana place the snuff on elaborately carved snuff trays with affinities to pre-Columbian Andean artifacts. Ceremonies of the Maué, Kaxúyana, Guahibo, and Tunebo, among others, are often night-long sessions accompanied by continuous use of snuff (Frikel 1961; Reichel-Dolmatoff 1944, 1978); on the other hand, Yanomamö and Tupari snuffing rituals are frequently diurnal.

The pipes and associated *Anadenanthera* seeds from Inca Cueva and Huachichocana in northwestern Argentina provide the earliest evidence for psychoactive plant use in all of South America. The archaeological context for these pipes has been dated at ca. 2130 B.C. and 1450 B.C., respectively. The earliest evidence for snuffing is provided by the Peruvian coastal sites of Huaca Prieta and Asia, both dated to ca. 1200 B.C. Further south, in the extreme north coast of Chile, several sites have yielded snuffing equipment dated to ca. 1000-800 B.C.

The highest concentration of archaeological evidence for the use of visionary snuffs is in the southern sector of the Central Andes. This area includes the Atacama Desert, the Puna de Jujuy, and the Quebrada de Humahuaca. In San Pedro de Atacama, the archaeological region with the highest incidence of snuffing paraphernalia, approximately 20 to 22 percent of the male population was using psychoactive snuffs between the third and the tenth centuries A.D. The Loa River basin of northern Chile and the Quebrada de Humahuaca in northwestern Argentina are the second and third areas with extensive and clear archaeological evidence for the use of snuffs. The plant source of the snuff used in this area is *Anadenanthera colubrina* var. *Cebil,* as demonstrated by the detection of bufotenine in archaeological snuff samples and by the presence of its seeds in archaeological contexts (Llagostera et al. 1988; Torres et al. 1991). The probable plant source for the snuff powder used at Huaca Prieta, Chavín de Huantar, as well as by the Muisca of the northern Andes, was *Anadenanthera peregrina.* This species was probably obtained from the tropical forest area, one of many tropical forest goods traded into the Andean highlands and the Pacific coast.

Indigenous use of psychoactive preparations from seeds of *Anadenanthera* species closely overlaps the geographical range of the genus. Those groups on the margins or beyond its distribution often engaged in trade to obtain these seeds. The Piaroa traded curare for *yopo* with the Guahibo, who did not prepare this dart poison (Reichel-Dolmatoff 1944). Yanomamö villages located near *Anadenanthera* groves will trade the seeds over a wide area (Chagnon 1992). In examining the ancient cultures of the Atacama and northwestern Argentina, the study of such trade relations could contribute to the understanding of patterns of ideological exchange.

A comparative review of the interaction between San Pedro de Atacama and northwestern Argentina raises pertinent questions regarding the spread of ideological traits. Mercantile exchange between these two areas is apparent in the frequent presence of ceramics, baskets, smoking pipes, and other artifacts. Objects from the Argentine northwest are frequent in San Pedro de Atacama and vice versa. However, two important features do not seem to correspond to the established trade patterns. First, it is known that the habitat of *A. colubrina* var. *Cebil* did not include the Atacama Desert. Available evidence points to the seeds of this leguminous tree as a primary component of snuff powder preparations. If the *cebil* seed trade was as important as the evidence suggests, certain elements of technique and iconography were not part of the exchange. In San Pedro de Atacama, smoking via ceramic or stone pipes disappeared from the archaeological record ca. A.D. 300, concurrent with an increase in the presence of snuffing paraphernalia. Visionary inhalants greatly lose importance in San Pedro de Atacama after A.D. 1000. In contrast, in neighboring northwestern Argentina, smoking was the preferred modality for the consumption of visionary substances since at least 2000 B.C., and snuffing did not acquire importance until after A.D. 900. Second, Tiwanaku iconography was of relative importance in San Pedro de Atacama, while in northwestern Argentina there is no evidence for this type of iconography. Given the extensive trade between these two areas ca. A.D. 100 to 900, which most probably included *cebil* seeds, it is notable that snuffing paraphernalia as well as Tiwanaku iconographic elements were apparently not present in northwestern Argentina during this period. The existence of diverse snuff powder recipes must be considered, not all of which may have been dependent on *A. colubrina*. Flora with psychoactive properties unknown to us might have provided the necessary ingredients for alternative formulas that might have been used by the people of San Pedro de Atacama. Notwithstanding this factor, it can be concluded that ideological exchange was not an indispensable part of mercantile exchange and in some instances remained autonomous and discreet.

The iconography related to psychoactive plant use in South America is composed of widespread themes and motifs that appear in every culture, as well as regional iconographic configurations that reflect the influence of the cultures within which these images were produced. Thematic units with a widespread geographical distribution include avian, feline, and ophidian representations, images that are closely related to the use of shamanic inebriants all over South America. Avian imagery is associated with snuffing in the form of bird bone tubes with feathers as cleaners or as ornamentation, even as part of the shamanic costume. Avian motifs are sometimes carved onto snuffing implements (e.g., the Maué and Tupari). Snuffs are kept in jaguar bones, and Guahibo shamans from the Colombian lowlands paint their faces with marks simulating a jaguar's skin, wear necklaces of jaguar teeth, and carry their snuffing paraphernalia in bags of jaguar fur (Reichel-Dolmatoff 1978). Regional and temporal variations of central Andean thematic units are seen in the profile and frontal staff-bearing figures represented on snuff trays incised with Tiwanaku motifs, and in the decapitation or Sacrificer theme that appears most frequently in northern Chile and northwestern Argentina.

The wide spatial and temporal distribution of the evidence for *Anadenanthera* ritual and visionary use attest to its importance in the construction and subsequent maintenance and modifications of pre-Columbian and postcontact indigenous ideologies. The study of the objects utilized in the manufacture and ingestion of *Anadenanthera* preparations by pre-Columbian cultures provides the opportunity to explore its role in the construction of complex iconographic systems and state formation in the central Andes. Throughout the pre-Hispanic world, psychoactive plants are considered intermediaries between the human and the supernatural realm; they are capable of participating in the interpretation and creation of cultural elements (see Bourne 1906; Colombo 1992; Frikel 1961; Las Casas 1909; Pané 1974; Reichel-Dolmatoff 1971).

The sources of snuff powders used in traditional healing practices throughout South America have been verified by chemical analysis. Although complicated by the occasional admixture of one or more plants to these preparations, the presence of large quantities of bufotenine is enough evidence to assign species of *Anadenanthera* as at least one ingredient of the snuff. The absence of bufotenine and the presence of a high concentration of 5-methoxy-*N,N*-dimethyltryptamine assigns one or more species of *Virola* as its source. Detection in Amazonian snuffs of the carboline alkaloids harmine, harmaline, and tetrahydroharmine suggest use of species of *Banisteriopsis* as snuff powder admixtures. Although traces of several reduced β-carboline alkaloids have been detected in *Anadenanthera,* these generally either lack a ring oxygen substituent or possess one at position 6, clearly different from the harmine class, which always has a methoxy or hydroxy group at position 7. The theory that admixtures of β-carbolines and tryptamines in the same psychoactive preparations gives rise to enhanced effects has been advanced. In the case of orally ingested ayahuasca preparations, the known MAO inhibitory effects of harmine and harmaline have been postulated to play a role in rendering the normally orally inactive dialkyltryptamines such as DMT far more centrally bioavailable (see Ott 1994 for a thorough discussion). A certain number of anecdotal reports would also suggest that ingestion of dialkyltryptamine/β-carboline preparations by smoking also leads to enhanced effects relative to the ingestion of DMT alone (Ott 1994). Several lines of reasoning suggest that such use might not be the case with either snuffed or smoked preparations of *Anadenanthera.* As mentioned, analytical encounters with snuff or smoking preparations containing harmine (from *Banisteriopsis*) and the dialkylated tryptamines (from *Anadenanthera*) are extremely rare. Given the common co-occurrence of these plants in the same geographical regions and the obvious general shamanic awareness of the properties of preparations of both plants, we can conclude that such snuff admixtures are not widely deemed necessary. The occasional finding of a snuff preparation of only the β-carboline–containing *Banisteriopsis* could suggest a local or temporary unavailability of *Anadenanthera* seed preparations. Although of possible pharmacological significance as pure compounds, the reduced β-carboline alkaloids found in *A. peregrina,* 2-methyl- and 1,2-dimethyl-6-methoxy-1,2,3,4-tetrahydro-β-carboline, were of very low concentration and were confined to the bark, a part of the plant known not to be employed in snuff preparations. A single reported occurrence of the third carboline alkaloid, 2-methyl-1,2,3,4-tetrahydro-β-carboline, in trace (<.01 percent) amounts in seeds of *A. peregrina* would be without physiological significance. Last, none of the three *Anadenanthera* carbolines have ever been detected in the snuff preparations themselves.

Laboratory work has confirmed that even over relatively short time periods, the chemical composition of the snuff powder preparations degrade. The only detectable alkaloid after a year's storage was bufotenine, perhaps reflecting its very high concentration in the original sample. However, alkaloids have been detected in snuff samples and seeds that have been stored for much longer periods. Snuff samples of more than a thousand years in age excavated in the Atacama Desert (Torres et al. 1991) and seeds from 120-year-old museum sources (Schultes et al. 1977) have also been found to contain bufotenine residues.

The biosynthetic sequences by which secondary metabolites such as the tryptamine alkaloids are formed have been extensively studied. At first glance, it might be assumed that small molecules such as bufotenine are formed through a simple, linear reaction pathway, much as they are synthesized in the laboratory. In certain plant species, this might be true, but in dealing with complex biological organisms, studying the number of variables in chemical reactions taking place in living cells can be daunting. Arriving at a complete picture of biosynthetic pathways involves understanding the role of enzymes and cofactors, reaction kinetics and chemical mechanisms, stoichiometry of reactions, and the relationships of intermediates to products. Although much useful information can be gained from precursor-product studies involving precursor feeding (balance studies) or radiolabeling experiments, enzymatic rate-limiting steps must be taken into account. Although complete biochemical studies with

Anadenanthera have not been reported, the information gleaned from several partial studies indicates that the "best guess" reaction sequence for the formation of bufotenine is: tryptophan → tryptamine → serotonin (5-HT) → *N*-methyl-5-hydroxytryptamine → bufotenine (Figure 4.6).

Of the dozen alkaloids found in *Anadenanthera,* many have significant biological effects in human beings and other animals. For example, numerous anecdotal (Ott 1994; Shulgin and Shulgin 1997) and a few clinical studies (Strassman and Qualls 1994; Strassman et al. 1994) have positively demonstrated the short-acting, powerful visionary effects of *N,N*-dimethyltryptamine (DMT). Fewer studies of its close analog, 5-methoxy-DMT (Shulgin and Shulgin 1997) have shown an even more powerful event, not universally appreciated. Serotonin (5-HT) is perhaps the most widely studied of the simple tryptamines by virtue of being a very important mammalian neurotransmitter involved in a variety of CNS functions such as sleep, appetite, sexual function, pain, and motor regulation. Outside of basic pharmacological experiments demonstrating simple effects on blood pressure, heart rate, and receptor binding properties, much less is known about the monoalkyl tryptamine *Anadenanthera* alkaloids, 5-methoxy-*N*-methyltryptamine and 5-hydroxy-*N*-methyltryptamine (*N*-methyl-serotonin). Next to nothing is known of the pharmacology of bufotenine *N*-oxide and the tetrahydro-β-carbolines. Some interest in the β-carbolines has been shown relative to their possible anxiogenic and MAO inhibitory properties, as well as their potential role as human pineal metabolites in the study of alcoholism. Except for a minor role as possible synergists to the effects of bufotenine, the presence of any of these compounds in snuff preparations is insignificant because of their very low concentrations. The main constituent and most centrally significant component of the *Anadenanthera* snuffs is bufotenine, 5-hydroxy-*N,N*-dimethyltryptamine.

There have been only a few reported human studies with pure bufotenine, and still fewer with authenticated *Anadenanthera* snuff preparations. None of these studies could be considered truly clinical because of the lack of blind, placebo-controlled, and random methods. Considering the often profound and prolonged central effects induced in humans by fully visionary substances such as LSD, mescaline, DOM, and psilocybin, a truly random study with such drugs would raise serious ethical and moral questions, especially with naive subjects, or even those whose sole idea of intoxication involves alcohol, marijuana, or cocaine. Such experimentation could only be approached with full disclosure and an enlightened informed consent, even with a group of veteran subjects, well-experienced with the nature and sequelae of visionary events.

Self-experiments using bufotenine free base have been reported (Ott 2001a, 2001b). Because of the sparse pharmacological information on bufotenine, Ott, with the cooperation of two well-informed and experienced volunteers, decided to investigate the intranasal activity of bufotenine free base. The alkaloid was isolated from *A. colubrina* var. *Cebil* seeds collected in Salta, Argentina. All bioassays were conducted outside the United States in countries in which bufotenine is not a controlled substance (only in the United States is bufotenine illegal). Self-experiments by Ott and one of the authors (Torres) demonstrated its marked visionary effects. Nasal inhalation of 100 mg bufotenine free base elicited brilliantly swirling geometric patterns accompanied by synesthesia at four minutes. There was noticeable heaviness in the limbs and slight pressure all over the body at 15 minutes. Geometric patterns subsided at approximately 25 minutes, after a period of pronounced spatial and temporal disorientation. The profound visionary stimuli that followed were not as colorful and full of light as those caused by psilocybin, mescaline, and LSD. Instead, the psychoptic space was dimly illuminated and completely removed from the familiar, its components barely visible in the threshold between light and dark. The body was relaxed, with no redness in the face present, nor cardiac nor respiratory distress experienced. Cessation of effects was abrupt at one hour and 50 minutes.

Enough information can be gleaned from the limited number of anecdotal studies with bufotenine to conclude that it is, indeed, a potent short-acting psychoactive compound possessing properties not unlike those of its close analog, *N,N*-dimethyltryptamine. It can also be concluded that bufotenine is largely responsible for the inebriating effects of *Anadenanthera* snuffs and fumatories. Although postulated to occur naturally in humans suffering from a variety of mental disorders, the verification of bufotenine as a causative factor in schizophrenia, bipolar disorder, chronic anxiety, or paranoid psychosis associated with violence has not been conclusively demonstrated.

Investigations of the basic pharmacology of bufotenine have shown that it is not a particularly remarkable substance. Although demonstrated to have partial to full agonist properties at a host of 5-HT (and possibly alpha-adrenergic) receptor subtypes, it does not appear to have a high specificity for any single receptor. Other effects of bufotenine on the serotonin neurotransmitter system include the release of 5-HT from synaptosomes and reuptake inhibition, effects possibly mediated by the serotonin active transport carrier. Bufotenine has also been shown to be a mild MAO inhibitor. These properties might partially account for the observed central effects of the drug in animals in which bufotenine has poor blood-brain barrier penetration. The major physiological actions of bufotenine in mammals include mild increases in both force and rate of heart contractions and pulmonary perfusion as a result of vasoconstriction. This property also gives rise to effects on temperature regulation. The acute toxicity of bufotenine appears to be rather low, with an LD_{50} in rodents of 200 mg/kg. Death occurs via respiratory arrest. The insect world seems to be remarkably sensitive to the application of bufotenine, perhaps reflecting the importance of 5-HT in the nervous systems of these organisms. Such effects as electrical activity in ant brain, diuresis in other insects, heart stimulation in the tobacco hornworm and certain crustaceans, nerve stimulation in snails, teratogenicity in the planarian worm, and stimulation of egg laying in butterflies have all been demonstrated.

We now conclude the story of *Anadenanthera* shamanic preparations and bufotenine. Undoubtedly, this monograph will not be the final word on topics that have occupied scientific interest for more than a century. Future avenues of research could include, for example, a clarification of the geographical distribution of the genus in the tropical forest area; *A. peregrina* var. *falcata* and *A. colubrina* var. *colubrina,* the two least known varieties, should be the subject of direct field studies. Andean archaeology would benefit by a thorough investigation of trade routes and patterns of interaction related to the trade in *Anadenanthera* seeds and related paraphernalia. The snuffing equipment was one of the carriers of ideology during the Middle Horizon period (ca. A.D. 200-900; Menzel 1964) of Andean cultural history, and it circulated over a wide geographical area. Such a study would allow us to better understand the exchange of complex ideologies between peripheral areas such as San Pedro de Atacama and

Niño Korin, with pre-Hispanic metropolitan centers in the Lake Titi-caca basin. A further study of bufotenine should include detailed in-vestigations of indigenous Mesoamerican, as well as Asian, use of cutaneous exudates of *Bufo* toad. We trust that the reader will be able to understand the complex role of *Anadenanthera* in New World ide-ologies that we have endeavored to chronicle. The twenty-first cen-tury will witness a further unfolding of our understanding of brain chemistry through the use of simple tryptamines such as bufotenine and its analogs as research tools.

Bibliography

Abramson, H. A. 1955. *Neuropharmacology,* Transactions of the Second Conference, Josiah Macy Jr. Foundation, New York.

Acosta, J. de. 1985. *Doctrina Cristiana y Catecismo para instrucción de los Indios.* Consejo Superior de Investigaciones Cientificas, Madrid (facsimile of trilingual text, orig. ed. 1584-1585, Antonio Ricardo Impresor, Lima, Peru).

Aghajanian, G. K., and H. J. Haigler. 1976. "Hallucinogenic indoleamines: Preferential action upon presynaptic serotonin receptors." *Psychopharmacology Communication,* (volume date 1975) 1, 6: 619-629.

Aguado, P. de. 1956. *Recopilación historial,* 4 vols. Biblioteca de la Presidencia de Colombia, Bogotá.

Aguerre, A. M., A. F. Distel, and C. A. Aschero. 1973. "Hallazgo de un sitio acerámico en la Quebrada de Inca Cueva (Provincia de Jujuy)." *Relaciones. Sociedad Argentina de Antropología* 8, new series: 197-231.

―――. 1975. "Comentarios sobre nuevas fechas en la cronología arqueológica precerámica de la Provincia de Jujuy." *Relaciones. Sociedad Argentina de Antropología* 9, new series: 211-214.

Agurell, S., B. Holmstedt, J. E. Lindgren, and R. E. Schultes. 1968. "Identification of two new ß-carbolines alkaloids in South American hallucinogenic plants." *Biochemical Pharmacology* 17: 2487-2488.

―――. 1969. "Alkaloids in certain species of *Virola* and other South American plants of ethnopharmacologic interest." *Acta Chemica Scandinavica* 23: 903-916.

Ahlborg, U., B. Holmstedt, and J. E. Lindgren. 1968. "Fate and metabolism of some hallucinogenic indolealkylamines." *Advances in Pharmacology* 6, B: 213-229.

Ahond, A., A. Cave, C. Kan-Fan, Y. Langlois, and P. Potier. 1970. "The fragmentation of *N,N*-Dimethyltryptamine oxide and related compounds: A possible implication in indole alkaloid biosynthesis." *Journal of the Chemical Society, Chemical Communications:* 517.

Alanís, R. 1947. *Material arqueológico de la civilización Diaguita.* Museo Arqueológico Regional "Inca Huasi," La Rioja, Argentina.

Alcalde Gonzáles, J. 1995. "Ocupación humana en el período temprano en el valle de Ilo: Chilatilla Bajo, Ilo, Perú." *Actas del XIII Congreso de Arqueología Chilena,* pp. 165-170 plus 3 figs. Universidad de Antofagasta, Chile.

Aldunate, C., J. Berenguer, V. Castro, L. Cornejo, J. L. Martínez, and C. Sinclaire. 1986. *Cronología y asentamientos en la región del Loa Superior.* Universidad de Chile, Santiago.

Allende, M. del Pilar. 1981. *La colección arqueológica "Emil de Bruyne" de Caspana.* Thesis for Licenciatura en Arqueología y Prehistória. Departamento de Ciencias Antropológicas y Arqueología, Universidad de Chile, Santiago.

Almaula, N., B. Ebersole, J. A. Ballesteros, H. Weinstein, and S. Sealfon. 1996. "Contribution of a helix 5 locus to selectivity of hallucinogenic and nonhallucinogenic ligands for the human 5-hydroxytryptamine$_{2A}$ and 5-hydroxytryptamine$_{2C}$ receptors: Direct and indirect effects on ligand affinity mediated by the same locus." *Molecular Pharmacology* 50: 34-42.

Almaula N., B. J. Ebersole, D. Zhang, H. Weinstein, and S. C. Sealfon. 1996. "Mapping the binding site pocket of the serotonin 5-Hydroxytryptamine$_{2A}$ receptor. Ser3.36(159) provides a second interaction site for the protonated amine of serotonin but not of lysergic acid diethylamide or bufotenin." *Journal of Biological Chemistry* 271, 25: 14672-14675.

Almeida Costa, O. de. 1970. "Farmaco-etnologia do Paricá e do Yákee." *Revista Brasileira de Farmacia* 51, 9-10: 273-299.

Alvares-Pereira, N., I. C. Marins, and H. Moussatche. 1963. "Some pharmacological studies on bufotenine and bufotenidine." *Revista Brasileira de Biologia* 23, 3: 211-222.

Alvarsson, J.-Å. 1988. *The Mataco of the Gran Chaco: An ethnographic account of change and continuity in Mataco socio-economic organization.* Almqvist and Wiksell International, Stockholm, Sweden.

————. 1995. "Tobacco, *Cebil* and shamanism among the Weenhayek: A few notes on the secular and ritual use of *Nicotiana tabacum* and *Anadenanthera colubrina* among the Weenhayek Indians of the Gran Chaco." *Acta Americana* 3, 2: 117-136, Sweden.

Ambrosetti, J. B. 1899. *Notas de arqueología Calchaquí.* Buenos Aires, Argentina.

————. 1902. *Antigüedades Calchaquíes. Datos arqueológicos de la provincia de Jujuy.* Imprenta y Casa Editora de Coni y Hermanos, Buenos Aires, Argentina.

————. 1906. "El hacha de Huaycama." *Anales del Museo Nacional de Buenos Aires,* vol. 16, 15-23, Argentina.

————. 1907-1908. *Exploraciones arqueológicas en la ciudad prehistórica de La Paya,* 2 vols. Facultad de Filosofía y Letras, publicaciones de la Sección de Antropología 3, Buenos Aires, Argentina.

Andary, C., G. Privat, J. J. Serrano, and C. Francois. 1978. "5-hydroxyindole derivatives of *Amanita:* Chemical and pharmacological study." *Collection de Medecine Legale et de Toxicologie Medicale* 106: 43-54.

Anden, N. E., H. Corrodi, and K. Fuxe. 1971. "Hallucinogenic drugs of the indolealkylamine type and central monoamine neurons." *Journal of Pharmacology and Experimental Therapeutics* 179, 2: 236-249.

Anglería, P. M. de. 1964-1965. *Décadas del Nuevo Mundo,* 2 vols. Porrúa, Mexico. English ed., Anghiera, Petro Martire d'. 1912. *De orbe novo decadas: The eight decades of Peter Martyr d'Anghera,* 2 vols. New York.

Anton, R., Y. Jiang, B. Weniger, J. P. Beck, and L. Rivier. 1993. "Pharmacognosy of *Mimosa tenuiflora* (Willd.) Poiret." *Journal of Ethnopharmacology* 38, 2-3: 153-157.

Arenas, P. 1992. "El *cebil* o el 'árbol de la ciencia del bien y del mal.'" *Parodiana* 7, 1-2: 101-114, Centro de Estudios Farmacológicos y Botánicos, Buenos Aires.

Ariens, E. J. 1954. "Affinity and intrinsic activity in the theory of competitive inhibition." *Archives of International Pharmacodynamics* 99: 32-55.

Arrom, J. J. 1975. *Mitología y artes Prehispánicas de las Antillas*. Siglo XXI Editores, Mexico City.

Aschero, C. A., and H. D. Yacobaccio. 1994. "20 años despues: Inca Cueva 7 reinterpretado." *Resumenes del XI Congreso Nacional de Arqueología Argentina*, San Rafael, Argentina.

Asociacion Contisuyo. 1997. *Contisuyo: Memorias de las culturas del Sur*, Moquegua, Peru.

Axelrod, J. 1961. "Enzymatic formation of psychomimetic metabolites from normally occurring compounds." *Science* 134: 343.

Axelsson, S., A. Bjorklund, and N. Seiler. 1971. "Identification of bufotenine in toad brain by chromatography and mass spectrometry of its 1-(dimethylamino)naphthalene-5-sulfonyl [DANS]-derivative." *Life Sciences* 10: 745-749.

Ayala, F. G. P. de. 1980. *El primer nueva corónica y buen gobierno*, ed. J. V. Murra and R. Adorno, trans. J. L. Uirioste. Colección América Nuestra—América Antigua, Siglo Veintiuno, Mexico City.

Bailey Kennedy, A. 1982. "*Ecce Bufo:* The toad in nature and in Olmec iconography." *Current Anthropology* 23, 3: 273-290.

Balzer, I., and R. Hardeland. 1992. "Effects of indoleamines and short photoperiods on the encystment of *Gonyaulax polyedra*." *Chronobiology International* 9: 260-265.

Barabas, A. M., and M. A. Bartolomé. 1979. "The mythic testimony of the Mataco." *Latin American Indian Literatures* 3, 2: 76-85, University Center for International Studies, University of Pittsburgh, Pennsylvania.

Barf, T. J., P. de Boer, H. Wikström, S. J. Peroutka, K. Svensson, M. D. Ennis, N. B. Ghazal, J. C. McGuire, and M. W. Smith. 1996. "5HT$_{1D}$ receptor agonist properties of novel 2-[5-[[(trifluoromethyl)sulfonyl]oxy]indolyl]ethylamines and their use as synthetic intermediates." *Journal of Medicinal Chemistry* 39: 4717-4726.

Barlow, R. B., and I. Khan 1959a. "Action of some analogs of tryptamine on the isolated rat uterus and on the isolated rat fundus strip preparations." *British Journal of Pharmacology* 14: 99-107.

————. 1959b. "Actions of some analogs of 5-hydroxytryptamine on the isolated rat uterus and the rat fundus strip preparations." *British Journal of Pharmacology* 14: 265-272.

Baron, A. M. 1979. *Excavación de un cementerio (Los Abuelos, Caspana); sus potencialidades*. Thesis for Licenciatura en Arqueología y Prehistória. Departamento de Ciencias Antropológicas y Arqueología, Universidad de Chile, Santiago.

———. 1984. "Craneos Atacameños y su asociación con tabletas para alucinógenos." *Culturas Atacameñas. Proceedings of the XLIV International Congress of Americanists.* Universidad del Norte, Antofagasta, Chile.

Barry, T. L., G. Petzinger, and S. W. Zito. 1996. "GC/MS comparison of the West Indian aphrodisiac 'Love Stone' to the Chinese medication 'Chan Su': Bufotenine and related bufadienolides." *Journal of Forensic Science* 41: 1068-1073.

Basar, E., C. Basar-Eroglu, B. Rosen, and A. Schutt. 1984. "A new approach to endogenous event-related potentials in man: Relation between EEG and P300 wave." *International Journal of Neuroscience* 24: 1-21.

Bather, P. A., J. R. Linsay-Smith, and R. O. C. Norman. 1971. "Amine oxidation. Part V. Reactions of some N-oxides, including heterocyclic-ring formation, with sulfur dioxide, acetic anhydride, and trifluoroacetic anhydride." *Journal of the Chemical Society (C):* 3060-3068.

Baumann, P., and N. Narasimhachari. 1973. "Identification of N,N-dimethyltryptamine, 5-methoxy-N,N-dimethyltryptamine, and bufotenine by cellulose TLC [thin-layer chromatography]." *Journal of Chromatography* 86, 1: 269-273.

Baxter, C., and M. Slaytor. 1972. "Biosynthesis and turnover of N,N-dimethyltryptamine and 5-methoxy-N,N-dimethyltryptamine in *Phalaris tuberosa*." *Phytochemistry* 11: 2767-2773.

Becher, H. 1960. "Die Surara und Pakidai. Zwei Yanonami-Stamme in Nordwestbrasilien." *Mitteilungen aus dem Museum für Völkerkunde in Hamburg* 26.

Becker-Donner, E. 1953. "Nichtkeramische Kulturfunde Nordwestargentiniens. Aus den Sammlungen der Wiener Museum für Völkerkunde." *Archiv für Völkerkunde* 3: 273-324, Wilhelm Braumuller, Universitats-Verlag, Vienna.

Belleau, B. 1964. "A molecular theory of drug action based on induced conformational perturbations of receptors." *Journal of Medicinal Chemistry* 7: 776-784.

Benington, F., R. D. Morin, and L. C. Clark. 1965. "5-Methoxy-N,N-dimethyltryptamine, a possible endogenous psychotoxin." *Alabama Journal of Medical Science* 2: 397-403.

Bennett, W. C., E. F. Bleiler, and F. H. Sommer. 1948. *Northwest Argentine archaeology.* Yale Publications in Anthropology 38, New Haven, Connecticut.

Benson, L. 1959. *Plant classification.* D.C. Heath and Co., Lexington, Massachusetts.

Bentham, G. 1840. "Contributions towards a flora of South America." *Hooker Journal of Botany* 2: 38-103, 127-146, 210-223, 286-324.

———. 1841-1842. "Notes on *Mimoseae,* with a short synopsis of species." *Hooker Journal of Botany* 4: 323-418.

———. 1874-1875. "Revision of the suborder *Mimoseae.*" *Transactions of the Linnean Society* 30: 335-664, London.

Bercht, F., E. Brodsky, J. A. Farmer, and D. Taylor. 1997. *Taíno. Pre-Columbian art and culture from the Caribbean.* El Museo del Barrio and The Monacelli Press, New York.

Berendsen, H. H. G., and C. L. E. Broekkamp. 1991. "A peripheral 5-HT$_{1D}$-like receptor involved in serotonergic induced hindlimb scratching in rats." *European Journal of Pharmacology* 194: 201-208.

Berendsen, H. H. G., F. Jenck, and C. L. E. Broekkamp. 1989. "Selective activation of 5HT$_{1A}$ receptors induces lower lip retraction in the rat." *Pharmacology Biochemistry and Behavior* 33: 821-827.

Berenguer, J. 1984. "Hallazgos arqueológicos La Aguada en San Pedro de Atacama, norte de Chile." *Gaceta Arqueológica Andina* 12: 12-14, Instituto Andino de Estudios Arqueológicos, Lima.

———. 1987. "Consumo nasal de alucinógenos en Tiwanaku: Una aproximación iconográfica." *Boletín del Museo Chileno de Arte Precolombino* 2: 33-53, Santiago, Chile.

———. 2001. "Evidence for snuffing and shamanism in Prehispanic Tiwanaku stone sculpture." *Eleusis* 5: 61-83, Telesterion and Museo Civico di Rovereto, Trento, Italy.

Berenguer, J., A. Deza, A. Roman, and A. Llagostera. 1986. "La secuencia de Myriam Tarragó para San Pedro de Atacama: Un test por termoluminiscencia." *Revista Chilena de Antropología* 5: 17-54, Facultad de Filosofía, Humanidades y Educación, Universidad de Chile, Santiago.

———. 1988. "Testing a cultural sequence for the Atacama Desert." *Current Anthropology* 29, 2: 341-346.

Berger, G., M. Maziere, C. Marazano, D. Comar, and J. Sastre. 1978. "Carbon-11 labeling of the psychoactive drug *O*-methyl bufotenine and its distribution in the animal organism." *European Journal of Nuclear Medicine* 3, 2: 101-104.

Berlin, J., C. Ruegenhagen, P. Dietze, L. F. Fecker, O. J. M. Goddijn, and J. H. C. Hoge. 1993. "Increased production of serotonin by suspension and root cultures of *Peganum harmala* transformed with a tryptophan decarboxylase cDNA clone from *Catharanthus roseus.*" *Transgenic Research* 2, 6: 336-344.

Bernauer, K. 1964. "Notiz uber Isolierung von Harmin und (+)-1,2,3,4-Tetrahydroharmin aus einer indianischen Schnupfdroge." *Helvetica Chimica Acta* 47: 1075.

Bertonio, L. 1984. *Vocabulario de la lengua Aymara.* Documentos Históricos 1, Ediciones CERES (orig. ed. 1612), Cochabamba, Bolivia.

Bhattacharya, S. K., A. Chakrabarti, M. Sandler, and V. Glover. 1996. "Effects of some anxiogenic agents on rat brain monoamine oxidase (MAO) A and B inhibitory (tribulin) activity." *Indian Journal of Experimental Biology* 34: 1190-1193.

Bhattacharya, S. K., A. Parikh, and S. Ghosal. 1971. "Effects of some indole-3-alkylamines on the melanophores of *Rana tigrina.*" *Indian Journal of Experimental Biology* 9: 400-401.

Bhattacharya, S. K., and A. K. Sanyal. 1971. "Anticholinesterase activity of bufotenine." *Indian Journal of Physiology and Pharmacology* 15, 3: 133-134.

Biocca, E., C. Galeffi, E. G. Montalvo, and G. B. Marini-Bettòlo. 1964. "Sulle sostanze allucinogene impiegate in Amazonia. Nota I. Osservazioni sul *Paricà* dei Tukano e Tariâna del bacino del Rio Uaupés." *Annali di Chimica* 54: 1175-1178.

Bird, J. B. 1943. "Excavations in northern Chile." *Anthropological Papers of the American Museum of Natural History* 38, 4, New York.

———. 1948. "Preceramic cultures in Chicama and Virú." In *A reappraisal of Peruvian Archaeology,* ed. W. C. Bennett, *Memoirs of the Society for American Archaeology* 4: 21-28, Menasha, Wisconsin.

Bird, J. B., and J. Hyslop. 1985. "The preceramic excavations at the Huaca Prieta, Chicama Valley, Peru." *Anthropological Papers of the American Museum of Natural History* 62, 1: 1-294, American Museum of Natural History, New York.

Bloom, B. M. 1970. "Receptor theories." In *Medicinal Chemistry,* 3rd ed., ed. A. Burger, 108-114, Wiley-Interscience, New York.

Boess, F. G., F. J. Monsma Jr., C. Carolo, V. Meyer, A. Rudler, C. Zwingelstein, and A. J. Sleight. 1997. "Functional and radioligand binding characterization of rat 5-HT$_6$ receptors stably expressed in HEK293 cells." *Neuropharmacology* 36: 713-720.

Boetzkes, M., W. Gockel, and M. Höhl. 1986. *Alt-peru. Auf den Spuren der Zivilisation. Herausgegeben anlasslich der Neuaufstellung der Alt-Peru-Sammlung des Roemer-Museums.* Roemer-Museum, Hildesheim, Germany.

Boman, E. 1908. *Antiquités de la región Andine de la Republique Argentine et du Désert d'Atacama,* 2 vols. Imprimerie National, Librairie H. Le Soudier, Paris.

Bongiorno de Pfirter, G. M., and E. L. Mandrile. 1983. "Active principles having hallucinogenic effects. II. Bufotenine and other tryptamines. Their presence in *Anadenanthera peregrina* (L.) Spegazzini (Leguminosae)." *Acta Farmaceutica Bonaerense* 2: 47-54.

Bonhour, A., E. Fischer, and M. C. Melgar. 1967. "Estudios psicofarmacológicos con bufotenina." *Revista de Psiquiatría y Psicología Médica* 8, 3: 123-143, Buenos Aires, Argentina.

Boulenguez, P., J. Chaveau, L. Segu, A. Morel, J. Lanoir, and M. Delaage. 1991. "A new 5-hydroxy-indole derivative with preferential affinity for 5-HT$_{1B}$ binding sites." *European Journal of Pharmacology* 194, 1: 91-98.

Bourne, E. G. 1906. "Columbus, Ramon Pane and the beginnings of American anthropology." *Proceedings of the American Antiquarian Society* 17, new series: 310-348, Worcester, Massachusetts.

Bradley, P., and J. Briggs. 1974. "Mode of action of psychotomimetic drugs. Antagonism of the excitatory actions of 5-hydroxytryptamine by methylated derivatives of tryptamine." *British Journal of Pharmacology* 50, 3: 345-354.

Bray, W. 1978. *The gold of El Dorado.* Times Newspapers Limited, London.

Brazier, J. D. 1958. "The anatomy of some timbers formerly included in *Piptadenia.*" *Tropical Woods* 108: 46-64, School of Forestry, Yale University.

Brenan, J. P. M. 1955. "Notes on Mimosoideae: I." *Kew Bulletin* 2: 161-191 (170-183 *Piptadenia*), Royal Botanical Garden, Kew, London.

Bresolin, S., and V. M. Vargas. 1993. "Mutagenic potencies of medicinal plants screened in the Ames test." *Phytotherapy Research* 7, 3: 260-262.

Brewer-Carias, C., and J. A. Steyermark. 1976. "Hallucinogenic snuff drugs of the Yanomamo Caburiwe-Teri in the Cauaburi River, Brazil." *Economic Botany* 30: 57-66.

Brimblecombe, R. 1967. "Hyperthermic effects of some tryptamine derivatives in relation to their behavioral activity." *International Journal of Neuropharmacology* 6: 423-429.

Brimblecombe, R. W., and R. M. Pinder. 1975. *Hallucinogenic agents.* Wright-Scientechnica, Bristol.

Brown, W. 1922. "Studies in the physiology of parasitism 8. On the exosmosis of nutrient substances from host tissue into the infection drop." *Annals of Botany (London)* 36: 101-119.

Brune, G. G., and H. E. Himwich. 1962. "Indole metabolites in schizophrenic patients." *Archives of General Psychiatry* 6: 324-328.

Budowski, J. de, G. B. Marini-Bettòlo, F. Delle Monache, and F. Ferrari. 1974. "On the alkaloid composition of the snuff drug *yopo* from Upper Orinoco (Venezuela)." *Il Farmaco, Edizione Scientifica* 29: 574-578, Istituto di Chimica Farmaceutica, Universitá di Pavia, Italy.

Bu'Lock, J. D. 1965. *The biosynthesis of natural products.* McGraw-Hill, London.

Bumpus, F. M., and I. Page. 1955. "Serotonin and its methylated derivatives in human urine." *Journal of Biological Chemistry* 212: 111.

Burger, R. L. 1995. *Chavín and the origins of Andean civilization.* Thames and Hudson, London.

Burkart, A. 1952. *Las leguminosas argentinas silvestres y cultivadas.* Ed. ACME, Buenos Aires (*Piptadenia* pp. 144-146).

Califano, M. 1976. "El chamanismo Mataco." *Scripta Ethnologica* 3, 3, part 2: 7-60, Centro de Estudios de Etnología Americana, Buenos Aires.

———. 1995. "Los rostros del chamán: Nombres y estados." In *Chamanismo en Latinoamerica: Una revisión conceptual,* ed. J. Galinier, I. Lagarriga, and M. Perrin, 103-142. Editorial Plaza y Valdés, Mexico.

Callaway, J. C. 1994. *Pinoline and other tryptamine derivatives: Formations and functions.* Kuopio University Publications A. Pharmaceutical Sciences 15, Kuopio, Finland.

Callaway, J. C., M. M. Airaksinen, and J. Gynther. 1995. "Endogenous β-carbolines and other indole alkaloids in mammals." Selected papers from the conference Plants, Shamanism and Altered States of Consciousness, San Luis Potosí, Mexico, *Integration* 5: 19-33, Bilwis-verlag, Knetzgau, Germany.

Caro Alvarez, J. A. 1977. *La Cohoba*. Museo del Hombre Dominicano, Santo Domingo, Dominican Republic.

Casanova, E. 1942. "El yacimiento arqueológico de Angosto Chico." *Relaciones de la Sociedad Argentina de Arqueología* 3: 73-87, plus 8 plates, Buenos Aires.

————. 1946. "The cultures of the Puna and the Quebrada de Humahuaca." *Handbook of South American Indians* 2: 619-632, Bureau of American Ethnology 143, Washington, DC.

————. 1950. *Restauración del Pucará (de Tilcara)*. Instituto de Antropología, Facultad de Filosofía y Letras, Universidad de Buenos Aires, Argentina.

Caspar, F. 1956. *Tupari*. G. Bell and Sons, London.

Cassels, B. K., and J. S. Gómez-Jeria. 1985. "A reevaluation of psychotomimetic amphetamine derivatives in humans." *Journal of Psychoactive Drugs* 17: 129-130.

Castillo, G. 1984. "Un cementerio del Complejo Las Animas en Coquimbo: Un ejemplo de relaciones con San Pedro de Atacama." *Estudios Atacaneños* 7: 264-277, Instituto de Investigaciones Arqueológicas y Museo R. P. Le Paige, San Pedro de Atacama, Chile.

————. 1992. "Evidencia sobre uso de narcóticos en el norte semiarido chileno: Catastro regional." *Boletín del Museo Regional de Atacama* 4: 105-160, Copiapó, Chile.

Cerletti, A., M. Taeschler, and H. Weidmann. 1968. "Pharmacologic studies on the structure-activity relationship of hydroxyindole alkylamines." *Advances in Pharmacology* 6(B): 233-246.

Chacama, J. 2001. "Tabletas, tubos y espatulas: Aproximación a un complejo alucinógeno en el área de Arica, extremo norte de Chile." *Eleusis* 5: 85-100 (thematic issue, *Archaeology of hallucinogens in the Andean region*), Telesterion and Museo Civico di Rovereto, Trento, Italy.

Chagnon, N. 1992. *Yanomamö: The last days of Eden*. First Harvest/Harcourt Brace Jovanovich, Orlando, Florida.

Chagnon, N. A., P. Le Quesne, and J. M. Cook. 1970. "Algunos aspectos de uso de drogas, comercio y domesticación de plantas entre los indígenas Yanomamö de Venezuela y Brasil." *Acta Científica Venezolana* 21: 186-193.

————. 1971. "Yanomamö hallucinogens: Anthropological, botanical, and chemical findings." *Current Anthropology* 12, 1: 72-74.

Chamakura, R. P. 1993. "Bufotenine." *Microgram* 26, 8: 185-192.

————. 1994. "Bufotenine—A hallucinogen in ancient snuff powders of South America and a drug of abuse on the streets of New York City." *Forensic Science Review* 6, 1: 1-18.

Chávez, S. J., and C. M. Torres. 1986. "Pukara style elements present on some snuff tablets from San Pedro de Atacama, northern Chile." Paper presented at the 28th annual meeting of the Institute of Andean Studies, Berkeley, California.

Chilton, W. S., J. Bigwood, and R. E. Jensen. 1979. "Psilocin, bufotenine and serotonin: Historical and biosynthetic observations." *Journal of Psychedelic Drugs* 11, 1-2: 61-69.

Choi, D.-S., G. Birraux, J.-M. Launay, and L. Maroteaux. 1994. "The human serotonin 5-HT$_{2B}$ receptor: Pharmacological link between 5-HT$_2$ and 5-HT$_{1D}$ receptors." *FEBS Letters* 352: 393-399.

Chweitzer, A., E. Geblewicz, and W. C. Liberson. 1937. "Action de la mescaline sur les ondes α (Rythme de Berger) chez l'homme." *Comptes Rendus des Seances de la Societe de Biologie et de Ses Filiales* 74: 1296-1299.

Ciruzzi, S. 1992. "Le lettere di Ernesto Mazzei a Paolo Mantegazza dall'America Meridionale." *Archivio per l'Antropologia e la Etnologia* 122: 207-227, Florence, Italy.

Clark, A. J. 1937. "General pharmacology." In *Handbuch der experimentellen Pharmakologie* 4, ed. A. Heffter, 4-190, Springer, Berlin.

Cobo, B. 1964. *Historia del Nuevo Mundo*, 2 vols. Biblioteca de Autores Españoles, vols. 91, 92, Ediciones Atlas, Madrid.

Colombo, F. 1992. *Historie, del S. D. Fernando Colombo; nelle quali s'ha particolare et vera relatione della vita et de' fatti dell'Ammiraglio Christoforo Colombo suo padre.* Translated from the original Spanish into Italian by Alfonso Ulloa (orig. ed. Apresso Francesco de' Franceschi Sanese, Venice, Italy, 1571), Isonomia, Este (PD), Italy.

"Conditions for investigational use of hallucinogenic drugs bufotenine, *N,N*-dimethyltryptamine, and ibogaine and their salts." 1968. *Federal Register* 33: 2384 (31 Jan.).

Conklin, W. J. 1983. "Pukara and Tiahuanaco tapestry: Time and style in a *Sierra* weaving tradition." *Ñawpa Pacha* 21: 1-44, Institute of Andean Studies, Berkeley, California.

Cooper, J. M. 1949. "Stimulants and narcotics." In *Handbook of South American Indians* 5, ed. J. Steward, 525-558. Smithsonian Institution, Bureau of American Ethnology Bulletin 143, Washington, DC.

Coppens, W., and J. Cato-David. 1971. "Aspectos etnográficos y farmacológicos: El *yopo* entre los Cuiva-Guajibo." *Antropológica* 28: 3-24, Fundación La Salle, Caracas, Venezuela.

Cordy-Collins, A. 1980. "An artistic record of the Chavín hallucinatory experience." *The Masterkey for Indian Lore and History* 54, 3: 84-93, The Southwest Museum, Los Angeles, California.

———. 1982. "Psychoactive painted Peruvian plants: The shamanism textile." *Journal of Ethnobiology* 2, 2: 144-153.

Correnti, G., and A. Eskin. 1982. "Transmitter-like action of serotonin in phase shifting a rhythm from the *Aplysia* eye." *American Journal of Physiology* 242: R333-R338.

Costa, M. A. 1988. "Reconstitución física y cultural de la población tardía del cementerio de Quitor 6 (San Pedro de Atacama)." *Estudios Atacameños* 8: 99-

126, Instituto de Investigaciones y Museo, Universidad del Norte, San Pedro de Atacama, Chile.

Costantini, E. S. 1975. "El uso de alucinógenos de orígen vegetal por las tribus indígenas del Paraguay actual." In *Etnofarmacología de plantas alucinógenas latinoamericanas,* ed. J. L. Diaz, Cuadernos Científicos CEMEF 4: 35-48, Centro Mexicano de Estudios en Farmacodependencia, Mexico.

Courvoisier, S., and O. Leau. 1958. "Protective action of parenterally administered 5-hydroxytryptamine (5-HT) toward bronchospasms induced in the guinea pig by (5-HT) aerosols; Specificity of this action." *Proceedings of the International Congress of Neuro-Pharmacology, Rome:* 303-307.

Cowen, M. A., H. Nishi, and D. Hammack. 1973. "An electrophysiological analysis of hallucinogens." *Biological Psychiatry* 5, 3: 239-256.

Crum Brown, A., and T. Fraser. 1889. "On the connection between chemical constitution and physiological action. Part I. On the physiological action of the salts of the ammonium bases, derived from *Strychnia, Brucia, Thebaia, Codeia, Morphia,* and *Nicotia.*" *Transactions of the Royal Society (Edinburgh)* 25: 151-203.

Dasso, M. C. 1985. "El chamanismo de los Mataco de la margen derecha del Río Bermejo (Provincia del Chaco, República Argentina)." *Scripta Ethnologica, Supplementa* 5: 9-35, Centro de Estudios de Etnología Americana, Buenos Aires.

Dauelsberg, P. 1985. "Faldas del Morro: Fase cultural agro-alfarera temprana." *Chungará* 14: 7-44, Instituto de Antropología, Universidad de Tarapacá, Arica, Chile.

Davis, W. 1988. *Passage of darkness: The ethnobiology of the Haitian zombie.* University of North Carolina Press, Chapel Hill.

Davis, W., and A. T. Weil. 1992. "Identity of a New World psychoactive toad." *Ancient Mesoamerica* 3: 51-59.

De Lima, C. G., C. M. Tereza, C. A. Schwartz, J. S. Cruz, and A. Sebben. 1991. "Utilization of o-phthalaldehyde-sulfuric acid as a spray reagent in thin-layer chromatographic detection of some indolealkylamines and application to cutaneous extracts of toad species." *Talanta* 38: 1303-1307.

Deadwyler, S. A., and R. E. Hampson. 1997. "The significance of neural ensemble codes during behavior and cognition." *Annual Review of Neuroscience* 20: 217-244.

Debenedetti, S. 1930. "Las ruinas del Pucará, Tilcara, Quebrada de Humahuaca (Prov. de Jujuy)." *Archivos del Museo Etnográfico* 2 (primera parte), Facultad de Filosofía y Letras, Universidad de Buenos Aires. Monograph.

Dewhurst, W. G., and E. Marley. 1965. "The effects of a-methyl derivatives of noradrenaline, phenylethylamine and tryptamine on the central nervous system of the chicken." *British Journal of Pharmacology* 25: 682-704.

Dieve, C. E. 1978. "El chamanismo Taíno." *Boletín del Museo del Hombre Dominicano* 7, 9: 189-207, Dominican Republic.

Dijour, E. 1933. "Las cérémonies d'expulsions des maladies chez les Matako." *Journal de la Sociétè des Américanistes* 25, new series: 212-217, Paris.

Doat, J. 1978. "Tannins in tropical woods." *Bois et Forets des Tropiques* 182: 37-54.

Dobritzhoffer, D. 1967. *Historia de los Abipones.* Universidad del Noreste, Resistencia, Argentina.

Dominguez, J. A., and R. Pardal. 1938. "El *hataj,* droga ritual de los indios Matako. Historia de su empleo en América." *Comisión Honoraria de Reducciones de Indios* 6: 35-48, Ministerio del Interior, Buenos Aires.

Domino, E. F., R. R. Krause, and J. Bowers. 1973. "Various enzymes involved with putative neurotransmitters." *Archives of General Psychiatry* 29: 195-201.

Don, N. S., B. E. McDonough, G. Moura, C. A. Warren, K. Kawanishi, H. Tomita, Y. Tachibana, M. Bohlke, and N. R. Farnsworth. 1998. "Effects of *Ayahuasca* on the human EEG." *Phytomedicine* 5: 87-96.

Donnan, C. B. 1976. *Moche art and iconography.* UCLA Latin American Center Publications, University of California, Los Angeles.

———. 1978. *Moche art of Peru: Precolumbian symbolic communication.* Museum of Cultural History, University of California, Los Angeles.

———. 1982. "La caza del venado en el arte Mochica." *Revista del Museo Nacional* 46: 235-251, Lima.

Donnan, C. B., and D. McClelland. 1999. *Moche fineline painting: Its evolution and its artists.* UCLA Fowler Museum of Cultural History, Los Angeles.

Dougherty, B. 1972. "Las pipas de fumar arqueológicas de la Provincia de Jujuy." *Relaciones. Sociedad Argentina de Antropología* VI, new series: 83-89, Buenos Aires.

Dromey, R. G., M. J. Stefik, T. C. Rindfleisch, and A. M. Duffield. 1976. "Extraction of mass spectra free of background and neighboring component contributions from gas chromatography/mass spectrometry data." *Analytical Chemistry* 48: 1368.

Ducke, A. 1938. "Plantes nouvelles." *Archivos del Instituto de Biología Vegetal* 4, 1: 3.

———. 1939. *As leguminosas da Amazônia brasileira.* Servicio de Publicidade Agricola, Rio de Janeiro, Brazil.

Duviols, P. 1967. "Un inédit de Cristóbal de Albornoz: 'La instrucción para descubrir todas las guacas del Pirú y sus camayos y haziendas.'" *Journal de la Société des Americanistes* 55, 2: 497-510, Musée de l'Homme, Paris.

Dyer, D. C. 1974. "Evidence for the action of d-lysergic acid diethylamide, mescaline, and bufotenine on 5-hydroxytryptamine receptors in umbilical vasculature." *Journal of Pharmacology and Experimental Therapeutics* 188, 2: 336-341.

Efron, D. H., B. Holmstedt, and N. Kline, eds. 1967. *Ethnopharmacologic search for psychoactive drugs.* Public Health Service Publication 1645, U.S. Department of Health, Education and Welfare, Washington, DC.

Eglen, R. M., L. Jakeman, and R. A. Alvarez. 1994. "The 5-hydroxytryptamine (5-HT)$_7$ receptor." *Expert Opinion on Investigational Drugs* 3: 175-177.

Eglen, R. M., L. A. Perkins, L. K. M. Walsh, and R. L. Whiting. 1992. "Agonist action of indole derivatives at 5-HT$_1$-like, 5-HT$_2$, 5-HT$_3$ and 5-HT$_4$ receptors in vitro." *Journal of Autonomic Pharmacology* 12, 5: 321-333.

Eliade, M. 1964. *Shamanism: Archaic techniques of ecstasy.* Bollingen Series 76, Princeton University Press, Princeton, New Jersey.

Elkin, K. L., L. Pierrou, U. G. Ahlborg, B. Holmstedt, and J.-E. Lindgren. 1973. "Computer-controlled mass fragmentography with digital signal processing." *Journal of Chromatography* 81: 47-55.

Engel, F. 1963. "A preceramic settlement in the central coast of Peru: Asia, Unit 1." *Transactions of the American Philosophical Society,* new series, vol. 53, part 3, Philadelphia.

Erspamer, V., and B. Asero. 1952. "Identification of enteramine, the specific hormone of the enterochromaffin cell system, as 5-hydroxytryptamine." *Nature* 169: 800-801.

Erspamer, V., T. Vitali, M. Roseghini, and J. M. Cei. 1967. "5-Methoxy- and 5-hydroxyindoles in the skin of *Bufo alvarius*." *Biochemical Pharmacology* 16: 1149-1164.

Ettlinger, M., and A. Kjaer. 1968. "Sulfur compounds in plants." In *Recent advances in phytochemistry,* ed. T. J. Mabry, R. E. Alston, and V. C. Runeckles, 61-62. Appleton-Century-Crofts, New York.

Evans, O. J., and J. Southward. 1914. "A further note on the occurrence of turquoise at Indio Muerto, northern Chile." *Man, a monthly record of anthropological science* 14: 37-39, Royal Anthropological Institute, London.

Evarts, E. V., W. Landau, W. H. Freygang Jr., and W. H. Marshall. 1955. "Some effects of lysergic acid diethylamide and bufotenine on electrical activity in the cat's visual system." *American Journal of Physiology* 182: 594-598.

———. 1956. "Some effects of bufotenine and lysergic acid diethylamide on the monkey." *Archives of Neurology and Psychiatry* 75: 49-53.

Fabian, S. M. 1992. *Space-time of the Bororo of Brazil.* University Press of Florida, Gainesville.

Fabing, H. D. 1956. "On going berserk: A neurochemical inquiry." *American Journal of Psychiatry* 113: 409-415.

Fabing, H. D., and J. R. Hawkins. 1956. "Intravenous bufotenine injection in the human being." *Science* 123: 886-887.

Fabing, H. D., E. Kropa, and J. R. Hawkins. 1956. "Bufotenine effects in humans." *Federation Proceedings* 15: 421.

Falkenberg, G. 1972. "Crystal and molecular structure of bufotenine, 5-hydroxy-N,N-dimethyltryptamine." *Acta Crystallography, Section B,* 28, Pt. 11: 3219-3228.

Farabee, W. C. 1922. "Indian tribes of eastern Peru." *Papers of the Peabody Museum of American Archaeology and Ethnology,* vol. X, Cambridge, Massachusetts.

Farber, N. B., J. Hanslick, C. Kirby, L. McWilliams, and J. Olney. 1998. "Serotonergic agents that activate 5HT$_{2A}$ receptors prevent NMDA antagonist neurotoxicity." *Neuropsychopharmacology* 18: 57-62.

Farnsworth, N. R. 1968. "Hallucinogenic plants." *Science* 162: 1086-1092.

Fellows, L. E., and E. A. Bell. 1971. "Indole metabolism in *Piptadenia peregrina*." *Phytochemistry* 10, 9: 2083-2091.

Fernández Distel, A. A. 1980. "Hallazgo de pipas en complejos precerámicos del borde de la Puna Jujeña (Republica Argentina) y el empleo de alucinógenos por parte de las mismas culturas." *Estudios Arqueológicos* 5: 55-75, Universidad de Chile, Antofagasta.

————. 1985. "Huachichocana: Informes específicos. Ficha tecnica de la Cueva CH III." *Paleoetnológica* 1, 1: 9-12, Centro Argentino de Etnología Americana, Buenos Aires.

Ferrari, M. D., and P. M. Saxena. 1995. "5-HT$_1$ receptors in migraine pathophysiology and treatment." *European Journal of Neurology* 2: 5-21.

Fewkes, J. W. 1907. "The aborigines of Porto Rico and neighboring islands." *Twenty-fifth Annual Report of the Bureau of American Ethnology to the Secretary of the Smithsonian Institution. 1903-1904,* 1-220, Government Printing Office, Washington, DC.

Fischer, E., T. Fernández Lagravere, A. J. Vasquez, and A. O. DiStefano. 1961. "Bufotenine-like substance in the urine of schizophrenics." *Journal of Nervous and Mental Disease* 133: 441-444.

Fish, M. S., and E. Horning. 1956. "Studies on hallucinogenic snuffs." *Journal of Nervous and Mental Disease* 124, 1: 33-37 (Special issue, Society of Biological Psychiatry Eleventh Annual Meeting).

Fish, M. S., N. Johnson, and E. C. Horning. 1955. "*Piptadenia* alkaloids. Indole bases of *P. peregrina* (L.) Benth. and related species." *Journal of the American Chemical Society* 77: 5892-5895.

————. 1956. "Tertiary-amine oxide rearrangements." *Journal of the American Chemical Society* 78: 3668-3671.

Fish, M. S., N. M. Johnson, E. P. Lawrence, and E. C. Horning. 1955. "Oxidative *N*-dealkylation." *Biochimica et Biophysica Acta* 18: 564-565.

Florey, E., and M. Rathmayer. 1978. "The effects of octopamine and other amines on the heart and on neuromuscular transmission in decapod crustaceans: Further evidence for a role as neurohormone." *Comparative Biochemistry and Physiology, C: Comparative Pharmacology* 61C, 1: 229-237.

Fozard, J. R., and A. T. M. Mobarok Ali. 1976a. "Inhibition of the stimulant effect of 5-hydroxytryptamine on cardiac sympathetic nerves by 5-hydroxytryptamine and related compounds." *British Journal of Pharmacology* 58: 416P-417P.

————. 1976b. "Evidence for tryptamine receptors on cardiac sympathetic nerves." *British Journal of Pharmacology* 58: 276P-277P.

Fozard, J. R., A. Mobarok, and T. M. Abu. 1978. "Dual mechanism of the stimulant action of *N,N*-dimethyl-5-hydroxytryptamine (bufotenine) on cardiac sympathetic nerves." *European Journal of Pharmacology* 49, 1: 25-30.

Franch, J. A. 1982. "Religiosidad, alucinógenos y patrones artísticos Taíno." *Boletín del Museo del Hombre Dominicano* 10, 17: 103-117, Dominican Republic.

Franzen, F. 1961. "The significance of endogenous proteinogenic amines in internal medicine with special reference to renal function." *Zeitschrift fur die Gesamte Innere Medizin und Ihre Grengebiete* 16: 214-218.

Fraser, D. 1966. "The Heraldic Woman: A study in diffusion." In *The many faces of primitive art,* ed. D. Fraser, 36-99, Prentice Hall, New Jersey.

Freedman, D. X. 1968. "On the use and abuse of LSD." *Archives of General Psychiatry* 18: 330-347.

Frikel, P. 1961. "*Morí-* a festa do rapé. Indios Kachúyana; Río Trombetas." *Boletim do Museu Paraense Emilio Goeldi,* Belem, Pará, Brasil.

———. 1970. *Os Kaxúyana, notas etno-historicas.* Publicaçoes avulsas no. 14, Museu Paraense Emilio Goeldi, Belem, Pará, Brasil.

Fritz, S. 1922. *Journal of the travels and labours of Father Samuel Fritz in the river of the Amazons between 1686 and 1723.* Trans. from the Evora ms. and edited by George Edmundson, The Hakluyt Society, London.

Fuller, R. W., H. Snoddy, and K. Perry. 1995. "Tissue distribution, metabolism and effects of bufotenine administered to rats." *Neuropharmacology* 34: 799-804.

Fung, R. 1972. "Las Aldas: Su ubicación dentro del proceso histórico del Perú antiguo." *Dédalo* 9-10, Museu de Arte e Arqueología, Universidade de Saô Paulo, Brazil.

Furst, P. T. 1972a. *Flesh of the gods.* Praeger, New York.

———. 1972b. "Ritual use of hallucinogens in Mesoamerica: New evidence for snuffing from the Preclassic and Early Classic." In *Religión en Mesoamerica. XII Mesa Redonda,* ed. U. J. Litvak and T. N. Castillo, 61-68, Sociedad Méxicana de Antropología, Mexico.

———. 1974a. "Archaeological evidence for snuffing in prehispanic Mexico." *Botanical Museum Leaflets* 24, 1: 1-28, Harvard University, Cambridge, Massachusetts.

———. 1974b. "Hallucinogens in Precolumbian art." In *Art and environment in native America,* ed. M. E. King and I. R. Traylor, 50-101, Museum of Texas Technological University, Lubbock, Texas.

Gaddum, J. H. 1953. "Tryptamine receptors." *Journal of Physiology* 119: 363-368.

Gaddum, J. H., and Z. P. Picarelli. 1957. "Two kinds of tryptamine receptor." *British Journal of Pharmacology* 12: 323-328.

Gallaher, T. K., K. Chen, and J. C. Shih. 1993. "Higher affinity of psilocin for human than rat 5-HT$_2$ receptor indicates binding site structure." *Medicinal Chemistry Research* 3: 52-66.

Gambier, M. 2001. "The southernmost archaeological evidence for snuffing in the Central Andes." *Eleusis* 5: 153-157 (thematic issue, *Archaeology of hallucino-*

gens in the Andean region), Telesterion and Museo Civico di Rovereto, Trento, Italy.

García Arévalo, M. 1982. *Arqueología Taína, Museo del Hombre Dominicano.* Catálogo de Exposición, Instituto de Cooperación Iberoamericana, Madrid.

García Arévalo, M., and L. Chanlatte. 1976. "Las espátulas vómicas sonajeras de la cultura Taína." Museo del Hombre Dominicano, Dominican Republic.

García Márquez, M., and R. Bustamante Montoro. 1990. "Arqueología del Valle de Majes." *Gaceta Arqueológica Andina,* V, 18/19: 25-40, Lima.

Gessner, P. K. 1970. "Pharmacological studies of 5-methoxy-*N,N*-dimethyltryptamine, LSD [*N,N*-diethyl-D-lysergamide], and other hallucinogens." In *Psychotomimetic drugs,* ed. D. H. Efron, 105-122, Raven Press, New York.

Gessner, P. K., D. D. Godse, A. H. Krull, and J. M. McMullan. 1968. "Structure-activity relationships among 5-methoxy-*N:N*-dimethyltryptamine, 4-hydroxy-*N:N*-dimethyltryptamine (psilocin) and other substituted tryptamines." *Life Sciences* 7: 267-277.

Gessner, P. K., P. A. Khairallah, W. M. McIsaac, and I. Page. 1960. "Relation between the metabolic fate and pharmacological actions of serotonin, bufotenine and psilocybin." *Journal of Pharmacology and Experimental Therapy* 130: 126-133.

Gessner, P. K., W. M. McIsaac, and I. Page. 1961. "Pharmacological actions of some methoxyindolealkylamines." *Nature* 190: 179-180.

Gessner, P. K., and I. Page. 1962. "Behavioral effects of 5-methoxy-*N,N*-dimethyltryptamine, other tryptamines, and lysergic acid diethylamide (LSD-25)." *American Journal of Physiology* 203: 167-172.

Getting, P. 1989. "Emerging principles governing the operation of neural networks." *Annual Review of Neuroscience* 12: 185-202.

Geyer, M. A., J. D. Warbritton, D. B. Menkes, J. Zook, and A. Mandell. 1975. "Opposite effects of intraventricular serotonin and bufotenin on rat startle responses." *Pharmacology Biochemistry and Behavior* 3: 687-691.

Gheerbrant, A. 1954. *Journey to the far Amazon: An expedition into unknown territory.* Simon and Schuster, New York.

Ghosal, S., and B. Mukherjee. 1966. "Indole-3-alkylamine bases of *Desmodium pulchellum.*" *Journal of Organic Chemistry* 31: 2284-2288.

Giesbrecht, A. M. 1960. "Sobre a ocorrência de bufotenine em semente *Piptadenia falcata* Benth." *Anais da Associação Brasileira de Química* 19: 117-119.

Gillin, J. C., J. Kaplan, R. Stillman, and R. J. Wyatt. 1976. "The psychedelic model of schizophrenia: The case of *N,N*-dimethyltryptamine." *American Journal of Psychiatry* 133: 203-208.

Gillin, J. C., J. Tinklenberg, D. M. Stoff, R. Stillman, J. S. Shortlidge, and R. J. Wyatt. 1976. "5-Methoxy-*N,N*-dimethyltryptamine: Behavioral and toxicological effects in animals." *Biological Psychiatry* 11, 3: 355-358.

Glen, R. C., G. R. Martin, A. P. Hill, R. Hyde, P. M. Woollard, J. A. Salmon, J. Buckingham, and A. D. Robertson. 1995. "Computer-aided design and synthesis of 5-substituted tryptamines and their pharmacology at the 5-HT$_{1D}$ receptor: Discovery of compounds with potential anti-migraine properties." *Journal of Medicinal Chemistry* 38: 3566-3580.

Glennon, R. A. 1974. "Quantum chemical investigation of the pi-electronic structure of the hallucinogenic *N,N*-dimethyltryptamines." *Research Communications in Chemical Pathology and Pharmacology* 9, 1: 185-188.

Glennon, R. A., P. K. Gessner, D. D. Godse, and B. J. Kline. 1979. "Bufotenine esters." *Journal of Medicinal Chemistry* 22, 11: 1414-1416.

Glennon, R. A., S.-S. Hong, M. Bondarev, H. Law, M. Dukat, S. Rakhit, P. Power, E. Fan, D. Kinneau, R. Kamboj, et al. 1996. "Binding of *O*-alkyl derivatives of serotonin at human 5-HT$_{1D\beta}$ receptors." *Journal of Medicinal Chemistry* 39: 314-322.

Glennon, R. A., M. Titeler, and J. McKenney. 1984. "Evidence for 5-HT$_2$ involvement in the mechanism of action of hallucinogenic drugs." *Life Sciences* 35, 25: 2505-2511.

Glennon, R. A., R. Young, F. Benington, and R. D. Morin. 1982. "Hallucinogens as discriminative stimuli: A comparison of 4-methoxy- and 5-methoxy-*N,N*-dimethyl tryptamine with their thiomethyl counterparts." *Life Sciences* 30, 5: 465-467.

Glennon, R. A., R. Young, and J. A. Rosecrans. 1983. "Antagonism of the effects of the hallucinogen DOM and the purported 5-HT agonist quipazine by 5-HT$_2$ antagonists." *European Journal of Pharmacology* 91, 2-3: 189-196.

Goebel, F. 1841. "Ueber das Harmalin." *Annalen der Chemie und Pharmazie* 38: 363-367.

Goi, S. R., S. Miana de Faria, and M. C. P. Neves. 1984. "Nitrogen fixation, nodule type, and occurence of ureides in woody legumes." *Pesquisa Agropecuaria Brasileira* 19 (special edition): 185-190.

Goldstein, L. 1975. "The effect of LSD and other hallucinogens on the electrical activity of the brain during wakefulness and sleep." In *LSD—A Total Study,* ed. D. V. Siva Sankar, 395-435. PJD Publications, New York.

Gómara, F. L. de. 1965-1966. *Historia general de las Indias,* 2 vols. Editorial Iberia, Barcelona.

Gomez-Jeria, J. S., B. K. Cassels, and J. C. Saavedra-Aguilar. 1987. "A quantum-chemical and experimental study of the hallucinogen (+/-)-1-(2,5-dimethoxy-4-nitrophenyl)-2-aminopropane (DON)." *European Journal of Medicinal Chemistry* 22: 433-437.

Gomide, J. L., N. P. Kutscha, J. E. Shottafer, and L. W. Zabel. 1972. "Kraft pulping and fiber characteristics of five Brazilian woods." *Wood and Fiber* 4, 3: 158-169.

Gonçalves de Lima, O. 1946. "Observações sôbre o 'vinho da Jurema' utilizado pelos índios Pancarú de Tacaratú (Pernambuco)." *Arquivos do Instituto de Pesquisas Agronómicas* 4: 45-80.

González, A. R. 1964. "La cultura de La Aguada del N.O. Argentino." *Revista del Instituto de Antropología* 2-3: 205-253, Universidad Nacional de Córdoba, Córdoba, Argentina.

Gragson, T. L. 1997. "The use of underground plant organs and its relation to habitat selection among the Pumé Indians of Venezuela." *Economic Botany* 51, 4: 377-384.

Granier-Doyeux, M. 1948. "El uso popular de la planta *niopo* o *yopo*." *Boletín de la Oficina Sanitaria Panamericana* 27: 156-158, Washington, DC.

———. 1965. "Native hallucinogenic drugs *Piptadenias*." *Bulletin on Narcotics* 17, 2: 29-38, Dept. of Social Affairs, United Nations, New York.

Grof, S. 1975. *Realms of the human unconscious: Observations from LSD research.* Viking, New York.

Grossa, N., F. delle Monache, F. Ferrari, and G. B. Marini-Bettòlo. 1975. "New observations on the alkaloid composition of hallucinogenic snuff drugs *yopo* and *epéna*." *Atti Accademia Nazionale dei Lincei* 58-II: 605-607.

Gumilla, J. 1984. *El Orinoco ilustrado; historia natural, civil y geográfica de las naciones situadas en las riveras del Río Orinoco.* Facsimile of 1791 ed. (Carlos Gibert y Tuto, Barcelona), Carvajal S.A., Cauca, Colombia (nonfacsimile edition published by Biblioteca de la Presidencia de Colombia, Editorial ABC, Bogotá, Colombia, 1955).

Gupta, M. P., T. D. Arias, J. Etheart, and G. M. Hatfield. 1979. "The occurrence of tryptamine and *N*-methyltryptamine in *Mimosa somnians*." *Journal of Natural Products* 42, 2: 234-236.

Habermehl, G., and H. J. Preusser. 1970. "Antimicrobial activity of amphibious cutaneous gland secretions. II. Compounds from Leptodactylus pentadactylus." *Zeitschrift für Naturforschung B* 25: 1451-1452.

Haefely, W., M. A. Ruch-Monachon, M. Jalfre, and R. Schaffner. 1976. "Interaction of psychotropic agents with central neurotransmitters as revealed by their effects on PGO waves in the cat." *Arzneimittel-Forschung* 26, 6: 1036-1039.

Hageman, W. E., D. G. Wentling, and T. P. Pruss. 1973. "Interaction of vasoactive agents and microemboli on the pulmonary circulation." *European Journal of Pharmacology* 22: 295-303.

Halifax, J. 1979. *Shamanic voices: A survey of visionary narratives.* E. P. Dutton, New York.

Handovsky, H. 1920. "Ein Alkaloid in Gifte von *Bufo vulgaris*." *Archiv Experimentellen Pathologie und Pharmakologie* 86: 138-158.

Harner, M. J. 1973. "The role of hallucinogenic plants in European witchcraft." In *Hallucinogens and shamanism,* ed. M. J. Harner, 125-150. Oxford University Press, New York.

Hartig, P. R. 1997. "Molecular biology and transductional characteristics of 5-HT receptors." *Handbook of Experimental Pharmacology* 129: 176-212.

Hartmann, T. 1982a. "Artefactos indígenas brasileiros em Portugal." *Boletim da Sociedade de Geografia de Lisboa* 175-182, Sociedade de Geografia de Lisboa, Portugal.

———. 1982b. "Contribuçao aos estudios de Henry Wassén e Otto Zerries." *Revista do Museu Paulista,* new series, 28: 191-202, São Paulo, Brazil.

Hashimoto, Y., K. Kawanishi, O. Hayaishi, and A. Ichiyama. 1970. "Amazonian hallucinogens: Their influence on the enzymic effects of serotonin biosynthesis and degradation." *Anais. Academia Brasileira de Ciencias* 42 (Supl): 377-390.

Hegnauer, R. 1962. *Chemotaxonomie der Pflanzen,* vol. 1. Birkhauser Verlag, Berlin.

Hegnauer, R., and R. J. Grayer-Barkmeijer. 1993. "Relevance of seed polysaccharides and flavanoids for the classification of the *Leguminosae:* A chemotaxonomic approach." *Phytochemistry* 34: 3-16.

Helms, M. W. 1986. "Art styles and interaction spheres in Central America and the Caribbean: Polished black wood in the Greater Antilles." *Journal of Latin American Lore* 12, 1: 25-43.

Henker, G. A., and M. J. Huston. 1950. "*Yopo,* a South American snuff." *Canadian Pharmaceutical Journal* 83, 18: 8-9.

Hensing, J. 1719. "The chemical examination of the brain and the unique phosphorus from it [which] ignites all combustibles." University Press, Geissen, Hesse.

Hernández de Alba, G. 1948a. "The Achagua and their neighbors." In *Handbook of South American Indians* 4, ed. J. Steward, 399-412. Smithsonian Institution, Bureau of American Ethnology Bulletin 143, Washington, DC.

———. 1948b. "The Betoi and their neighbors." In *Handbook of South American Indians* 4, ed. J. Steward, 393-398. Smithsonian Institution, Bureau of American Ethnology Bulletin 143, Washington, DC.

Herrera, F. L. 1934. "Botánica etnológica. Filología Quechua, III. 1. Nombres simples de algunas plantas indígenas del departamento del Cuzco." *Revista del Museo Nacional de Lima* 3: 39-62, Peru.

Hieronymus, G. 1882. *Plantae diaphoricae florae argentinae.* G. Kraft, Buenos Aires.

Himwich, H. E. 1967. "Comparative neurophysiological studies of psychotomimetic *N*-dimethylamines and *N*-diethylamines and their nonpsychotomimetic congeners devoid of the *N*-dimethyl or *N*-diethyl configurations." In *Amines and Schizophrenia,* ed. H. E. Himwich, S. S. Kety, and J. R. Smythies, 137-149. Pergamon, Oxford.

Hinestrosa, J. de. 1965. "La descripción que se hizo en la Provincia de Xauxa." In *Relaciones geográficas de Indias* 1, ed. M. J. de la Espada, 167-175. Biblioteca de Autores Españoles, vol. 183, Ediciones Atlas, Madrid.

Ho, B. T., W. M. McIsaac, R. An, R. T. Harris, K. E. Walker, P. Kralik, and M. M. Airaksinen. 1970. "Biological activities of some 5-substituted *N,N*-dimethyltryptamines, α-methyltryptamines, and gramines." *Psychopharmacologia* 16: 385-394.

Hochstein, F. A., and A. M. Paradies. 1957. "Alkaloids of *Banisteria caapi* and *Prestonia amazonicum.*" *Journal of the American Chemical Society* 79: 5735.

Hoehne, F. C. 1939. *Plantas e substancias vegetais toxicas o medicinais do Brasil.* Jardim Botanico, São Paulo.

Hoffer, A., and H. Osmond. 1967. *The hallucinogens.* Academic Press, New York.

Hofmann, A. 1980. *LSD, my problem child*. McGraw-Hill, New York.

Hollister, L. E. 1962. "Drug-induced psychoses and schizophrenic reactions. A critical comparison." *Annals of the New York Academy of Science* 96: 80-92.

Holmes, J. C., and F. A. Morell. 1957. "Oscillographic mass spectrometric monitoring of gas chromatography." *Applied Spectroscopy* 11: 86-87.

Holmstedt, B. 1965. "Tryptamine derivatives in epená an intoxicating snuff used by some South American Indian tribes." *Archives internationales de Pharmacodynamie et de Thérapie* 156, 2: 285-305.

Holmstedt, B., and J. E. Lindgren. 1967a. "Chemical constituents and pharmacology of South American snuffs." In *Ethnopharmacologic search for psychoactive drugs,* ed. D. H. Efron et al., 339-373. Public Health Service Publication 1645, U.S. Department of Health, Education and Welfare, Washington, DC.

———. 1967b "Discussion on the psychoactive action of various tryptamine derivatives." In *Ethnopharmacologic search for psychoactive drugs*, ed. D. H. Efron et al., 377. Public Health Service Publication 1645, U.S. Department of Health, Education and Welfare, Washington, DC.

———. 1967c. "Gas chromatographic analysis of some psychoactive indole bases." In *Amines and schizophrenia,* ed. H. E. Himwich, S. S. Kety, and J. R. Smythies, 151-166. Pergamon, Oxford.

———. 1972. "Alkaloid analysis of botanical material more than a thousand years old." *Etnologiska Studier* 32: 139-144, Göteborgs Etnografiska Museum, Gothenburg, Sweden.

Holmstedt, B., J. E. Lindgren, T. Plowman, L. Rivier, R. E. Schultes, and O. Tovar. 1980. "Indole alkaloids in Amazonian *Myristicaceae:* Field and laboratory research." *Botanical Museum Leaflets* 28: 215-234, Harvard University.

Hoshino, T., and K. Shimodaira. 1936. "Uber die Synthese des Bufotenin-methylathers (5-methoxy-*N*-dimethyl-tryptamin) und Bufotenins. (Synthesen in der indol-gruppe). XV." *Bulletin of the Chemical Society of Japan* 11: 221-224.

Hoyer, D., D. E. Clarke, J. R. Fozard, P. R. Hartig, G. R. Martin, E. J. Mylecharane, P. R. Saxena, and P. A. Humphrey. 1994. "International Union of Pharmacology classification of receptors for 5-hydroxytryptamine (serotonin)." *Pharmacology Review* 46: 157-203.

Humboldt, A. von, and A. Bonpland. 1971. *Personal narrative of travels to the equinoctial regions of America, during the years 1799-1804,* trans. and ed. T. Ross. Reprint of the 1852-1853 ed. in 3 volumes by Benjamin Blom, New York.

Humphrey, P. P. A. 1991. "5-Hydroxytryptamine and the pathophysiology of migraine." *Journal of Neurology* 238: S38-S44.

Hunziker, A. T. 1973. "El *cebil (Anadenanthera colubrina,* var. *cebil)* en la provincia de Córdoba." *Kurtziana* 7: 265, Buenos Aires.

Hutchinson, J. 1964. *The genera of flowering plants (Angiospermae)*. Bd. 1, S. 277, Clarendon Press, Oxford.

Iacobucci, G., and E. Ruveda. 1964. "Bases derived from tryptamine in Argentine *Piptadenia* species." *Phytochemistry* 3, 3: 465-467, Buenos Aires (see also *Chemistry Abstracts* 61, 1964).

Isbell, B. J. 1978. *To defend ourselves: Ecology and ritual in an Andean village.* Institute of Latin American Studies, University of Texas, Austin.

Isbell, W. H., and G. McEwan, eds. 1991. *Huari administrative structure: Prehistoric monumental architecture and state government.* Dumbarton Oaks Research Library and Collection, Washington, DC.

Jacob, J., and J. M. Robert. 1966. "Hyperthermic response to intravenous and intracisternal administered tryptamine, serotonin, and their *N*- and *O*-methylated derivatives, in rabbits pretreated with a monoamine oxidase inhibitor." *Comptes Rendus Hebdomadaires des Seances de L'Academie des Sciences, Serie D: Sciences Naturelles* 263: 300-303.

Jakab, R. L., and P. S. Goldman-Rakic. 1998. "5-Hydroxytryptamine$_{2A}$ serotonin receptors in the primate cerebral cortex: Possible site of action of hallucinogenic and antipsychotic drugs in pyramidal cell apical dendrites." *Proceedings of the National Academy of Science USA* 95: 735-740.

Jerina, D. M., J. Daly, and B. Witkop. 1971. "The NIH shift and a mechanism of enzymatic oxygenation." *Medical Research* 5: 413-476.

Jimenez de la Espada, M., ed. 1965. *Relaciones geográficas de Indias,* 3 vols. Biblioteca de Autores Españoles, vols. 183-185, Ediciones Atlas, Madrid.

Jin, H., O. Oksenberg, A. Ashkenazi, S. J. Peroutka, A. M. Duncan, R. Rozmahel, Y. Yang, G. Mengod, J. M. Palacios, and B. F. Dowd. 1992. "Characterization of the human 5-hydroxytryptamine$_{1B}$ receptor." *Journal of Biological Chemistry* 267: 5735-5738.

Johnson, J. V., and R. A. Yost. 1985. "Tandem mass spectrometry for trace analysis." *Analytical Chemistry* 57: 758a-760a.

Johnson, J. V., R. A. Yost, and K. F. Faull. 1984. "Tandem mass spectrometry for the trace determination of tryptolines in crude brain extracts." *Analytical Chemistry* 56: 1655-1661.

Johnson, M. P., R. J. Loncharich, M. Baez, and D. L. Nelson. 1994. "Species variations in transmembrane region V of the 5-hydroxytryptamine type 2A receptor alter the structure activity relationship of certain ergolines and tryptamines." *Molecular Pharmacology* 45: 277-286.

Kapfhammer, W. 1997. *Große Schlange und Fliegender Jaguar. Zur mythologischen Grundlage des rituellen Konsums Halluzinoger Drogen in Südamerika.* Völkerkundliche Arbeiten Band 6 (Dissertation 1996, Ludwig-Maximilians-Universität, Munich), Holos-Verlag, Bonn.

Karkkainen, J. M., and M. Raisanen. 1992. "Nialamide, an MAO inhibitor, increases urinary excretion of endogenously produced bufotenin in man." *Biological Psychiatry* 32: 1042-1048.

Karkkainen, J., M. Raisanen, M. O. Huttunen, E. Kallio, H. Naukkarinen, and M. Virkkunen. 1995. "Urinary excretion of bufotenin (*N,N*-dimethyl-5-hydroxytryptamine) is increased in suspicious violent offenders: A confirmatory study." *Psychiatry Research* 58: 145-152.

Kaubisch, N., J. W. Daly, and D. Jerina. 1972. "Arene oxides as intermediates in the oxidative metabolism of aromatic compounds: Isomerization of methyl-substituted arene oxides." *Biochemistry* 11, 16: 3080-3088.

Keane, P. E., and P. Soubrie. 1997. "Animal models of integrated serotonergic functions: Their predictive value for the clinical applicability of drugs interfering with serotonergic transmission." *Handbook for Experimental Pharmacology* 129: 707-725.

Kerchache, J. 1994. *L'Art des sculpteurs Taïnos. Chefs-d'œuvre des Grandes Antilles Precolombiennes.* Exhibition catalog (24 Feb.-29 May, 1994), Musée du Petit Palais, Editions des musées de la Ville de Paris, France.

Kermack, W. D., W. H. Perkin, and R. Robinson. 1921. "Harmine and harmaline. V. Synthesis of Norharman." *Journal of the Chemical Society* 119: 1602-1642.

Kirchhoff, P. 1948. "Food-gathering tribes of the Venezuelan Llanos." In *Handbook of South American Indians* 4, ed. J. Steward, 445-455. Smithsonian Institution, Bureau of American Ethnology Bulletin 143, Washington, DC.

Kline, T. B., F. Benington, R. D. Morin, and J. M. Beaton. 1982. "Structure-activity relationships in potentially hallucinogenic *N,N*-dialkyltryptamines substitued in the benzene moiety." *Journal of Medicinal Chemistry* 25, 8: 908-913.

Knobloch, P. J. 2000. "Wari ritual power at Conchopata: An interpretation of *Anadenanthera colubrina* iconography." *Latin American Antiquity* 11, 4: 387-402. Society for American Archaeology, Washington, DC.

Koch-Grünberg, T. 1909-1910. *Zwei Jahre unter den Indianern: Reisen in nordwest-Brasilien 1903/1905.* 2 vols., Ernst Wasmuth, Berlin.

⸻. 1917-1928. *Vom Roroima zum Orinoco: Ergebnisse einer Reise in Nordbrasilien und Venezuela in den Jahren 1911-1913.* 5 vols., D. Reimer, Berlin. Vols. 2-5 have imprint: Strecker und Schröeder, Stuttgart. Spanish version, *Del Roraima al Orinoco,* 3 vols. 1979, Ediciones del Banco Central de Venezuela, Caracas.

Koella, W. P., and C. H. Wells. 1959. "Influence of LSD-25 on optically evoked potentials in the nonanesthetized rabbit." *American Journal of Physiology* 196: 1181-1184.

Korolkovas, A. 1970. *Essentials of molecular pharmacology.* Wiley-Interscience, New York.

Koschitzky, M. von. 1992. *Las telas de malla de los Wichí/Mataco: Su elaboración, su función y una posible interpretación de los motivos.* Colección Mankacén, Centro Argentino de Etnología Americana, Buenos Aires.

Kostowski, W., W. Rewerski, and T. Piechocki. 1972. "Effects of some hallucinogens on aggressiveness of mice and rats." *Pharmacology* 7, 4: 259-263.

Krapovickas, P. 1958-1959. "Arqueología de la Puna Argentina." *Anales de Arqueología y Etnología* 14-15: 53-113, Universidad Nacional de Cuyo, Facultad de Filosofía y Letras, Mendoza, Argentina.

Krauss, G. J., and H. Reinbothe. 1970. "Polychromatic detection of amino acids with different ninhydrin spray reagents after separation on MN 300 HR-cellulose thin layers. Further occurences of Mimosacean amino acids." *Biochemie und Physiologie der Pflanzen* 161, 6: 577-592.

———. 1973. "Free amino acids in *Mimosaceae* seeds." *Phytochemistry* 12, 1: 125-142.

Krebs-Thomson, K., M. P. Paulus, and M. A. Geyer. 1998. "Effects of hallucinogens on locomotor and investigatory activity and patterns: Influence of 5-HT$_{2A}$ and 5-HT$_{2C}$ receptors." *Neuropsychopharmacology* 18: 339-351.

Ku, B. S., and H. Takeuchi. 1984. "Identification and pharmacological characteristics of the two giant neurons, v-RPLN and V-VNAN, on the ventral surface in the suboesophageal ganglia of the African giant snail (*Achinata fulica* Férussac)." *Comparative Biochemistry and Physiology C* 77: 315-321.

Kulkarni, A. S. 1973. "Scratching response induced in mice by mescaline and related amphetamine derivatives." *Biological Psychiatry* 6: 177.

Kunike, H. 1916. "Goldaltertumer der Chibcha." *Internationales Archiv für Etnographie* 24: 23-32, plus plates, Leiden, Netherlands.

La Condamine, C.-M. 1778. *Rélation abrégéed'un voyage fait dans l'intérieur de l'Amérique Méridionale. Depuis de la Côte de la Mer du Sud, jusqu'aux Côtes du Brésil & de la Guiane, en descendant la riviere des Amazones.* J.-E. Dufour & P. Roux Publishers, Maestricht, The Netherlands.

LaBarre, W. 1972. "Hallucinogens and the shamanic origins of religion." In *Flesh of the gods,* ed. P. T. Furst, 261-278. Praeger, New York.

Lafón, C. R. 1954. *Arqueología de la Quebrada de La Huerta (Quebrada de Humahuaca, Prov. de Jujuy).* Publicaciones del Instituto de Arqueología 1, Facultad de Filosofía y Letras, Universidad de Buenos Aires, Argentina.

Lai, A., M. Tin-Wa, E. S. Mika, G. J. Persinos, and N. R. Farnsworth. 1973. "Phytochemical investigation of *Virola peruviana,* a new hallucinogenic plant." *Journal of Pharmaceutical Sciences* 62, 9: 1561-1563.

Langley, J. N. 1905. "On the reaction of cells and of nerve-endings to certain poisons, chiefly as regards the reaction of striated muscle to nicotine and to *curari.*" *Journal of Physiology (London)* 33: 374-413.

Larraín Barros, H. 1976. "La *Vilca* o *Paricá (Anadenanthera* spp.): ¿Purga o estímulante indigena? Alguna referencias etnohistóricas." *Sarance: Revista del Instituto Otavaleño de Antropología* 2, 3: 27-49, Otavalo, Ecuador.

Las Casas, B. de. 1909. *Apologética historia de Las Indias: Historiadores de Indias* 1, Nueva Biblioteca de Autores Españoles. Bailly, Bailliere e Hijos, Editores, Madrid.

Latcham, R. E. 1938. *Arqueología de la región Atacameña.* Prensas de la Universidad de Chile, Santiago.

Lavalle, J. A. 1984. *Huari.* Colección Arte y Tesoros del Perú, Banco de Credito del Perú, Lima.

Le Cointe, P. 1947. "Arvores e plantes uties brasiliana." *Bibliotecha Pedagogica Brasileira, Sera 5a,* 251: 389.

Le Paige, G. 1959. "Les tablettes à offrande de Caspana." *Bulletin, Société Suisse des Americanistes* 9, 17: 3-5, Geneva.

————. 1964. "El preceramico en la Cordillera Atacameña y los cementerios del período agroalfarero de San Pedro de Atacama." *Anales de la Universidad del Norte* 3, Antofagasta, Chile.

————. 1965. "San Pedro de Atacama y su zona." *Anales de la Universidad del Norte* 4, Antofagasta, Chile.

————. 1972. "Tres cementerios indígenas en San Pedro de Atacama y Toconao." *Actas del VI Congreso Nacional de Arqueología Chilena* (1971), 163-187, Museo Nacional de Historia Natural, Santiago.

————. 1974. "El yacimiento de Tchaputchayna." *Estudios Atacameños* 2: 59-74, Museo de Arqueología, San Pedro de Atacama.

Lee, M. S., and R. A. Yost. 1988. "Rapid identification of drug metabolites with tandem mass spectrometry." *Biomedical and Environmental Mass Spectrometry* 15: 193-204.

Legler, G., and R. Tschesche. 1963. "Die Isolierung von *N*-Methyltryptamin, 5-Methoxy-N-methyltryptamin und 5-Methoxy-*N,N*-dimethyltryptamin aus der Rinde von *Piptadenia peregrina* Benth." *Die Naturwissenschaften* 50: 94-95, Springer-Verlag, Berlin.

Lehmann-Nitsche, R. 1902. *Catalogo de las antigüedades de la Provincia de Jujuy.* Talleres de Publicaciones del Museo de La Plata, Argentina.

Lemaire, D., P. Jacob, and A. T. Shulgin. 1985. "Ring-substituted β-methoxyphenethylamines: A new class of psychotomimetic agents active in man." *Journal of Pharmacy and Pharmacology* 37: 575-577.

Lenicque, P. M. 1973. "Morphologenetic actions of 5-hydroxytryptamine and some analogous substances on the regeneration of the planarian worm *Dugesia tigrina*." *Acta Zoologica* 34: 131-137.

Lévi-Strauss, C. 1948. "Tribes of the right bank of the Guaporé River." In *Handbook of South American Indians* 3, ed. J. Steward, 371-379. Smithsonian Institution, Bureau of American Ethnology Bulletin 143, Washington, DC.

————. 1979. *The origin of table manners: Introduction to a science of mythology* 3. Harper and Row, New York.

Lewin, L. 1924. *Phantastica—Die Betaubenden und Erregenden Genussmittel fur Arzte und Nichtarzte.* Georg Stilke Verlag, Berlin.

Leysen, J. E., W. Gommeren, L. Heylen, W. H. M. L. Luyten, I. Van de Weyer, P. Vanhoenacker, G. Haegeman, A. Schotte, P. Van Gompel, R. Wouters, and A. S. Lesage. 1996. "Alnitidan, a new 5-hydroxytryptamine$_{1D}$ agonist and migraine-abortive agent: Ligand-binding properties of human 5-hydroxytryptamine$_{1Da}$, human 5-hydroxytryptamine$_{1D\beta}$, and calf 5-hydroxytryptamine$_{1D}$ receptors investigated with [^{3}H]5-hydroxytryptamine and [^{3}H]alnitidan." *Molecular Pharmacology* 50: 1567-1580.

Libro del árbol. Esencias forestales indígenas de la Argentina de aplicación industrial, vol. 2, 2nd ed. 1976. Celulosa Argentina S.A.

228   Anadenanthera: *Visionary Plant of Ancient South America*

Lindgren, J.-E. 1995. "Amazonian psychoactive alkaloids: A review." In *Ethnobotany: Evolution of a discipline,* ed. R. E. Schultes and S. von Reis, 343-348. Dioscorides Press, Portland, Oregon.

Linnaeus, C. von. 1753. *Caroli Linnæ Species plantarum. Exhibentes plantas rite cognitas ad genera relatas, cum differentiis specificis, nominibus trivialibus, synonymis selectis, locis natalibus, secundum systema sexuale digestas.* Impensis Laurentii Salvii, Holmiæ, Stockholm, Sweden.

Llagostera, A. 1995. "El componente cultural Aguada en San Pedro de Atacama." *Boletín del Museo Chileno de Arte Precolombino* 6: 9-34, Santiago.

Llagostera, A., and M. A. Costa. 1984. *Museo Arqueológico R. P. Le Paige, S. J.* Serie Patrimonio Cultural Chileno, Colección Museos Chilenos. Departamento de Extensión Cultural del Ministerio de Educación, Santiago.

Llagostera, A., C. M. Torres, and M. A. Costa. 1988. "El complejo psicotrópico en Solcor-3 (San Pedro de Atacama)." *Estudios Atacameños* 9: 61-98, Instituto de Investigaciones Arqueológicas, Universidad del Norte, San Pedro de Atacama.

Lovén, S. 1935. *Origins of the Tainan culture.* Elanders Boktryckeri Aktiebolag, Gothenburg, Sweden.

Lozano, P. 1941. *Descripción chorográfica del terreno, ríos, árboles y animales de las dilatadissimas provincias del Gran Chaco, Gualamba, y de los ritos y costumbres de las innumerables naciones barbaras é infieles, que le habitan.* Facsimile of 1733 edition, Universidad Nacional de Tucumán, San Miguel de Tucumán, Argentina.

Luchins, D., T. A. Ban, and H. E. Lehmann. 1978. "A review of nicotinic acid, N-methylated indoleamines and schizophrenia." *International Pharmacopsychiatry* 13: 16-33.

Luscombe, G., P. Jenner, and C. D. Marsden. 1982. "Myoclonus in guinea pigs is induced by indole-containing but not piperazine-containing 5HT agonists." *Life Sciences* 30: 1487-1494.

———. 1984. "5-hydroxytryptamine (5HT)-dependent myoclonus in guinea pigs is induced through brainstem 5-HT-1 receptors." *Neuroscience Letters* 44: 241-246.

Lyttle, T., D. Goldstein, and J. Gartz. 1996. "Bufo toads and bufotenine: Fact and fiction surrounding an alleged psychedelic." *Journal of Psychoactive Drugs* 28: 267-290.

Mabry, T. J., and J. A. Mears. 1970. "Alkaloids and plant systematics." In *Chemistry of the alkaloids,* ed. S. W. Pelletier, 719-746. Van Nostrand Reinhold, New York.

Maddrell, S. H. P., D. E. M. Pilcher, and B. O. C. Gardiner. 1969. "Stimulatory effect of 5-hydroxytryptamine (serotonin) on secretion by Malpighian tubules of insects." *Nature* 222: 784-785.

Mahler, D. J., and F. L. Humoller. 1959. "Effect of lysergic acid diethylamide (LSD) and bufotenine on performance in trained rats." *Proceedings of the Society for Experimental Biology and Medicine* 102: 697-701.

Mandell, A. J., and M. A. Geyer. 1976. "Hallucinations: Chemical and physiological." In *Biological foundations of psychiatry,* ed. R. A. Grenell and S. Gabay, 730. Raven Press, New York.

Mandell, A. J., and M. Morgan. 1971. "Indole(ethyl)amine *N*-methyltransferase in human brain." *Nature* 230: 85-87.

Mandell, A. J., and D. S. Segal. 1973. "The psychobiology of dopamine and the methylated indoleamines with particular reference to psychiatry." In *Biological psychiatry,* ed. J. Mendels, 89-112. Wiley, New York.

Mandell, A. J., and C. E. Spooner. 1969. "*N, N*-indole transmethylation theory of the mechanism of MAOI-indole amino acid load behavioral activation." *Schizophrenia,* ed. D. V. Siva Sankar, 496-507. PJD Publishers, New York.

Manske, R. 1931. "A synthesis of the methyl-tryptamines and some derivatives." *Canadian Journal of Research* 5: 592-600.

Marek, G. J., and G. K. Aghajanian. 1998. "Indoleamine and the phenethylamine hallucinogens: Mechanisms of psychotomimetic action." *Drug Alcohol Dependence* 51: 189-198.

Marengo, C. 1954. *El Antigal de Los Amarillos (Quebrada de Yacoraite, Prov. de Jujuy).* Publicaciones del Instituto de Arqueología 2, Facultad de Filosofía y Letras, Universidad de Buenos Aires, Argentina.

Marini-Bettòlo, G. B., E. Biocca, C. Galeffi, F. delle Monache, and E. G. Montalvo. 1965. "Allucinogi impiegati dagli Indi del Bacino Amazonico e dell'Alto Orinoco." *Annali, Istituto Superiore di Sanità* 1: 784-792, Rome.

Marini-Bettòlo, G. B., F. Delle Monache, and E. Biocca. 1964. "Sulle sostanze allucinogene dell'Amazonica. Nota II. Osservazione sull'Epena degli Yanoama del bacino del Rio Negro e dell'Alto Orinoco." *Annali di Chimica* 48: 1179-1186.

Marques de Melo, C. F., H. Bernardo de Souza, M. de F. Alves, and M. de L. Duarte. 1971. "Tropical woods reforestation, cellulose and paper." *Instituto de Pesquisas e Experimentaçao Agropecuarias do Norte, serie Tecnologia* 2, 1, Brazil.

Márquez, M. E. 1979. *Los Tunebo: Una cosmogonía precolombina.* Editorial Copymundo, Medellín, Colombia.

Matsumoto, H., and I. Pietruszewska. 1978. "Urinary excretion of bufotenine, *N,N*-dimethyltryptamine and 3,4-dimethoxyphenylethylamine, and the clinical picture of mental disorders." *Psychiatria Polska* 12, 2:189-197 (English summary p. 196).

McBride, M. C., 2000. "Bufotenine: Toward an understanding of possible psychoactive mechanisms." *Journal of Psychoactive Drugs* 32, 3: 321-331.

McClue, S. J., C. Brazell, and S. M. Stahl. 1989. "Hallucinogenic drugs are partial agonists of the human platelet shape change response: A physiological model of the 5-HT$_2$ receptor." *Biological Psychiatry* 26, 3: 297-302.

McClure, W. O. 1973. "Butterflies of the soul: Drugs and mental illness." In *Wednesday night at the lab: Antibiotics, bioengineering, contraceptives, drugs and ethics,* ed. K. L. Rinehardt, W. O. McClure, and T. L. Brown, 151-163. Harper and Row, New York.

McFadden, W. 1973. *Techniques of combined gas chromatography/mass spectrometry: Applications in organic analysis.* Wiley-Interscience, New York.

McFarlane, I., and M. Slaytor. 1972. "The role of *N*-acetyl amines in tetrahydro-β-carboline and tetrahydroisoquinoline biosynthesis." *Phytochemistry* 11: 229-234.

McGowan, K., A. Kane, N. Asarkof, J. Wicks, V. Guerina, J. Kellum, S. Baron, A. R. Gintzler, and M. Donowitz. 1983. "*Entamoeba histolytica* causes intestinal secretion: Role of serotonin." *Science* 221: 762-764.

MChAP (Museo Chileno de Arte Precolombino). 1984. *Tesoros de San Pedro de Atacama.* Museo Chileno de Arte Precolombino, Santiago, Chile.

———. 1994. *La cordillera de los Andes: Ruta de encuentros.* Museo Chileno de Arte Precolombino, Santiago, Chile.

McKenna, D. J., L. E. Luna, and G. H. N. Towers. 1986. "Ingredientes biodinámicos en las plantas que se mezclan al *ayahuasca:* Una farmacopea tradicional no investigada." *América Indígena* 46, 1: 73-99, Instituto Indigenista Interamericano, Mexico City.

McKenna, D. J., D. B. Repke, L. Lo, and S. J. Peroutka. 1990. "Differential interactions of indolealkylamines with 5-hydroxytryptamine receptor subtypes." *Neuropharmacology* 29: 193.

McKenna, D. J., G. H. N. Towers, and F. S. Abbott. 1984. "Monoamine oxidase inhibitors in South American hallucinogenic plants. Part 2: Constituents of orally-active Myristicaceous hallucinogens." *Journal of Ethnopharmacology* 12, 2: 179-211.

McKenzie, E., L. Nettleship, and M. Slaytor. 1975. "New natural products from *Peganum harmala.*" *Phytochemistry* 14: 273-275.

McLeod, W. R., and B. R. Sitaram. 1985. "Bufotenine reconsidered." *Acta Psychiatrica Scandinavica* 72, 5: 447-450.

Mears, J. A., and T. J. Mabry. 1971. "Alkaloids in the *Leguminosae.*" In *Chemotaxonomy of the Leguminosae,* ed. J. B. Harborne, D. Boulter, and B. L. Turner, 73-178. Academic Press, New York.

Meckes-Lozoya, M., X. Lozoya, R. J. Marles, C. Soucy-Breau, A. Sen, and J. T. Arnason. 1990. "*N,N*-dimethyltryptamine alkaloid in *Mimosa tenuiflora* bark *(tepescohuite).*" *Archivos de Investigación Médica* 21, 2: 175-177.

Medhurst, A. D., and A. J. Kaumann. 1993. "Characterization of the 5-HT$_4$ receptor mediating tachycardia in piglet isolated right atrium." *British Journal of Pharmacology* 110: 1023-1030.

Meister, A. 1965. *Biochemistry of the amino acids.* Academic Press, New York.

Mell, C. D. 1930. "Interesting sources of natural dyestuffs: Tannin and dyes from *cojoba.*" *Textile Colorist* 52: 754.

Mengod, G., J. M. Palacios, K. H. Wiederhold, and D. Hoyer. 1997. "5-Hydroxytryptamine receptor histochemistry: Comparison of receptor mRNA distribution and radioligand autoradiography in the brain." *Handbook of Experimental Pharmacology* 129: 213-237.

Menzel, D. 1964. "Style and time in the Middle Horizon." *Ñawpa Pacha* 2: 1-105, plus plates, Institute of Andean Studies, Berkeley, California.

Métraux, A. 1939. "Myths and tales of the Matako Indians." *Etnologiska Studier 9*: 1-127, Göteborgs Etnografiska Museum, Gothenburg, Sweden.

———. 1946. "Ethnography of the Chaco." In *Handbook of South American Indians* 1, ed. J. H. Steward, 197-370. Smithsonian Institution, Bureau of American Ethnology Bulletin 143, Washington, DC.

———. 1947. "Rubber." In *Handbook of South American Indians* 5, ed. J. Steward, 227-228. Smithsonian Institution, Bureau of American Ethnology Bulletin 143, Washington, DC.

———. 1948a. "Tribes of Eastern Bolivia and Madeira headwaters." In *Handbook of South American Indians* 3, ed. J. Steward, 381-463. Smithsonian Institution, Bureau of American Ethnology Bulletin 143, Washington, DC.

———. 1948b. "Tribes of the middle and upper Amazon River." In *Handbook of South American Indians* 3, ed. J. Steward, 687-712. Smithsonian Institution, Bureau of American Ethnology Bulletin 143, Washington, DC.

Meyer, K. 1966. "Cardiotoxic steroids from toads." *Memórias do Instituto Butantan* 33: 433-440, São Paulo.

Migliaccio, G. P., T.-L. N. Shieh, S. R. Byrn, B. A. Hathaway, and D. E. Nichols. 1981. "Comparison of solution conformational preferences for the hallucinogens bufotenin and psilocin using 360-MHz proton NMR spectroscopy." *Journal of Medicinal Chemistry* 24: 206-209.

Miyauchi, Y., T. Yoshimoto, and K. Minami. 1976. "Extractives from the heartwood of *Piptadenia* sp." *Mokuzai Gakkaishi* 22, 1: 47-50.

Monnier, M., P. Krupp, and S. Graber. 1960. "Electrophysiological classification of central nervous system drugs. II. Action of hallucinogenic, psychotogenic and analeptic drugs on the mechanisms of arousal and relaxation." *Archiv Internale Pharmacodynamie* 127: 337-360.

Monroe, P. J., D. L. Smith, G. M. Williams, and D. J. Smith. 1994. "Bufotenine has a parachloroamphetamine-like action on the storage and release of serotonin in rat spinal cord synaptosomes." *Biogenic Amines* 10: 273-284.

Montell, G. 1926. "An archaeological collection from the Loa Valley, Atacama." *Oslo Etnografiske Museums Skrifter,* vol. 5, Hefte 1, Oslo.

Moraes, E. H. F. de, M. A. Alvarenga, Z. M. G. S. Ferreira, and G. Akisue. 1990. "Nitrogenated bases of *Mimosa scabrella*." *Quimica Nova* 13, 4: 308-309.

Morner, A. 1959. "Catalogue of the Silva Castro Collection." *Revista de Museu Paulista,* XI new series: 133-176, São Paulo, Brazil.

Moro, G. A., M. N. Graziano, and J. D. Coussio. 1975. "Alkaloids of *Prosopis nigra*." *Phytochemistry* 14: 827.

Mostny, G. 1958. "Máscaras, tubos y tabletas para rapé y cabezas trofeo entre los atacameños." *Miscellanea Paul Rivet, octogenario dicata* 2: 379-392, Universidad Nacional Autónoma de México, Mexico City.

Mostny, G., and H. Niemeyer. 1983. *Arte rupestre chileno.* Series *El Patrimonio Cultural Chileno,* Departamento de Extensión Cultural del Ministerio de Educación, Santiago, Chile.

Mulvany de Peñaloza, E. 1984. "Motivos fitomorfos de alucinógenos en Chavín." *Chungará* 12: 57-80, Instituto de Antropología y Arqueolología, Universidad de Tarapacá, Arica, Chile.

Mulvena, D. P., and M. Slaytor. 1983. "*N*-methyltransferase activities in *Phalaris aquatica.*" *Phytochemistry* 22: 47-48.

Murphy, D. L., and R. Weiss. 1972. "Reduced monoamine oxidase activity in blood platelets from bipolar depressed patients." *American Journal of Psychiatry* 128: 1351-1357.

Narasimhachari, N., D. Callison, and R. L. Lin. 1979. "Effect of MAO inhibitors on the tissue distribution of dimethyltryptamine, 5-methoxydimethyltryptamine and bufotenine after their intraperitoneal administration in rat." *Research Communications in Psychology, Psychiatry and Behavior* 4: 257-268.

Naville, R. 1959. "Tablettes et tubes a aspirer du rapé." Société Suisse des Americanistes. *Bulletin* 17: 1-3, Musee et Institut d'Ethnographie de la Ville de Geneve, Switzerland.

Nettleship, L., and M. Slaytor. 1974. "Limitations of feeding experiments in studying alkaloid biosynthesis in *Peganum harmala* callus cultures." *Phytochemistry* 13: 735-742.

Nichols, D. E. 1997. "Role of serotonergic neurons and 5-HT receptors in the action of hallucinogens." *Handbook of Experimental Pharmacology* 129: 563-585.

Nies, A., D. S. Robinson, C. L. Ravaris, and J. M. Davis. 1971. "Amines and monoamine oxidase in relation to ageing and depression in man." *Psychosomatic Medicine* 33: 470.

Nimuendajú, C. 1948a. "The Maué and Arapium." In *Handbook of South American Indians* 3, ed. J. Steward, 245-254. Smithsonian Institution, Bureau of American Ethnology Bulletin 143, Washington, DC.

———. 1948b. "The Mura and Piraha." In *Handbook of South American Indians* 3, ed. J. Steward, 255-269. Smithsonian Institution, Bureau of American Ethnology Bulletin 143, Washington, DC.

Nir, I., C. P. Weller, and F. G. Sulman. 1974. "Behavioral effect of intraventricular application of methoxyindolealkylamines in the rat." *Psychopharmacologia* 39: 323-329.

Nishida, R., T. Ohsugi, and H. Fukami. 1990. "Oviposition stimulant activity of tryptamine analogs on a Rutaceae-feeding swallowtail butterfly, *Papilio xuthus.*" *Agricultural and Biological Chemistry* 54: 1853-1855.

Nordenskiöld, E. 1930. The use of enema tubes and enema syringes among Indians. *Comparative Ethnographical Studies* 8: 184-195, Gothenburg, Sweden.

Northrup, J. K., and T. Mansour. 1978. "Adenylate cyclase from *Fasciola hepatica* 1. Ligand specificity of adenylate cyclase-coupled serotonin receptors." *Molecular Pharmacology* 14: 804-819.

Núñez, L. 1963. "Problemas en torno a la tableta de rapé." *Anales de la Universidad del Norte* 2: 149-168, Antofagasta, Chile.

————. 1964. "El Sacrificador: Un elemento co-tradicional andino." *Noticiero Mensual,* Museo Nacional de Historia Natural 8: 96, Santiago de Chile.

————. 1969. "Informe arqueológico sobre una muestra de posible narcótico, del sitio Patillos-1 (Prov. de Tarapacá, Norte de Chile)," with additional notes by S. H. Wassén and B. Luning. *Årstryck 1967-1968,* 83-95, Göteborgs Etnografiska Museum, Gothenburg, Sweden.

————. 1976. *Registro regional de fechas radiocarbónicas del norte de Chile. Estudios Atacameños* 4: 74-123, Museo Arqueológico de San Pedro de Atacama, Universidad del Norte, Chile.

————. 1994. "Cruzando la cordillera por el norte: Señoríos, caravanas y alianzas." In *La cordillera de los Andes: Ruta de encuentros,* 9-21, Museo Chileno de Arte Precolombino, Santiago.

Oblitas Poblete, E. 1963. *Cultura Callawaya.* La Paz, Bolivia.

Ohsugi, T., R. Nishida, and H. Fukami. 1991. "Multi-component system of oviposition stimulants for a *Rutaceae*-feeding swallowtail butterfly, *Papilio xuthus (Lepidoptera: Papilionidae)."* *Applied Entemology and Zoology* 26: 29-40.

Ondegardo, P. de. 1916. "Informaciones acerca de la religión y gobierno de los Incas." In *Colección de libros y documentos referentes a la historia del Perú,* ed. H. H. Urteaga, Sanmarti y Compañia Lima.

Osmond, H. 1956. "Research on schizophrenia." In *Neuropharmacology,* ed. H. A. Abramson, 183-233. Madison Printing, Princeton, New Jersey.

Osmond, H., and J. Smythies. 1952. "Schizophrenia, a new approach." *Journal of Mental Science:* 309-315.

Ott, J. 1985. *The Cacahuatl eater: Ruminations of an unabashed chocolate addict.* Natural Products Company, Vashon, Washington.

————. 1994. *Ayahuasca analogues: Pangæan entheogens.* Natural Products Company, Kennewick, Washington.

————. 1996. *Pharmacotheon: Entheogenic drugs, their plant sources and history,* 2nd ed. Natural Products Company, Kennewick, Washington.

————. 2001a. "Pharmañopo-psychonautics: Human intranasal, sublingual, intrarectal, pulmonary and oral pharmacology of bufotenine." *Journal of Psychoactive Drugs* 33, 3: 273-281.

————. 2001b. *Shamanic snuffs or entheogenic errhines.* Entheobotanica, Solothurn, Switzerland.

Ovalle, A. de. 1888. *Historia del Reyno de Chile y de las misiones y ministerios que ejercita en el la Compañia de Jesus.* Colección de Historiadores de Chile, 12, 13, Santiago.

Oviedo y Valdés, G. F. de. 1959. *Historia general y natural de la Indias,* Biblioteca de Autores Españoles, vols. 117-121, Ediciones Atlas, Madrid. (*Historia general y natural de la Indias, islas y tierra firme del mar océano,* ed. J. A. de los Ríos, 4 vols. Imprenta de la Real Academia de la Historia, Madrid, 1851-1855.)

Oyarzún, A. 1931. "Las tabletas y los tubos para preparar y aspirar la *paricá* en Atacama." *Revista Chilena de Historia y Geografía* 68, 72: 68-76, Santiago.

Pachter, I. J., D. E. Zacharias, and O. Ribeiro. 1959. "Indole alkaloids of *Acer saccharinum* (the silver maple), *Dictyoloma incanescens, Piptadenia colubrina* and *Mimosa hostilis.*" *Journal of Organic Chemistry* 24: 1285-1287.

Pagés Larraya, F. 1959. "La cultura del *Paricá.*" *Acta Neuropsiquiátrica Argentina* 5: 375-383, Buenos Aires.

Palavecino, E. 1979. "The magic world of the Mataco." *Latin American Indian Literatures* 3, 2: 61-75, University Center for International Studies, University of Pittsburgh, Pennsylvania.

Pané, F. R. 1974. *Relación acerca de las antigüedades de los indios.* New version with notes, maps, and appendixes by J. J. Arrom, Siglo Veintiuno Editores, Mexico City.

Pardal, R. 1937. *Medicina aborígen americana* ("Las *Piptadenias,*" 333-341). Colección Humanior, Biblioteca del Americanista Moderno, Sección C, 3, Buenos Aires.

Pardo, L. L., and E. Ricci. 1956. "Estudio sistemático de la riqueza en taninos de diversas especies indígenas." *Anales de la administración nacional de bosques:* 7-17, Buenos Aires, Argentina.

Paris, R., A. Saint-Firmin, and S. Etchepare. 1967. "Sur les alcaloïdes et les flavonoïdes d'une légumineuse d'Haïti: *Piptadenia peregrina* Benth. Absence d'alcaloïdes chez le *Piptadenia africana.* Hook. f." *Annales Pharmaceutiques Françaises* 25, 7-8: 509-513.

Parkinson, B., J. Hemmen, and K. Groh. 1987. *Tropical landshells of the world.* Verlag Christa Hemmen, Wiesbaden, Alemania.

Paton, W. D. M. 1967. "Kinetic theories of drug action with special reference to the acetylcholine group of agonists and antagonists." *Annals of the New York Academy of Science* 144: 869.

Paulson, J. C., and W. O. McClure. 1974. "Lack of correlation between hallucinogenesis and inhibition of axoplasmic transport." *Molecular Pharmacology* 10, 3: 419-424.

Pauwels, P. J., C. Palmier, T. Wurch, and F. C. Colpaert. 1996. "Pharmacology of cloned human 5-HT$_{1D}$ receptor-mediated functional responses in stably transfected rat C6-glial cell lines: Further evidence differentiating human 5-HT$_{1D}$ and 5-HT$_{1B}$ receptors." *Naunyn-Schmiedeberg's Archives of Pharmacology* 353: 144-156.

Pelletier, S. W. 1970. *Chemistry of the alkaloids.* Van Nostrand Reinhold, New York.

Perdomo, D. P. 1978. *Nuevas pictografías en la isla de Santo Domingo: Las cuevas de Borbón.* Ediciones Museo del Hombre Dominicano, Santo Domingo, Dominican Republic.

Pérez, J. A. 1978. "Concerning the archaeology of the Humahuaca Quebrada." In *Advances in Andean archaeology,* ed. D. Browman, 513-524. Mouton Publishers, The Hague.

Pérez de Barradas, J. 1958. *Orfebrería Prehispánica de Colombia: Estilos Calima y Muisca,* 2 vols. Banco de la República, Bogotá, Colombia.

Pérez Gollán, J. A., and I. Gordillo. 1994. *"Vilca/Uturuncu.* Hacia una arqueología del uso de alucinógenos en las sociedades prehispánicas de los Andes del Sur." *Cuicuilco* 1, 1: 99-140, Mexico.

Perkin, W. H., Jr., and R. Robinson. 1919. "Harmine and harmaline. Part III." *Journal of the Chemical Society:* 933, London.

Peroutka, S. J. 1994. "Pharmacological differentiation of human 5-HT$_{1B}$ and 5-HT$_{1D}$ receptors." *Biological Signals* 3: 217-222.

Peroutka, S. J., and T. A. Howell. 1994. "The molecular evolution of G-protein coupled receptors: Focus on 5-hydroxytryptamine receptors." *Neuropharmacology* 33: 319-324.

Petroff, G., J. Doat, and M. Tissot. 1967. "Papermaking characteristics of some tropical reforestation trees. II." *Centre Technique Forestier Tropical* 29: 1-177.

Phelps, S. 1976. *Art and artefacts of the Pacific, Africa and the Americas: The James Hooper Collection.* Hutchinson, London.

Phisalix, M., and G. Bertrand. 1893. "Toxicite comparee du sang et du venin de crapaud commun *(Bufo vulg.),* consideree au point de vue de la secretion interne des glandes cutanees de cet animal." *Comptes Rendus Hebdomadaires des Seance de L'Academie des Sciences* 116: 1080-1082.

Platt, N., and S. Reynolds. 1986. "The pharmacology of the heart of a caterpillar, the tobacco hornworm, *Manduca sexta." Journal of Insect Physiology* 32: 221-230.

Plazas, C. and A. M. Falchetti. 1979. *La orfebreria prehispánica de Colombia.* Museo del Oro, Banco de la República, Bogotá.

Plotkin, M. J. 1993. *Tales of a shaman's apprentice: An ethnobotanist searches for new medicines in the Amazon rain forest.* Viking, New York.

Plouvier, V. 1962. "The cyclitols in some botanical groups: L-inositol of the composites and D-pinitol of the legumes." *Comptes Rendus Hebdomadaires des Seance de L'Academie des Sciences* 255: 1770-1772.

Polia Meconi, M. 1996. *"Despierta, remedio, cuenta . . .": Adivinos y médicos del Ande,* 2 vols. Fondo Editorial, Pontificia Universidad Católica del Perú, Lima.

———. 1999. *La cosmovisión religiosa Andina en los documentos inéditos del Archivo Romano de la Compañia de Jesús.* Fondo Editorial, Pontificia Universidad Católica del Perú, Lima.

Polonovski, M. 1927. "Sur les aminoxydes des alcaloides 3. Action des anhydrides et chlorures d'acides organiques. Preparation des bases nor." *Bulletin de la Societe Chimique de France* 1927: 1190.

Polykrates, G. 1960. "Einige Holzschnitzereien der Kashuiéna-Indianer." *Folk, Dansk Etnografisk Tidsskrift* 2: 115-120, Danish Ethnographical Association, Copenhagen.

Pompeiano, M., J. M. Palacios, and G. Mengod. 1994. "Distribution of the serotonin 5-HT$_2$ receptor family mRNAs: Comparison between 5-HT$_{2A}$ and 5-HT$_{2C}$ receptors." *Molecular Brain Research* 23: 163-178.

Port, G. N. J., and B. Pullman. 1974. "*Ab initio* SCF MO study of the conformation of serotonin and bufotenine." *Theoretica Chimica Acta* 33, 3: 275-278.

Posnansky, A. 1945. *Tiahuanacu, the cradle of American man*, vols. 1 and 2 (English/Spanish edition). J. J. Augustin Publisher, New York.

————. 1957. *Tiahuanacu, the cradle of American man*, vols. 3 and 4 (English/Spanish edition). Ministerio de Educación, La Paz, Bolivia.

Poulton, J. E. 1981. "Transmethylation and demethylation reactions in the metabolism of secondary plant products." In *The biochemistry of plants* 7, ed. E. E. Conn, 667-723. Academic Press, New York.

Prado, L. L., and E. Ricci. 1956. "Systematic study of the tannin content of various indigenous species." *Anales de la Administracíon Nacional de Bosques, Rep. Argentina* 1956: 7-17.

Prance, G. T. 1970. "Notes on the use of plant hallucinogens in Amazonian Brazil." *Economic Botany* 24: 62-68.

————. 1972. "Ethnobotanical notes from Amazonian Brazil." *Economic Botany* 26, 3: 221-237.

Preuss, K. T. 1974. *Arte monumental prehistórico: Excavaciones hechas en el Alto Magdalena y San Agustín, Colombia*. Dirección de Divulgación Cultural de la Universidad Nacional, Bogotá, Colombia (Translation of *Monumentale Vorgeschichtliche Kunst*, Göttingen. 1929).

Primo, B. L. 1945. "Tannin content of certain Brazilian vegetable products." *Anais. Associaçao Brasileira de Quimica* 4: 117-120.

Prous, A. 1974. "Les sculptures préhistoriques du sud-brésilien." *Bulletin de la Societé Préhistorique Française* 71, C.R.S.M. no. 7: 210-217.

Raffauf, R. F. 1970. *A handbook of alkaloids and alkaloid-containing plants*. Wiley-Interscience, New York.

Räisänen, M. 1985. *Studies on the synthesis and excretion of bufotenin and N,N-dimethyltryptamine in man*. Dissertation, Department of Medical Chemistry, University of Helsinki, Finland.

Räisänen, M., M. Virkkunen, M. Huttunen, and B. Furman. 1984. "Increased urinary excretion of bufotenin by violent offenders with paranoid symptoms and family violence." *Lancet*, Sept. 22: 700-701.

Rangel, J. L. 1943. "Goma de angico." *Revista de Química Industrial* 12: 16-18, Rio de Janeiro, Brazil.

Rapport, M. M., A. A. Green, and I. H. Page. 1948. "Serum vasoconstrictor (serotonin) IV. Isolation and characterization." *Journal of Biological Chemistry* 176: 1243-1251.

Ratcliffe, F. 1971. "Effect of mescaline and bufotenine on some central actions of noradrenaline." *Archives Internationales de Pharmacodynamie et de Therapie* 194, 1: 147-157.

Rätsch, C. 1996. "Eine Erfahrung mit dem Mataco-Schnupfpulver *Hataj*." *Yearbook for Ethnomedicine and the Study of Consciousness* 5: 59-65, Verlag für Wissenschaft und Bildung, Berlin.

Rauzzino, F., and J. Seifter. 1967. "Potentiation and antagonism of biogenic amines." *Journal of Pharmacology and Experimental Therapeutics* 157: 143-148.

Raymond-Hamet, M. 1956. "Some physiological properties of a remarkable South American stimulant: *Piptadenia peregrina*." *Comptes Rendus Hebdomadaires des Seance de L'Academie des Sciences* 243: 512-514.

Record, S. J., and C. D. Mell. 1924. *Timbers of tropical America.* Yale University Press, New Haven.

Reichel-Dolmatoff, G. 1944. "La cultura material de los indios Guahibo." *Revista del Instituto Etnológico Nacional,* I, 2: 437-506, Bogotá.

———. 1965. *Colombia.* Praeger, New York.

———. 1971. *Amazonian cosmos: The sexual and religious symbolism of the Tukano Indians.* University of Chicago Press, Chicago.

———. 1972. "The feline motif in prehistoric San Agustín sculpture." In *The cult of the feline: A conference on Precolumbian iconography,* ed. E. P. Benson, 51-68. Dumbarton Oaks, Washington, DC.

———. 1978. *El chamán y el jaguar: Estudio de las drogas narcóticas entre los indios de Colombia.* Siglo Veintiuno Editores, Mexico (Spanish version of *The shaman and the jaguar.* Temple University Press, Philadelphia, 1975).

Reimann, W., and F. Schneider. 1993. "The serotonin receptor agonist 5-methoxy-*N,N*-dimethyltryptamine facilitates noradrenaline release from rat spinal cord slices and inhibits monoamine oxidase activity." *General Pharmacology* 24, 2: 449-453.

Reis Altschul, S. von. 1964. "A taxonomic study of the genus *Anadenanthera*." *Contributions from the Gray Herbarium of Harvard University* 193: 3-65, Cambridge, Massachusetts.

———. 1967. "*Vilca* and its use." In *Ethnopharmacologic search for psychoactive drugs,* ed. D. H. Efron et al., 307-314. Public Health Service Publication 1645, U.S. Department of Health, Education and Welfare, Washington, DC.

———. 1972. *The genus Anadenanthera in Amerindian cultures.* Botanical Museum, Harvard University, Cambridge, Massachusetts.

———. 1976. "*Anadenanthera*: Source of the classic tryptamine-containing snuffs of the New World." *Psychopharmacology Bulletin* 12, 4: 10-12, U.S. Department of Health, Education and Welfare, Washington, DC. Abridged proceedings of the fourteenth annual meeting of the American College of Neuropsychopharmacology (San Juan, Puerto Rico, December 16-19, 1975).

Reiter, R. J. 1980. "The pineal and its hormones in the control of reproduction in mammals." *Endocrinology Review* 1: 109-131.

————. 1985. "Action spectra, dose-response relationships, and temporal aspects of light's effects on the pineal gland." *Annals of the New York Academy of Science* 453: 215-230.

Rendón, P. 1999. La tableta de rapé de Amaguaya. Unpublished manuscript. Museo Tiwanaku, La Paz, Bolivia.

Rendón, W. J. 1984. "Obtención de la Bufotenina de la semilla de *Piptadenia macrocarpa* Benth." *Revista Boliviana de Química* 5, 1: 39-43.

Repke, D. B., W. J. Ferguson, and D. K. Bates. 1981. "Psilocin analogs II. Synthesis of 3-[2-(dialkylamino)ethyl]-, 3-[2-(*N*-methyl-*N*-alkylamino)ethyl]-, and 3-[2-(cycloalkylamino)ethyl]indol-4-ols." *Journal of Heterocyclic Chemistry* 18: 175-179.

Repke, D. B., D. B. Grotjahn, and A. T. Shulgin. 1985. "Psychotomimetic *N*-methyl-*N*-isopropyltryptamines: Effects of variation of aromatic oxygen substituents." *Journal of Medicinal Chemistry* 28: 892.

Repke, D. B., D. T. Leslie, D. M. Mandell, and N. G. Kish. 1977. "GLC-mass spectral analysis of psilocin and psilocybin." *Journal of Pharmacy Science* 66: 743.

Repke, D. B., D. M. Mandell, and J. H. Thomas. 1973. "Alkaloids of *Acacia baileyana*." *Lloydia* 36: 211-213.

Rhyage, R. 1964. "Use of mass spectrometer as a detector and analyzer for effluents emerging from high temperature gas liquid chromatography column." *Analytical Chemistry* 36: 759-764.

Rhyage, R., and S. Wikstrom. 1971. *Gas chromatography–mass spectrometry.* Wiley, New York.

————. 1973. "Integrated gas chromatography–mass spectrometry." *Quarterly Reviews of Biophysics* 6: 311-335.

Rivero, J. 1956. *Historia de las misiones de los Llanos de Casanare y los ríos Orinoco y Meta.* Biblioteca de la Presidencia de Colombia, Empresa Nacional de Publicaciones, Bogotá.

————. 1980. "Indole protoalkaloids metabolism in *Anadenanthera peregrina* seeds." *Planta Medica* 39: 215B.

Rivier, L. 1994. "Ethnopharmacology of LSD and related compounds." In *50 years of LSD: Current status and perspectives of hallucinogens,* ed. A. Pletscher and D. Ladewig, 43-55. Parthenon, New York.

Rivier, L., and J.-E. Lindgren. 1971. "*Ayahuasca,* the South American hallucinogenic drink: An ethnobotanical and chemical investigation." *Economic Botany* 25: 101-129.

Rivier, L., and P.-E. Pilet. 1971. "Composes hallucinogenes indoliques naturels." *Annee Biologique* 3-4: 130-149.

Roseghini, M., R. Endean, and A. Temperilli. 1976. "New and uncommon indole and imidazole alkylamines in skins of amphibians from Australia and Papua New Guinea." *Zeitschrift für Naturforsch Cung* 31, 3-4: 118-120.

Roseghini, M., G. F. Erspamer, C. Severini, and M. Simmaco. 1989. "Biogenic amines and active peptides in extracts of the skin of thirty-two European amphibian species." *Comparative Biochemistry and Physiology C: Comparative Pharmacology and Toxicology* 94C, 2: 455-460.

Roseghini, M., V. Erspamer, and R. Endean. 1976. "Indole-, imidazole- and phenyl-alkylamines in the skin of one hundred amphibian species from Australia and Papua New Guinea." *Comparative Biochemistry and Physiology* 54C, 1: 31-43.

Roseghini, M., V. Erspamer, G. F. Erspamer, and J. M. Cei. 1986. "Indole-, Imidazole- and phenyl-alkylamines in the skin of one hundred and forty American amphibian species other than bufonids." *Comparative Biochemistry and Physiology C: Comparative Pharmacology and Toxicology* 85C: 139-147.

Rosen, E. von. 1924. *Popular account of archaeological research during the Swedish Chaco-Cordillera expedition, 1901-1902.* Bonniers Boktryckeri, Stockholm.

Rosenthal, F. R. T. 1955. "Constitution of some Brazilian vegetal gums." *Revista de Quimica Industrial* 24, 276: 17-19, Rio de Janeiro.

Roth, B. L., M. S. Choudhary, N. Khan, and A. Uluer. 1997. "High-affinity agonist binding is not sufficient for agonist efficacy at 5-hydroxytryptamine$_{2A}$ receptors: Evidence in favor of a modified ternary complex model." *Journal of Pharmacology and Experimental Therapeutics* 280: 576-583.

Rouse, I. 1964. "Prehistory of the West Indies." *Science* 144: 499-513.

———. 1992. *The Tainos: Rise and decline of the people who greeted Columbus.* Yale University Press, New Haven.

Ruch-Monachon, M., M. Jalfre, and W. Haefely. 1976. "Drugs and PGO waves in the lateral geniculate body of the curarized cat. II. PGO wave activity and brain 5-hydroxytryptamine." *Archives of International Pharmacodynamic Therapy* 219: 269-286.

Russell, M. G. N., and R. Dias. 2002. "Memories are made of this (perhaps): A review of serotonin 5-HT$_6$ receptor ligands and their biological functions." *Current Topics in Medicinal Chemistry* 2, 6: 643-654.

Ryden, S. 1944. *Contributions to the archaeology of the Rio Loa Region.* Elanders Boktryckeri Aktiebolag, Gothenburg, Sweden.

Safford, W. E. 1916. "Identity of *cohoba*, the narcotic snuff of ancient Haiti." *Journal of the Washington Academy of Sciences* 6: 547-562.

Sai-Halász, A., G. Brunecker, and S. Szára. 1958. "Dimethyltryptamin: Ein neues Psychoticum." *Psychiatria et Neurologia* 135: 285-301.

Salas, A. M. 1945. *El Antigal de Ciénaga Grande (Quebrada de Purmamarca, Prov. de Jujuy).* Publicaciones del Museo Etnográfico de la Facultad de Filosofía y Letras, Serie A.V., Universidad de Buenos Aires, Argentina.

Salmoiraghi, G. C., and I. Page. 1957. "Effects of LSD-25, BOL148, bufotenine, mescaline and ibogaine on the potentiation of hexobarbital hypnosis produced by serotonin and reserpine." *Journal of Pharmacology and Experimental Therapeutics* 120: 20-25.

Salomon, F., and G. L. Urioste, eds. 1991. *The Huarochirí manuscript: A testament of ancient and colonial Andean religion.* University of Texas Press, Austin.

Sanders, E., and M. T. Bush. 1967. "Distribution, metabolism, and excretion of bufotenine in the rat with preliminary studies of its *O*-methyl derivative." *Journal of Pharmacology and Experimental Therapeutics* 158: 340-352.

Sanders-Bush, E., J. A. Oates, and M. T. Bush. 1976. "Metabolism of bufotenine-2-14C in human volunteers." *Life Sciences* 19, 9: 1407-1411.

Santa Cruz de Pachacuti, J. de. 1993. *Relación de antigüedades deste Reyno del Piru.* Edición facsimilar y transcripción paleográfica del Codice de Madrid. Travaux de l'Institut Français D'Etudes Andines 74, Centro de Estudios Regionales Andinos Bartolomé de Las Casas, Cuzco, Peru.

Santos Biloni, J. 1990. *Árboles autóctonos Argentinos.* Tipográfica Editora Argentina, Buenos Aires.

Sasse, F., U. Heckenberg, and J. Berlin. 1982. "Accumulation of β-carboline alkaloids and serotonin by cell cultures of *Peganum harmala.*" *Zeitschrift fur Pflanzenphysiologie* 105S: 315-322.

Saunders, N. J., and D. Gray. 1996. "*Zemís,* trees, and symbolic landscapes: Three Taíno carvings from Jamaica." *Antiquity* 70: 801-812.

Saxena, P. R., P. de Vries, J. P. C. Heiligers, A. M. VanDenBrink, W. Bax, T. Barf, and H. Wikström. 1996. "Investigations with GMC2021 in experimental models predictive of antimigraine activity and coronary side-effect potential." *European Journal of Pharmacology* 312: 53-62.

Schleiffer, H., ed. 1973. *Sacred narcotic plants of the New World Indians: An anthology of texts from the sixteenth century to date (Anadenanthera* spp. refs.: 76-93). Hafner Press, Macmillan, New York.

Schmidt, J., and H. Lang. 1955. "Paper technological properties of various tropical woods." *Das Papier* 9: 575-584.

Schneider, H. S. 1937. "Angico gum." *Revista de Quimica Industrial* 6: 286-290, Rio de Janeiro.

Schooley, C. M. 1994. The Tiwanaku camelid image on the snuff trays and tubes of San Pedro de Atacama, Chile. Master's thesis, University of New Mexico, Albuquerque.

Schultes, R. E. 1954. "A new narcotic snuff from the northwest Amazon." *Botanical Museum Leaflets* 16: 241-260, Harvard University, Cambridge, Massachusetts.

———. 1957. "The identity of the malpighiaceous narcotics of South America." *Botanical Museum Leaflets* 18: 1-56, Harvard University, Cambridge, Massachusetts.

———. 1963. "Botanical sources of the New World narcotics." *Psychedelic Review* 1: 145-166.

———. 1967. "The botanical origin of South American snuffs." *Ethnopharmacologic search for psychoactive drugs,* ed. D. H. Efron et al., 291-306. Public Health Service Publication 1645, U.S. Department of Health, Education, and Welfare, Washington, DC.

———. 1970. "The plant kingdom and hallucinogens." *Bulletin on Narcotics* 22, 1: 25-53.

———. 1972. "*Ilex guayusa* from 500 A.D. to the present." *Etnologiska Studier* 32: 115-138, Göteborgs Etnografiska Museum, Gothenburg, Sweden.

———. 1976. "Indole alkaloids in plant hallucinogens." *Planta Medica* 29: 330-342; see also *Journal of Psychedelic Drugs* 8, 1976: 7-25.

———. 1979a. "Evolution of the identification of the myristicaceous hallucinogens of South America." *Journal of Ethnopharmacology* 1: 211-239.

———. 1979b. "Evolution of the identification of the major South American narcotic plants." *Journal of Psychedelic Drugs* 11, 1-2: 119-134.

———. 1984. "Fifteen years of study of psychoactive snuffs of South America: 1967-1982—A review." *Journal of Ethnopharmacology* 11, 1: 17-32.

_____. 1990. "*De plantis toxicariis e mundo novo tropicale commentationes* XXXVI. *Justicia (Acanthaceae)* as a source of an hallucinogenic snuff." *Economic Botany* 44, 1: 61-70.

Schultes, R. E., and A. Bright. 1979. "Ancient gold pectorals from Colombia: Mushroom effigies?" *Botanical Museum Leaflets* 27, 5-6: 113-141, Harvard University, Cambridge, Massachusetts.

Schultes, R. E., and A. Hofmann. 1979. *Plants of the gods.* McGraw-Hill, New York.

———. 1980. *The botany and chemistry of hallucinogens.* Charles C Thomas, Springfield, Illinois.

Schultes, R. E., and B. Holmstedt. 1968. "*De plantis toxicariis e mundo novo tropicale commentationes* II. The vegetal ingredients of the myristicaceous snuffs of the northwest Amazon." *Rhodora* 70: 113-160.

Schultes, R. E., B. Holmstedt, and J.-E. Lindgren. 1969. "*De plantis toxicariis e mundo novo tropicale commentationes* III. Phytochemical examination of Spruce's original collection of *Banisteriopsis caapi.*" *Botanical Museum Leaflets* 22: 121-132, Harvard University, Cambridge, Massachusetts.

Schultes, R. E., B. Holmstedt, J.-E. Lindgren, and L. Rivier. 1977. "*De plantis toxicariis e mundo novo tropicale commentationes* XVIII. Phytochemical examination of Spruce's ethnobotanical collection of *Anadenanthera peregrina.*" *Botanical Museum Leaflets* 25: 273-287, Harvard University, Cambridge, Massachusetts.

Scripps. n.d. *Archives of the Scripps Institution of Oceanography.* http://scilib.ucsd.edu/sio/archives/siohstry/alphahelix-hist.html.

Seeman, G., and G. Brown. 1985. "Indolealkylamines and prolactin secretion: A structure-activity study in the central nervous system of the rat." *Neuropharmacology* 24: 1195-1200.

Seitz, G., J. 1967. "*Epená,* the intoxicating snuff powder of the Waika Indians and the Tucano medicine-man Agostino." In *Ethnopharmacologic search for psychoactive drugs,* ed. D. H. Efron et al., 315-338. Public Health Service Publication no. 1645, U.S. Department of Health, Education and Welfare, Washington, DC.

———. 1969. "Die Waikas und ihre Drogen." *Zeitschrift für Ethnologie* 94: 266-283.

Serrano, A. 1934. "El uso del tabaco y vegetales narcotizantes entre los indígenas de America." *Revista Geográfica Americana* 2, 15: 415-429, Buenos Aires.

———. 1941. "Los recipientes para *paricá* y su dispersión en América del Sud." *Revista Geográfica Americana* 15, 251-257, Buenos Aires.

Sharon, D. 2000. *Shamanism and the sacred cactus: Ethnoarchaeological evidence for San Pedro use in northern Peru.* San Diego Museum Papers 37, San Diego Museum of Man, San Diego, California (reprinted with revisions in *Eleusis* 5: 13-59 (thematic issue, *Archaeology of Hallucinogens in the Andean Region*), Telesterion and Museo Civico di Rovereto, Trento, Italy.

Sharon, D., and C. Donnan. 1974. "Shamanism in Moche iconography." In *Ethnoarchaeology,* Monograph IV, ed. C. Donnan and C. W. Clewlow, Institute of Archaeology, University of California, Los Angeles. Monograph.

Shulgin, A. 1976. "Profiles of psychedelic drugs, 1. DMT." *Journal of Psychedelic Drugs* 8: 167-168.

———. 1981a. "Chemistry of psychotomimetics." In *Handbook of experimental pharmacology* 55, ed. F. Hoffmeister and G. Stille, 3. Springer-Verlag, Berlin.

———. 1981b. "Profiles of psychedelic drugs, 11. Bufotenine." *Journal of Psychoactive Drugs* 13: 389.

Shulgin, A., and A. Shulgin. 1991. *Pihkal: A chemical love story.* Transform Press, Berkeley.

———. 1997. *Tihkal: The continuation.* Transform Press, Berkeley.

Simón, P. 1882-1892. *Noticias historiales de la conquista de Tierra Firme en las Indias Occidentales,* 5 vols. Bogotá, Colombia.

Sitaram, B. R., L. Lockett, G. L. Blackman, and W. R. McLeod. 1987. "Urinary excretion of 5-methoxy-*N,N*-dimethyltryptamine, *N,N*-dimethyltryptamine and their *N*-oxides in the rat." *Biochemical Pharmacology* 36: 2235-2237.

Sitaram, B. R., L. Lockett, M. McLeish, Y. Hayasaka, G. L. Blackman, and W. R. McLeod. 1987. "Gas chromatographic-mass spectroscopic characterization of the psychotomimetic indolealkylamines and their in vivo metabolites." *Journal of Chromatography* 422: 13-23.

Sitaram, B. R., R. Talomsin, G. L. Blackman, and W. R. McLeod. 1987. "Study of the metabolism of psychotomimetic indolealkylamines by rat tissue extracts, using liquid chromatography." *Biochemical Pharmacology* 36: 1503-1508.

Slaytor, M., and I. J. McFarlane. 1968. "The biosynthesis and metabolism of harman in *Passiflora edulis.* I." *Phytochemistry* 7: 605-611.

Sloviter, R. S., E. G. Drust, B. P. Damiano, and J. D. Connor. 1980. "A common mechanism for lysergic acid, indolealkylamine and phenethylamine hallucinogens: Serotonergic mediation of behavioral effects in rats." *Journal of Pharmacology and Experimental Therapeutics* 214, 2: 231-238.

Smet, P. A. G. M. de. 1983. "A multidisciplinary overview of intoxicating enema rituals in the Western Hemisphere." *Journal of Ethnopharmacology* 9: 129-166.

———. 1985. *Ritual enemas and snuffs in the Americas.* Latin American Studies Series, Foris Publications, Dordrecht, Holland.

Smet, P. A. G. M. de, and L. Rivier. 1985. "Intoxicating snuffs of the Venezuelan Piaroa Indians." *Journal of Psychoactive Drugs* 17, 2: 93-103.

———. 1987. "Intoxicating *paricá* seeds of the Brazilian Maué Indians." *Economic Botany* 41, 1: 12-16.

Smith, T. A. 1977. "Tryptamines and related compounds in plants." *Phytochemistry* 16: 171-175.

Snethlage, E. H. 1937. *Atiko y. Meine Erlebnisse bei den Indianern des Guaporé.* Klinkhardt and Biermann, Berlin.

Sotelo de Narvaez, P. 1965. "Relación de las Provincias de Tucumán." In *Relaciones geográficas de Indias* 1, ed. M. J. de la Espada, 390-396. Biblioteca de Autores Españoles 183, Ediciones Atlas, Madrid.

Spahni, J. C. 1964. "Le cimitière Atacamenien du Pucará de Lasana, vallée du Rio Loa (Chili)." *Journal de la Société des Américanistes* 53: 147-159, Paris.

———. 1967. "Recherches archeologiques a l'embouchure du Rio Loa (Côte du Pacifique, Chili)." *Journal de la Societé des Américanistes* 56, 1: 179-251, Paris.

Speeter, M. E., and W. C. Anthony. 1954. "The action of oxalyl chloride on indoles: A new approach to tryptamines." *Journal of the American Chemical Society* 76: 6208-6210.

Spegazzini, C. 1922. "Algunas observaciones relativas al suborden de las *Mimosoideas.*" *Physis* 6: 308-315, Argentina.

Spencer, D. G., T. Glaser, and J. Traber. 1987. "Serotonin receptor subtype mediation of the interoceptive discriminative stimuli induced by 5-methoxy-N,N-dimethyltryptamine." *Psychopharmacology* 93: 158-166.

Spencer, D. G., and J. Traber. 1987. "The interoceptive discriminative stimuli induced by the novel putative anxiolytic TVX Q 7821: Behavioral evidence for the specific involvement of serotonin $5HT_{1A}$ receptors." *Psychopharmacology* 91: 25-29.

Spix, C. F. P. von, and J. B. von Martius. 1823-1831. *Reise in Brasilien auf Befehl Sr. Majestat Maximilian Joseph I., Königs von Baiern, in den jahren 1817 bis 1820 gemacht und beschrieben,* 3 vols. and atlas of 41 pls., 7 maps, M. Lindauer and I. J. Lentner, Munich; Bei dem verfasser, Leipzig, in Comm. bei Friedr. Fleischer. Portuguese ed. *Viagem pelo Brasil,* 3 vols. 1981, 4th ed. (orig. ed. 1938, Imprensa Nacional, Rio de Janeiro), Editora Itatiaia, Editora da Universidade de São Paulo, Brazil.

Sprouse, J. S., and G. Aghajanian. 1988. "Electrophysiological responses of serotonergic dorsal raphe neurons to $5\text{-}HT_{1A}$ and $5\text{-}HT_{1B}$ agonists." *Synapse* 1: 3-9.

Spruce, R. 1970. *Notes of a botanist in the Amazon and the Andes.* Johnson reprint, New York (orig. ed. Macmillan 1908, London).

Stagno D'Alcontres, G., and G. Cuzzocrea. 1956-1957. "Active principles of *Piptadenia peregrina.*" *Attidella Societa Peloritana di Scienze Fisiche, Matematiche, e Naturali* 3: 167-177.

Stahl, P. W. 1985. "The hallucinogenic basis of Early Valdivia Phase ceramic bowl iconography." *Journal of Psychoactive Drugs* 17, 2: 105-123.

Stefanescu, P. 1968. "Synthesis of new indole compounds analogous to bufotenine." *Revista de Chimie* 19, 11: 639-642, Bucharest.

Stevens-Arroyo, A. 1988. *Cave of the Jagua: The mythological world of the Taínos.* University of New Mexico Press, Albuquerque.

Steward, J. H., and A. Métraux. 1948. "Tribes of the Peruvian and Ecuadorian Montaña." In *Handbook of South American Indians* 3, ed. J. Steward, 535-656. Smithsonian Institution, Bureau of American Ethnology Bulletin 143, Washington, DC.

Stoff, D. M., D. A. Gorelick, T. Bozewicz, W. H. Bridger, J. C. Gillin, and R. J. Wyatt. 1978. "The indole hallucinogens, *N,N*-dimethyltryptamine (DMT) and 5-methoxy-*N,N*-dimethyltryptamine (5-MeO-DMT), have different effects from mescaline on rat shuttlebox avoidance." *Neuropharmacology* 17, 12: 1035-1040.

Stolle, K., and D. Groger. 1968. "Untersuchungen zur Biosynthese des Harmins." *Archiv der Pharmazie* 301: 561-571.

Stolpe, H. 1927. *Collected essays in ornamental art.* Aftonbladets Tryckeri, Stockholm, Sweden.

Stothert, K., and I. Cruz Cevallos. 2001. "Making spiritual contact: Snuff tubes and other mortuary objects from coastal Ecuador." In *Mortuary practices and ritual associations: Shamanic elements in prehistoric funerary contexts in South America,* ed. J. E. Staller and E. Currie, 51-56. BAR International Series 9982, Oxford.

Strassman, R. J. 1994. "Human psychopharmacology of LSD, dimethyltryptamine and related compounds." In *50 years of LSD: Current status and perspectives of hallucinogens,* ed. A. Pletscher and D. Ladewig, 145-174. Parthenon, New York.

Strassman, R. J., and C. R. Qualls. 1994. "Dose-response study of *N,N*-dimethyltryptamine in humans. I. Neuroendocrine, autonomic, and cardiovascular effects." *Archives of General Psychiatry* 51 (Feb.): 85-97.

Strassman, R. J., C. R. Qualls, E. H. Uhlenhuth, and R. Kellner. 1994. "Dose-response study of *N,N*-dimethyltryptamine in humans. II. Subjective effects and preliminary results of a new rating scale." *Archives of General Psychiatry* 51: 98-108.

Stromberg, V. L. 1954. "The isolation of bufotenine from *Piptadenia peregrina.*" *Journal of the American Chemical Society* 76: 1707.

Stucker, G. V., and M. Paya. 1938. *Investigaciones del laboratorio de química biológica,* vol. 2. Facultad de Ciencias Médicas, Universidad Nacional de Cordoba.

Swinburne, T. 1976. "Stimulants of germination and appressoria formation by *Colletotrichum musae* (Berk. and Curt) Arx. in banana leachate." *Phytopathologische Zeitschrift* 87: 74-90.

Szára, S. I. 1956. "Dimethyltryptamine: Its metabolism in man; the relation of its psychotic effect to the serotonin metabolism." *Experientia* 15, 6: 441-442.

———. 1957. "The comparison of the psychotic effect of tryptamine derivatives with the effects of mescaline and LSD-25 in self-experiments." In *Psychotropic drugs,* ed. S. Garattini and V. Ghetti, 460-467. Elsevier, New York.

———. 1961. "Hallucinogenic effects and metabolism of tryptamine derivatives in man." *Federation Proceedings* 20: 885-888.

Taborsky, R. G., P. Delvigs, D. Palaic, and F. M. Bumpus. 1967. "Synthesis and pharmacology of some hydroxylated tryptamines." *Journal of Medicinal Chemistry* 10, 3: 403-407.

Takahashi, T., K. Takahashi, T. Ido, K. Yanai, R. Iwata, K. Ishiwata, and S. Nozoe. 1985. "Carbon-11-labeling of indolealkylamine alkaloids and the comparative study of their tissue distributions." *International Journal of Applied Radiation and Isotopes* 36: 965-969.

Takeda, N. 1994. "Serotonin-degradative pathways in the toad *(Bufo japonicus)* brain: Clues to the pharmacological analysis of human psychiatric disorders." *Comparative Biochemistry and Physiology. C: Comparative Pharmacology and Toxicology* 107C: 275-281.

Takeda, N., R. Ikeda, K. Ohba, and M. Kondo. 1995. "Bufotenine reconsidered as a diagnostic indicator of psychiatric disorders." *NeuroReport* 6: 2378-2380.

Tarragó, M. N. 1968. "Secuencias culturales de la etapa agroalfarera de San Pedro de Atacama (Chile)." *Actas del XXXVII Congreso Internacional de Americanistas,* 2: 119-145, Buenos Aires, Argentina.

———. 1977. "Relaciones prehispánicas entre San Pedro de Atacama (norte de Chile) y regiones aledañas: La Quebrada de Humahuaca." *Estudios Atacameños* 5: 51-63, San Pedro de Atacama, Chile.

———. 1980. "Los asentamientos aldeanos tempranos en el sector septentrional del Valle Calchaquí, Provincia de Salta, y el desarrollo agrícola posterior." *Estudios Arqueológicos* 5: 29-53, Universidad de Chile, Antofagasta.

———. 1989. Contribución al conocimiento arqueológico de las poblaciones de los oasis de San Pedro de Atacama en relación con los otros pueblos puneños, en especial, el sector septentrional del Valle Calchaquí. PhD dissertation, Facultad de Humanidades y Artes, Universidad Nacional de Rosario, Rosario, Argentina.

Toledo, J. B., C. Zimmerman, and J. M. Rodriguez Vaquero. 1970. "Aporte al estudio farmacológico de las *Piptadenias* a propósito de su uso como alucinógeno por indígenas americanos." *Tribuna Farmaceutica* 3: 45-50, San Miguel de Tucumán, Argentina.

Torres, C. M. 1981. "Evidence for snuffing in the Prehispanic stone sculpture of San Agustín, Colombia." *Journal of Psychoactive Drugs* 13, 1: 53-60.

————. 1987a. "The iconography of the Prehispanic snuff trays from San Pedro de Atacama, northern Chile." *Andean Past* 1: 191-245, Latin American Studies Program, Cornell University, Ithaca, New York.

————. 1987b. "The iconography of South American snuff trays and related paraphernalia." *Etnologiska Studier* 37, Göteborgs Etnografiska Museum, Gothenburg, Sweden.

Torres, C. M., and W. J. Conklin. 1995. "Exploring the San Pedro de Atacama/Tiahuanaco relationship." In *Andean art—Visual expression and its relationship with Andean values and beliefs,* ed. P. Dransart, 78-108. Worldwide Archaeology Series 13, Avebury Press, Great Britain.

Torres, C. M., and D. Repke. 1996. "The use of *Anadenanthera colubrina* var. *Cebil* by Wichi (Mataco) shamans of the Chaco central, Argentina." *Yearbook for Ethnomedicine and the Study of Consciousness* 5: 41-58, Verlag für Wissenschaft und Bildung, Berlin.

Torres, C. M., D. Repke, K. Chan, D. McKenna, A. Llagostera, and R. E. Schultes. 1991. "Snuff powders from pre-Hispanic San Pedro de Atacama: Chemical and contextual analysis." *Current Anthropology* 32, 5: 640-649.

Torres, W. 1994. "Waji: 'Rezo' chamanístico Sikuani." *Boletín* 37: 34-51, Museo del Oro, Banco de la República, Bogotá.

Tortorelli, L. A. 1948. "The Argentine *Piptadenia* timbers." *Tropical Woods* 94: 1-27, School of Forestry, Yale University, New Haven.

Tower, D. B. 1983. *Hensing, 1719: An account of the first chemical examination of the brain and the discovery of phosphorus therein.* Raven Press, New York.

Trease, G. E., and W. C. Evans. 1971. *Pharmacognosy,* 10th ed. Williams and Wilkins, Baltimore.

Turner, W. B. 1971. *Fungal metabolites.* Academic Press, London.

Turner, W. J., and S. Merlis. 1959. "Effect of some indolealkylamines on man." *A.M.A. Archives of Neurology and Psychiatry* 81: 121-129.

Tyler, V. E., L. R. Brady, and J. E. Robbers. 1981. *Pharmacognosy.* Lea and Febiger, Philadelphia.

Tylor, E. B. 1913. *Primitive culture: Researches into the development of mythology, philosophy, religion, language, art and custom.* Murray, London.

Uhle, M. 1898. "A snuffing tube from Tiahuanaco." *Bulletin of the Museum of Science and Art* 1, 4: 158-177, University of Pennsylvania, Philadelphia.

————. 1912. "Las relaciones prehistóricas entre el Perú y la Argentina." *Proceedings of the XVII International Congress of Americanists:* 509-540. Buenos Aires, Argentina.

————. 1913. "Tabletas de madera de Chiu-Chiu." *Revista Chilena de Historia y Geografía* 8, 12: 454-458, Santiago.

————. 1915. "Los tubos y tabletas de rapé en Chile." *Revista Chilena de Historia y Geografía* 16, 20: 114-136, Santiago.

Uluitu, M., M. Lazar, and G. Catrinescu. 1976. "The influence of bufotenine on the feeding behavior and cerebral serotonin content in rats." *Revue Romaine de Morphologie d'Embryologie et de Physiologie, Physiologie* 13: 145-153.

Uscátegui, N. 1961. "Distribución actual de las plantas narcóticas y estimulantes usadas por las tribus indígenas de Colombia." *Revista de la Academia Colombiana de Ciencias* 11, 43: 215-228, Bogotá (see also *Botanical Museum Leaflets* 18: 273-304, Harvard University, 1959).

Vane, J. R. 1959. "Relative activities of some tryptamine analogs on the isolated rat stomach fundus strip preparation." *British Journal of Pharmacology* 14: 87-98.

Vargas Machuca, B. de. 1892. *Milicia y descripción de Las Indias,* 2 vols. Colección de Libros Raros o Curiosos Que Tratan de las Americas, vols. 8 and 9, Vi Suarez, Madrid.

Velez Salas, F. 1944. "*Piptadenias,* plantas usadas por nuestros aborígenes como ilusionógenas y para aumentar la fuerza en los combates." In *Revista Farmacéutica* 86, 12: 505-511, Caracas.

Vescelius, G. 1960. "Rasgos naturales y culturales de la costa extremo sur." In *Antiguo Perú: Espacio y tiempo,* ed. J. Mejia Baca, 381-383. Universidad de San Marcos, Instituto de Etnología y Arqueología, Lima.

Vigdorchik, M. M., K. F. Turchin, T. Gus'kova, L. Yakubovich, L. S. Krasavina, O. Lukin, N. Lutsenko, and N. Suvorov. 1984. "Identification of *N, N*-dimethyl-*O*-(β-glucopyranuronosyl)-5-hydroxytryptamine as a bufotenine metabolite in rabbits." *Bioorganicheskaya Khimiya* 10: 260-264.

Vollenweider, F. X. 1998. "Recent advances and concepts in the search for biological correlates of hallucinogen-induced altered states of consciousness." *Heffter Review* 1: 21-32.

Wassén, S. H. 1964. "Some general viewpoints in the study of native drugs especially from the West Indies and South America." *Ethnos* 29, 1-2: 97-120, Ethnographical Museum of Sweden, Stockholm.

———. 1965. "The use of some specific kinds of South American Indian snuffs and related paraphernalia." *Etnologiska Studier* 28, Göteborgs Etnografiska Museum, Gothenburg, Sweden.

———. 1967a. "Anthropological survey of the use of South American snuffs." In *Ethnopharmacologic search for psychoactive drugs,* ed. D. H. Efron et al., 233-289. Public Health Service Publication 1645, U.S. Department of Health, Education and Welfare, Washington, DC.

———. 1967b. "Om nagra Indianska droger och especiellt om snus samt tillbehör." *Årstryck 1963-1966,* 97-140, Göteborgs Etnografiska Museum, Gothenburg, Sweden.

———. 1970. "A naturalist's lost ethnographic collection from Brazil—or the case from 1786. A contribution to the study of South American Indian drugs." *Årstryck 1969,* 32-52, Göteborgs Etnografiska Museum, Gothenburg, Sweden.

———. 1972a. "The anthropological outlook for Amerindian medicinal plants." In *Plants in the development of modern medicine,* ed. T. Swain, 1-65. Harvard University Press, Cambridge, Massachusetts.

————. 1972b. "A medicine-man's implements and plants in a Tiahuanacoid tomb in highland Bolivia." *Etnologiska Studier* 32: 7-114, Göteborgs Etnografiska Museum, Gothenburg, Sweden.

————. 1973. "Ethnobotanical follow-up of Bolivian Tiahuanacoid tomb material and of Peruvian shamanism, psychotropic plant constituents, and *espingo* seeds." *Årstryck 1972,* 35-52, Göteborgs Etnografiska Museum, Gothenburg, Sweden.

————. 1985. "Convergent approaches to the analysis of hallucinogenic snuff trays." *Årstryck 1983-1984,* 26-37, Göteborgs Etnografiska Museum, Gothenburg, Sweden.

Wassén, S. H., and B. Holmstedt. 1963. "The use of *paricá,* an ethnological and pharmacological review." *Ethnos* 28, 1: 5-45, Ethnographical Museum of Sweden, Stockholm.

Wassicky, R. 1944. "The problem of quinine alkaloids in Brazil." *Revista Brasileira de Quimica* 18: 265-266, 322-324, São Paulo.

Wassicky, R., C. Ferreira, and E. de Camarago Fonseca. 1945. "A new method of determination of saponins with an antifoaming agent." *Anaisda Faculdade de Farmacia e Odontologiada Universidade de São Paulo* 4: 230-274.

Wasson, R. G. 1961. "The hallucinogenic fungi of Mexico: An inquiry into the origins of the religious idea among primitive peoples." *Botanical Museum Leaflets* 19, 7: 137-162, Harvard University, Cambridge, Massachusetts.

————. 1971. *Soma: Divine mushroom of immortality.* Harcourt Brace Jovanovich, New York.

Wasson, R. G., C. Ruck, and A. Hofmann. 1978. *The road to Eleusis.* Harcourt Brace Jovanovich, New York.

Weidmann, H., and A. Cerletti. 1959. "Pharmacodynamic differentiation of the 4-hydroxyindole derivatives psilocybin and psilocin in comparison with the 5-hydroxyindole derivatives serotonin and bufotenine." *Helvetica Physiologica et Pharmacologica Acta* 17: 46-48.

————. 1960. "Psilocybin and related compounds 1. Structure/activity relation of hydroxy-indole derivatives with regard to their effect on the knee jerk of spinal cats." *Helvetica Physiologica et Pharmacologica Acta* 18: 174-182.

Welsh, J. H. 1966. "Serotonin and related tryptamine derivatives in snake venoms." *Memórias do Instituto Butantan* 33: 509-518.

Westfall, C. 1993-1994. "Pipas prehispánicas de Chile: Discusión en torno a su distribución y contexto." *Revista Chilena de Antropología* 12: 123-161, Facultad de Ciencias Sociales, Universidad de Chile, Santiago.

Whiffen, T. W. 1915. *The northwest Amazons: Notes of some months spent among cannibal tribes.* Constable, London.

Whitaker, P. M., and P. Seeman. 1977. "Hallucinogen binding to dopamine/neuroleptic receptors." *Journal of Pharmacy and Pharmacology* 29, 8: 506-507.

Whitelock, O. v. St., and F. N. Furness. 1957. "The pharmacology of psychotomimetic and psychotherapeutic drugs." *Annals of the New York Academy of Science* 66, Art. 3: 417-840.

Wieland, H., W. Konz, and H. Mittasch. 1934. "Die Konstitution von Bufotenine und Bufotenidine. Uber Kroten-Giftstoffe. VII." *Justus Liebigs Annalen der Chemie* 513: 1.

Wieland, T., and W. Motzel. 1953. "Uber das Vorkommen von Bufotenin im gelben Knollenblatterpilz." *Justus Liebigs Annalen der Chemie* 581: 10.

Wilbert, J. 1958. "Datos antropológicos de los indios Piaroa." *Memoria de la Sociedad de Ciencias Naturales de La Salle* 18: 155-183, Caracas.

————. 1963. *Indios de la región Orinoco-Ventuari.* Monografía 8, Fundación La Salle de Ciencias Naturales, Caracas.

————. 1987. *Tobacco and shamanism in South America.* Yale University Press, New Haven.

Wilkinson, S. 1958. "5-Methoxy-*N*-methyltryptamine: A new indole alkaloid from *Phalaris arundinaceae* L." *Journal of the Chemical Society* 1958: 2079.

Willaman, J. J., and B. G. Schubert. 1961. "Alkaloid bearing plants and their contained alkaloids." *ARS, USDA, Tech Bull. 1234,* Government Printing Office, Washington, DC.

Williams, L. T., and R. J. Lefkowitz. 1979. "Methodological approach to radioligand binding studies of adrenergic receptors." In *Advances in pharmacology and therapeutics,* Vol. 1, *Receptors,* ed. J. Jacob, 223-232. Pergamon Press, Oxford.

Wing, L. L., G. S. Tapson, and M. Geyer. 1990. "5-HT$_2$ mediation of acute behavioral effects of hallucinogens in rats." *Psychopharmacology* 100, 3: 417-425.

Winocur, G., S. P. Bagchi, and P. Hubbard. 1971. "Effects of bufotenine and p-chlorophenylalanine and stress-induced behavior." *Psychopharmacologia* 22: 100-110.

Winter, J. C. 1972. "Xylamidine tosylate: Differential antagonism of the hypothermic effects of *N,N*-dimethyltryptamine, bufotenine, and 5-methoxytryptamine." *Archives Internationales de Pharmacodynamie et de Therapie* 198: 61-68.

Wittliff, J. L. 1968. "Separation of toad venom constituents on silica gel-impregnated glass filter paper." *Toxicon* 6: 73-74.

Wooley, D., and E. Shaw. 1954. "A biochemical and pharmacological suggestion about certain mental disorders." *Proceedings of the National Academy of Science* 40: 228-231.

Wurdack, J. J. 1958. "Indian narcotics in southern Venezuela." *Garden Journal of the New York Botanical Garden* (July-August): 116-118, New York.

Yacovleff, E., and F. Herrera. 1934-1935. "El mundo vegetal de los antiguos peruanos." *Revista del Museo Nacional* 3, 2: 243-322; 4, 1: 31-102, Lima, Peru.

Yamasato, S., K. Kawanishi, A. Kato, and Y. Hashimoto. 1972. "Organic bases from Brazilian *Piptadenia* species." *Phytochemistry* 11, 2: 737-739.

Zeidler, J. A. 1988. "Feline imagery, stone mortars, and Formative Period interaction spheres in the northern Andean area." *Journal of Latin American Lore* 14, 2: 243-283.

Zerda, L. 1972. *El Dorado,* 2 vols. Biblioteca Banco Popular, Bogotá, Colombia.

Zerries, O. 1964. "Ausgewählte Holzschnitzarbeiten der Brasilien-Samnlung Spix und Martius von 1817/20 im Völkerkunde-Museum zu München." In *Völkerkundliche Abhandlungen,* Vol. I, *Beiträge zur Völkerkunde Südamerikas,* ed. H. Beche, 353-366, Kommissionsverlag Munstermann-Druck, Hanover.

———. 1980. *Unter Indianern Brasiliens: Samnlung Spix und Martius, 1817-1820.* Museum für Völkerkunde, Munich, Pinguin-Verlag, Innsbruck, Germany.

———. 1981. "Atributos e instrumentos rituoais do xama na America do Sul nao-Andina e o seu significado." In *Contribuçoes a antropologia em homenagem ao Professor Egon Schaden,* ed. T. Hartmann, 319-360. Coleçao Museu Paulista, Série Ensaios 4, Fundo de Pesquisas do Museu Paulista, São Paulo, Brasil.

———. 1985. "Morteros para *paricá,* tabletas para aspirar y bancos zoomorfos." *Indiana* 10: 421-441, Gedenkschrift Gerdt Kutscher Teil 2, Gbr. Mann Verlag, Berlin.

———. 1988. "Reptiliforme schnupfbretter aus Amazonien." In *Münchner Beitrage zur Völkerkunde, Festschrift László Vajda,* vol. 1: 257-268, Claudius Müller and Hans-Joachim Paproth, eds. Hirmer Verlag, Munich.

Zuidema, R. T. 1979. "El puente del río Apurímac y el origen mítico de la *Villca (Anadenanthera colubrina)." Collectanea Instituti Anthropos* 21: 322-324, Anthropos Institute, S. Augustin, Bonn.

Index

Page numbers followed by the letter "f" indicate figures.

Order a copy of this book with this form or online at:
http://www.haworthpress.com/store/product.asp?sku=5377

ANADENANTHERA
Visionary Plant of Ancient South America

_____ in hardbound at $59.95 (ISBN-13: 978-0-7890-2641-5; ISBN-10: 0-7890-2641-4)

_____ in softbound at $34.95 (ISBN-13: 978-0-7890-2642-2; ISBN-10: 0-7890-2642-2)

Or order online and use special offer code HEC25 in the shopping cart.

COST OF BOOKS_____

POSTAGE & HANDLING_____
*(US: $4.00 for first book & $1.50
for each additional book)*
*(Outside US: $5.00 for first book
& $2.00 for each additional book)*

SUBTOTAL_____

IN CANADA: ADD 7% GST_____

STATE TAX_____
*(NJ, NY, OH, MN, CA, IL, IN, PA, & SD
residents, add appropriate local sales tax)*
FINAL TOTAL_____
*(If paying in Canadian funds,
convert using the current
exchange rate, UNESCO
coupons welcome)*

☐ **BILL ME LATER:** (Bill-me option is good on
US/Canada/Mexico orders only; not good to
jobbers, wholesalers, or subscription agencies.)
☐ Check here if billing address is different from
shipping address and attach purchase order and
billing address information.

Signature_____

☐ **PAYMENT ENCLOSED: $**_____

☐ **PLEASE CHARGE TO MY CREDIT CARD.**

☐ Visa ☐ MasterCard ☐ AmEx ☐ Discover
☐ Diner's Club ☐ Eurocard ☐ JCB

Account # _____

Exp. Date_____

Signature_____

Prices in US dollars and subject to change without notice.

NAME_____

INSTITUTION_____

ADDRESS_____

CITY_____

STATE/ZIP_____

COUNTRY_____ COUNTY (NY residents only)_____

TEL_____ FAX_____

E-MAIL_____

May we use your e-mail address for confirmations and other types of information? ☐ Yes ☐ No
We appreciate receiving your e-mail address and fax number. Haworth would like to e-mail or fax special
discount offers to you, as a preferred customer. **We will never share, rent, or exchange your e-mail address
or fax number.** We regard such actions as an invasion of your privacy.

Order From Your Local Bookstore or Directly From
The Haworth Press, Inc.
10 Alice Street, Binghamton, New York 13904-1580 • USA
TELEPHONE: 1-800-HAWORTH (1-800-429-6784) / Outside US/Canada: (607) 722-5857
FAX: 1-800-895-0582 / Outside US/Canada: (607) 771-0012
E-mail to: orders@haworthpress.com

For orders outside US and Canada, you may wish to order through your local
sales representative, distributor, or bookseller.
For information, see http://haworthpress.com/distributors

(Discounts are available for individual orders in US and Canada only, not booksellers/distributors.)
PLEASE PHOTOCOPY THIS FORM FOR YOUR PERSONAL USE.
http://www.HaworthPress.com   BOF04